Lifestyle Fitness Coaching

James Gavin, PhD
Concordia University, Montreal

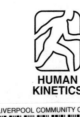

HUMAN KINETICS

Library of Congress Cataloging-in-Publication Data

Gavin, James, 1942-
 Lifestyle fitness coaching / James Gavin.
   p. cm.
 Includes bibliographical references and index.
 ISBN 0-7360-5206-2 (soft cover)
 1. Physical fitness. 2. Personal coaching. 3. Health promotion. 4. Lifestyles. I. Title.
 RA776.G289 2005
 613.7'1--dc22

                              2005000208

ISBN: 0-7360-5206-2

The Web addresses cited in this text were current as of January 10, 2005, unless otherwise noted.

Acquisitions Editor: Michael S. Bahrke, PhD; **Developmental Editor:** Maggie Schwarzentraub; **Assistant Editors:** Amanda M. Eastin and Carmel Sielicki; **Copyeditor:** Bob Replinger; **Proofreader:** Red Inc.; **Indexer:** Sharon Duffy; **Permission Manager:** Dalene Reeder; **Graphic Designer:** Nancy Rasmus; **Graphic Artist:** Denise Lowry; **Photo Manager:** Kelly J. Huff; **Cover Designer:** Keith Blomberg; **Photographer (cover):** Jimmy Chin/National Geographic/Getty Images; **Photographer (interior):** © Human Kinetics, photo on pg. 18 © Photodisc; **Art Manager:** Kelly Hendren; **Illustrator:** Accurate Art, Keri Evans, Kareema McLendon; **Printer:** Versa Press

Printed in the United States of America   10   9   8   7   6   5   4   3   2   1

Human Kinetics
Web site: www.HumanKinetics.com

United States: Human Kinetics, P.O. Box 5076, Champaign, IL 61825-5076
800-747-4457
e-mail: humank@hkusa.com

Canada: Human Kinetics, 475 Devonshire Road Unit 100, Windsor, ON N8Y 2L5
800-465-7301 (in Canada only)
e-mail: orders@hkcanada.com

Europe: Human Kinetics, 107 Bradford Road, Stanningley, Leeds LS28 6AT, United Kingdom
+44 (0) 113 255 5665
e-mail: hk@hkeurope.com

Australia: Human Kinetics, 57A Price Avenue, Lower Mitcham, South Australia 5062
08 8277 1555
e-mail: liaw@hkaustralia.com

New Zealand: Human Kinetics, Division of Sports Distributors NZ Ltd., P.O. Box 300 226 Albany, North Shore City, Auckland
0064 9 448 1207
e-mail: blairc@hknewz.com

Contents

Contents

Preface

Awareness of what people need to pursue active and healthy lifestyles has given birth to a number of new career paths in the past quarter century. Lifestyle fitness coaching is a recent arrival in the professional arena related to health and fitness. Its emergence is in response to previously unaddressed needs of both active and inactive individuals.

Careers in the fitness industry are rapidly evolving. In the past few decades, we have witnessed thousands of occasional group fitness instructors and floor monitors in fitness centers throughout North America transform their part-time roles into full-time careers. Perhaps the most dramatic expansion has occurred in the role of personal trainer, in which numbers have climbed substantially as represented by membership in professional associations (S. Webster, personal communication, October 9, 2003).

For those who exercise regularly, growth in the fitness industry translates into more options and services. Compared with fitness centers of the 1980s in which equipment was limited and high-impact aerobics formed the mainstay of group exercise, centers today offer a myriad of high-tech machines and a dazzling array of classes ranging from spinning, step, and cardio boxing to such formerly esoteric exercise forms as Pilates and yoga.

Paradoxically, public participation rates have not paralleled growth in the fitness industry. In fact, statistics suggest a flattening of participation at around 20% of the North American population (Centers for Disease Control and Prevention, 2003; Dishman, 1988; Hellmich, 2003), along with some alarming indicators of declines in activity level among baby boomers and increases in obesity level among children and adolescents (Brownlee, 2002; Nash, 2003).

Industry response to participation statistics has been to turn up the volume through better marketing and diversified programming. Health fitness professionals per se have responded to the challenge by widening their skill bases so that they can engage groups normally not considered club goers, such as those with long-term disabilities or chronic medical conditions (Chapman & Osterweil, 2001; Coven, 2003; Durrett, 2002).

A principal learning from all the efforts to attract and retain fitness participants is that social support and technical guidance are key (Dowda et al., 2003; Fraser & Spink, 2002; Gavin & Spitzer, 2002; Griffin, 1998; Resnick et al., 2002). With ever expanding options for active people and an increasingly sophisticated knowledge base about what works, what doesn't, what's helpful, and what's harmful, novices and even long-term exercisers rely increasingly on the help and advice of qualified professionals.

In this light, we can readily understand a recent trend among health fitness professionals to pursue certification in programs broadly defined as life coaching (Cantwell, 2003; Cantwell & Rothenberg, 2000; McMillan, 2001; Perina, 2002). People have long recognized that health fitness professionals who work on a one-to-one basis with clients are likely to be seen as friendly helpers with generalized wisdom that extends beyond the gym (Atkins, 2002; Gavin, 1991; Rupp et al., 1999). As such, they are willingly or otherwise engaged by clients in discussions far afield from the realm of physical training and sport. Professional associations such as the American College of Sports Medicine (ACSM) and IDEA Heath and Fitness Association (IDEA) have, for decades, worked on codes of conduct that delineate health fitness roles so as to declare out of bounds such interactions as counseling or nutritional advising, unless the professional has the requisite allied professional certifications (IDEA Code of Ethics, 2002; Johnson, 1997). Interest in life coaching is a strategic response by health fitness professionals to address some critical dynamics within the profession and among clients whom they serve.

Health fitness professionals want to have more engaging (defined in terms of number of paid hours per week) and lasting (defined as duration over one's working life) careers in the fitness industry. A 30-year-old personal trainer can expect changing capacities and interests over the lifespan. In preparation she may pursue the development of parallel or related areas of competency that will permit her to remain connected to the fitness world, rather than having to switch, for financial or physical reasons, to another industry or career. With this agenda in mind, increasing numbers of trainers and instructors are enrolling in courses in counseling, coaching, and nutrition, as well as other certification programs in allied helping professions (Lidane, 2003). Seemingly, the most noticeable trend in professional development has been that of life coaching.

Life coaching is a process of guidance and support for clients who desire assistance in strategizing, planning, and implementing self-change and personal improvement programs. Working with clients who are considered to be psychologically well adjusted (Martin, 2001; Whitworth, Kimsey-House, & Sandahl, 1998; Williams & Davis, 2002), coaches serve to motivate, guide, inform, and support personal change processes. Cantwell and Rothenberg (2000) identified common interests of coaching clients, including weight management, improved nutrition, stress reduction, self-care, and creating personal boundaries. In this respect, life coaching provides important assistance for clients who want to be more successful and happy in their lives, without purporting to provide deep-level psychological care or technical advice (such as dietary information) beyond the bounds of the coach's certifications.

Saying that the growth of life coaching derives largely from its connections to the fitness industry would be inaccurate. Although personal trainers and other fitness professionals have expressed keen interest in this field (Cantwell, 2003), the origins of life coaching have multiple roots—some in sports coaching, some in management consulting, and many in the fields of counseling and psychotherapy. With its diverse clientele, coaching has evolved a number of subspecialties. Perhaps the most notable one to date is that of executive coaching (Fitzgerald & Berger, 2002), which focuses on an organizational leader or manager's performance within the system in which she or he is employed.

In the fitness world the need for nontechnical professional assistance in reaching personal and health-related goals has been evident at least since the advent of personal training as a profession. Although some clients hire personal trainers for technical performance coaching, most clients are people who need the support of wise and personable professionals as

they engage the challenge of exercising regularly. Over time, expertise attributed to trainers in the physical realm may generalize to other domains of life, especially when trainers earn clients' respect by assisting them in achieving valued goals. Trainers have been highly cognizant of the conflict between client needs and professional boundaries (Atkins, 2002; Rupp et al., 1999). Thus, when the field of life coaching began to emerge, many trainers perceived a viable resolution to this conflict through certification as a life coach. Coaching certification was considered a legitimate way of working with clients on their broader life agendas while still permitting trainers to function within a sport and fitness context.

The Move Toward Lifestyle Fitness Coaching

Generalists and specialists work in all professional arenas. As suggested earlier, the role of life coach has an exceptionally broad agenda. Recognizing this, health fitness professionals who take on certification as life coaches may opt to channel their coaching agendas to issues more aligned with their expertise in sports and physical activity.

The concept of lifestyle fitness coaching as distinguished from life coaching implies a process of working with clients within parameters of the fitness world, while at the same time encompassing the wholeness of clients. Lifestyle fitness coaching has the further characteristic of emphasizing the pursuit of wide-ranging personal and lifestyle goals (or ends) through means of rationally defined and intentionally planned physical activity engagements. Unlike typical fitness prescriptions in which goals involve changes along physical parameters (e.g., weight, body composition, or aerobic capacity), lifestyle fitness coaching accepts as legitimate objectives changes in personal skills, character development, psychological and social functioning, and other lifestyle and learning intentions.

Although this wider benefit package emphasized in lifestyle fitness coaching is not entirely new, it is not commonly addressed. Undoubtedly, some fitness instructors and personal trainers design fitness programs with awareness of the multidimensional needs and interests of their clients. Health fitness professionals might direct clients who want to avoid social isolation while training toward group-based activities. They may guide those complaining of career-related stress toward activities in which enjoyment and relaxation predominate. Yet even in these examples, concerns about program adherence rather than conscious intentions to integrate physical with personal and lifestyle gains may determine the strategy of health fitness professionals.

Most academic and professional programs in the health fitness field emphasize the diagnosis of physical characteristics far more than they do the identification of relevant personal and social factors. Trainers and instructors who incorporate variables beyond PAR-Q, $\dot{V}O_2$max, percentage of body fat, or strength and flexibility measures in their profiling of clients (Cotton & Anderson, 1999) stand a far greater chance of creating programs that reflect and influence clients' lifestyles, personal habits, needs, and interests.

Although health fitness professionals can invent their own strategies for working with the whole client, an easier and more reliable path of learning can be found in a well-articulated, professionally developed, systematic approach to understanding and coaching clients in the world of sport and fitness. Indeed, the process of lifestyle fitness coaching described in this book offers exactly this.

Lifestyle fitness coaching is embedded in the world of sport, fitness, and active living. It assumes essential competencies and knowledge bases appropriate to fitness assessment and programming. These include demonstrated understanding and skill in such areas as human anatomy, physiology, kinesiology, program design, instructional technique, and communication. Individuals who wish to function as lifestyle fitness coaches would need certification as health fitness professionals or be in the process of completing such certification before undertaking this further development of knowledge and skill. In other words, lifestyle fitness coaching is not a stand-alone skill base, as life coaching might be.

The definition of this new role in the fitness industry will no doubt evolve over time, but at this point it can best be expressed as follows:

LIFESTYLE FITNESS COACHING is an ongoing and guided process of dialogue between a client and health fitness professional. It is informed by comprehensive fitness-related data about client needs, interests, and personal orientations, and it is directed toward broad-based goals of personal and health gains. Clients are to attain these goals through sustained involvement in physical activities, adjusted periodically according to the client's evolving life agendas.

What You Will Find in This Text

This book provides a systematic approach to understanding lifestyle fitness coaching and a presentation of the necessary skills for professional development. Moreover, it offers a methodology for gathering and analyzing personal information about clients that enables coaches to engage in dialogue about the means and ends of clients' sport and fitness programming. The following chapter overview summarizes core learnings:

- Chapter 1 makes the case for the emerging field of lifestyle fitness coaching.
- Chapter 2 explores the potential of sport and physical activity for fostering personal development.
- Chapter 3 examines the core dynamics of coaching relationships and what coaches must do to build trust and client confidence.
- Chapter 4 delves into four cornerstones of effective coaching relationships: goals, contracts, ethics, and boundaries.
- Chapter 5 addresses the theme of change from three perspectives: how the coaching process progresses, clients' stages of readiness for change, and the inside experiences of a person in a process of change.
- Chapter 6, the first of three chapters that emphasize skill development, highlights rapport building and information gathering skills.
- Chapter 7 offers rich insights into coaching skills directed toward the development of insight and understanding.
- Chapter 8 focuses on skill development for organizing, influencing, and guiding change processes.
- Chapter 9 provides sample dialogues with two clients over a series of coaching sessions to promote the understanding of skill usage and coaching processes.
- Chapter 10 focuses on the use of questionnaires and other sources of data that coaches can use. In particular, the chapter introduces the MAPS Inventory, contained on the accompanying CD-ROM.
- Chapter 11 offers dialogues between a coach and client involving questionnaires such as those included in the MAPS Inventory. Through these dialogues, the reader can

gain a deeper appreciation of using assessment tools in a coaching process.

- Chapter 12 concludes with some perspectives of the future for lifestyle fitness coaching along with suggestions for continuing professional development.

Each chapter of the book sets the stage for the next. The book orients the reader to this emerging field and then connects it to more established traditions of helping relationships, especially through an appreciation of time-tested values and qualities of effective helpers. Discussions of goals, boundaries, ethics, and contracting in coaching relationships provide a further foundation. The core dynamic of change is then presented from different perspectives—inside the client and between coach and client. A special feature of this book is its dissection of coaching skills in a language that incorporates the historical roots of coaching found in counseling, psychotherapy, and other helping arts. By developing the reader's appreciation for key communication processes, the book makes possible a readiness for understanding the flowing and evolving dialogues between coach and client. Finally, the unique assessment tools (MAPS Inventory) that accompany this book provide guides to understanding client interests, motivations, and lifestyle patterns.

The book maintains a strong focus within the fitness world by continually referring to coaching processes that take place in the arena in which health fitness professionals have training and certification. While acknowledging diverse dimensions and needs of clients, the lifestyle fitness coach confines the prescriptive process of dialogue between coach and client to sport, fitness, and other active-living engagements.

Through reading this book, you will obtain core understanding of lifestyle fitness coaching methods, along with the tools for appreciating client interests and profiles.

This book alone cannot make you a good coach, but if you are able to demonstrate in your practice the thought processes and skills described here, you will successfully embody the professional competencies of a lifestyle fitness coach. In this respect, this book relies on your willingness to assimilate the materials presented, to practice in supervised sessions the skills required, and to seek feedback from peers and supervisors concerning your enactment of coaching behaviors.

Tools for the Lifestyle Fitness Coach

Although health fitness professionals typically gather appropriate medical and physical data about their clients, few systematic assessment devices are available for obtaining other fitness-related information about clients. This book offers a set of questionnaires in the MAPS Inventory. MAPS is an acronym for *matching activities and personal styles*. Developed and applied extensively within the fitness industry, the questionnaires are available to you on an accompanying CD-ROM. When clients complete the MAPS Inventory, a report is automatically generated for discussions in the coaching process. Information contained in this report includes the following:

1. Client reasons and motivations for exercising
2. Background information including client experiences with exercise
3. Client lifestyle and exercise style profiles related to fitness programming
4. Ratings of 50 sports and fitness activities according to the degree to which they match client profiles
5. Recommendations of sports and fitness activities that have high probability for client enjoyment and adherence

The MAPS profiling system is a tool that has merit in and of itself. Yet in a world in which people are bombarded with advice and recommendations about health and fitness, the tool becomes most valuable when it is incorporated in a process of lifestyle fitness coaching.

Lifestyle Fitness Coaching offers you dynamic ingredients for enriched and rewarding interactions with committed exercisers who want the most from their physical activities and with novices who struggle at the edges of the fitness world. It is not just a book of ideas and generic advice—it is a guide to success.

The book gives equal emphasis to theory and practice. Good practitioners need to understand what they are doing as much as they need to be skillful in applying knowledge. Too often, people can articulate theories and concepts but cannot skillfully apply their knowledge base. Deep learning occurs most reliably through the integration of theoretical understanding, practical application, feedback, and reflection on experience. Although the written word may be rich and exciting, its meaning expands greatly through practice. I encourage you to practice as you read. If you are reading this book as part of a course, your coursework may include practice components. If you are reading this on your own, find colleagues with whom you can collaborate in a learning enterprise.

You will find references to other books and materials throughout the chapters. You may wish to investigate these resources in the future. For now, may this book provide you with the fundamental building blocks of information and skill for your career endeavors as a lifestyle fitness coach.

Acknowledgments

This work is the result of more than 30 years of thought and research. In another sense, it is the merger of two lifelong loves—one for helping others move toward their dreams and visions, and the other for the joy of movement that I have experienced throughout my life as a competitive swimmer, triathlete, modern dancer, aikidoist, yoga teacher, and on and on. In this respect, my first thank-you, following the inestimable love and appreciation that I feel for my parents, Mary O'Donnell and Paddy Gavin, goes to Joe Steady, my first swim coach. My second, then, belongs to Dorothea McCandless, a professor of psychology at Fordham University, who unwittingly opened the door to graduate studies for me. My particular orientation in psychology was most influenced by Dr. Carl Rogers, whose works I avidly read as a graduate student and with whom I had the privilege of working during the summers of 1970 and 1971.

From an academic perspective, this work officially began in dialogues with Dr. Richard Suinn, a colleague of mine at Colorado State University, some 30 years ago. We had been discussing the emerging research on the effects of aerobic exercise on mood states, and because many of these studies centered on runners, my curiosity was piqued. I wondered whether different sports would have different kinds of effects. In those years, I was training in modern dance, studying mime, and doing tai chi and yoga while continuing to run, bike, and swim. I credit Dixie Hays-Menzer, Dale Lee Nivens, and Deborah Gomes with opening my mind and heart to the nonlinearity of movement after I stumbled unwittingly into their modern dance studio in Fort Collins, Colorado. I thank them profoundly. My cognitive awareness of the importance of different movement processes and correlated physical developments owes acknowledgement to Dr. Ken Dychtwald, whose workshops and seminal work, *Bodymind*, were of immense value.

My personal understanding of physical activity as a powerful influence on personal development has continued to grow over the years. In this latest period of my life, I have turned to the study of aikido to foster my learning. In this regard, I have been blessed by the sensitive, humorous, insightful, and always centered teachings of my sensei, Pierre Bohemier. His lessons framed within the study of aikido have had wide application to most domains of my life.

This work would not have occurred without the support, feedback, and encouragement of many people who have worked with me at my university and in fitness centers with which I have been associated. I am deeply grateful to Claude Bastien, Avi Spitzer, Francine Gauvin, Madeleine Mcbrearty, Claudette Rouisse, Mario D'Urso, Frederic Boisrond, and Stephane Vaillaincourt for all the ways in which they have helped me advance this work.

I thank Drs. Rainer Martens and Mike Bahrke at Human Kinetics for believing in this work and for shepherding it through the various phases of publication, and I thank Ms. Maggie Schwarzentraub, whose insightful editing of the work greatly augmented its clarity.

Finally, I want to thank my greatest cheerleaders—my children, Jessica, Jacob, and Susannah—who in random moments always seem to offer morsels of wisdom or humor or encouragement that serve to nourish and inspire.

Making the Case for Lifestyle Fitness Coaching

*"Of all the powers
we have as human beings,
none is as powerful and profound
as our power of choice—the core
gift of human experience.... And
none is as misunderstood."*

Carolyn Myss

By the last quarter of the 20th century, health scientists had little doubt about the profound and multidimensional benefits of sport and physical activity. Although debate persists concerning the relative amounts and types of activity needed (American College of Sports Medicine, 2000), by the turn of the century a solid foundation was in place for advocating exercise as a cornerstone of healthy living.

In spite of this, statistics continue to reflect low levels of participation in physical activity across North America, and health fitness professionals seem at a loss to explain why their powerful message fails to influence close to 80% of the population (Centers for Disease Control and Prevention, 2003). Low participation rates seem unlikely to be due to lack of awareness. Popular magazines faithfully promote the latest exercise fads, the no-strain–no-pain workouts, and innumerable tips for tighter abs, firmer buttocks, and bigger biceps. Meanwhile, scientists weigh in with the heavy artillery, detailing frightening declines in youth fitness, unprecedented increases in adult obesity, and documented disease risks of inactivity (Katzmarzyk, Gledhill, & Shephard, 2002; Lawrence, 2002; Lee, 1995; Morgan, 1997; Nash, 2003). Nothing seems to work. The beat goes on—without the dancers.

1

Mindless of the problem, regular exercisers rack up miles on treadmills, cry out under weighted bars, delight themselves in group fitness classes, and, in so doing, keep a growing number of health fitness professionals employed. After all, the 20% of the population who do exercise are a significant number.

What Do We Know?

Innumerable studies published in the past 25 years have created an information base about those who exercise regularly and those who don't (Dishman, 1988; Katzmarzyk, Glendhill, & Shephard, 2002; Martin Ginis et al., 2003; O'Brien Cousins, 2000). In simplified terms, studies and observations of active and inactive populations suggest the following:

- **A one-size-fits-all approach to fitness is ineffective.** Individual needs, capacities, and preferences require some attempt to match personal attributes to fitness prescriptions (Arnot & Gaines, 1984; Griffin, 1998; Heyward, 2002).

- **Biomechanical criteria are necessary but not sufficient for good programming.** Knowing individuals' biomechanical characteristics is an essential starting place for formulating sound fitness prescriptions, yet personality traits, attitudes, belief systems, lifestyles, sociocultural factors, and values must also be part of any prescriptive process (Gavin, 2003; Hays, 2002).

- **Life stages and phases must be accounted for in "talking the talk" and "walking the walk" of fitness.** The study of life-span development (Feldman, 2000) informs us that people experience predictable changes over a lifetime and that those changes influence needs and preferences, as well as capacities. Motivational strategies for encouraging people to exercise will vary depending on the age grouping or even the unique constellation of life challenges an individual is confronting at a particular time.

- **Not all fads are created equal; some endure because they captivate human interest and address personal styles.** Step aerobics continues, whereas few remember slide (Lofshult, 2003). Walking and running will likely remain core fitness activities. The five-thousand-year-old practice of yoga shows a reawakened presence in North America (Corliss, 2001). When activities match the needs or interests of large segments of the population, they thrive; otherwise, they fade from existence.

- **A carrot is better than a stick; positive appeals work better than fear-based incentives.**

Fear is a great motivator—for a while. Confronting people with the full range of consequences of inactivity may get them to the point of considering or even beginning to exercise (Prochaska, Norcross, & DiClemente, 1995). Maintaining the exercise habit (Gavin, 1992), however, is another story. What works best for the long run are positive incentives (Kazdin, 2001; Skinner, 1938; Wolpe, 1990), and although some of these might apply to large segments of the population, identifying a person's specific interests and motivations is critical and indeed one of the reasons why the lifestyle fitness coaching approach will be invaluable.

- **Social support is crucial for initiating and maintaining exercise commitment.** A small percentage of the population is so committed to their individual exercise regimens that virtually nothing, including injury, will discourage their continuance. But for most people, social experience is pivotal in maintaining exercise involvement (Dowda et al., 2003; Fraser & Spink, 2002; Gavin & Spitzer, 2002; Griffin, 1998; Resnick et al., 2002). Family members can either reward or punish fitness interests. Friends can lead one another either to the mall or to the gym. Health fitness professionals can function as fitness technicians, or they can embrace all the **bio-psycho-socio-cultural** contributors to health and illness (Donatelle, Davis, Munroe, & Munroe, 2001; N. Johnson, 2003) of their clients. If they address the latter, a major component of their roles will be encouraging, motivating, and supporting their clients while simultaneously providing the requisite technical guidance.

- **Information is power, especially when it pertains to an increasingly diverse and sophisticated exercise world.** One need only look at current lists of contraindicated exercises to know that we have come a long way. A great deal of information is now available about biomechanics and proper exercise techniques. In the past, people with certain chronic conditions including coronary heart disease or osteoarthritis were discouraged from exercising, whereas with our present information base we are able to say to these individuals that they can exercise in particular ways or with certain restrictions (Cotton & Andersen, 1999). Moreover, speaking to people in "languages" that they understand implies knowing what they need based not only on physical characteristics but also on their history, cultural heritage, education, and personal visions.

- **Ultimately, we need to embrace a holistic model of fitness; motivating the body is not enough.** Images of fitness often emphasize end products. Magazines endlessly portray highly sculpted bodies, washboard abs, and curvaceous shapes. When we look at the means to these ends, we may see some strange piece of equipment on a TV ad or a combination of weight rooms and cardio exercise areas at a local fitness center. The means are far less appealing than the ends. Yet, if our quest relates to active living, then we need to broaden the images of means to incorporate ways of moving, ways of being, ways of standing, and ways of sitting. We need to merge the experiences of living with the experiences of fitness. As health fitness professionals we must address all that a person is, all that a person does, and all that a person desires (Eickhoff-Shemek, 1997; Peterson & Bryant, 2001).

Forces and Counterforces for Active Living

Can we invent a better mousetrap? Can we discover a magic pill that makes people leap from bed into their sweat suits? Can we find a hacker to turn off all the computers each day until users complete a minimum of 10 minutes of cardio exercise? Although seasoned professionals may occasionally have such fantasies, even they recognize that there is no easy solution. Perhaps the best we can do is find ways to make exercise and sport more attractive, interesting, relevant, and beneficial to larger numbers of people through all the stages of their lives.

Sport sciences in conjunction with the fitness industry have produced more knowledge and program options than ever before, yet we need to go beyond the creation of new programs or fitness classes. To address all the ages and stages of a person's life, to attract people of diverse backgrounds and interests, and to motivate sustained participation across the life span, we need to consider new strategies to guide and support fitness involvement according to a person's unique and evolving lifestyle.

Moving beyond what we are doing now requires us to reflect on who our clients are, what they want versus what they need, and how physically active clients differ from those whom we hope to entice into the fitness experience. We need to take stock of knowledge that we can trust and the skill base on which we currently rely. Then, we need to look toward the future, anticipate changes coming our way, and develop new skills and knowledge to enable us to be more effective with both active and inactive populations.

What supports people in being active, and what keeps inactive people from doing what most health experts say they should do? A dazzling array of options and program possibilities support fitness devotees. Advice on what to do and how to do it abounds. Biomechanical knowledge serves as a powerful ally in program and machine design. Many highly qualified personal trainers are available to assist with the latest techniques. Fitness centers keep their doors open 24 hours a day.

Reinforcing the inactive are traps and snares far more insidious than those offered by any Harlequin romance novel. Computer-based activities confront us wherever we go. Adrenaline-fueled crowds pour out of Hollywood's latest action blockbusters, with moviegoers living vicariously through their favorite action heroes and heroines. If you can't order it on the Internet, drive-to and drive-up options are available for the rest of your needs. Perhaps most pernicious of all is the fact that physical education in the formative years of primary and secondary schooling has become largely extinct (Fay & Doolittle, 2002).

So, what's the big picture? A perspective of participation since the beginning of the fitness revolution (circa 1965) might be portrayed as follows: We made great headway for about a decade, maintained progress for a couple more decades, perhaps lost some ground toward the end of the 20th century, and currently have to work hard to keep the aging active baby boomers from falling off the treadmill onto the couch.

For every new incentive we have for active living, an equally strong force seems to oppose action. Yes, health scientists have made a strong case for active living, but the world has changed, and it increasingly promotes sedentary lifestyles.

Conclusion? We need to identify the factors that people describe as getting in the way of their fitness involvements and address them as best we can. We need to appreciate the processes and challenges of change. Further, we need to increase the forces and supports for active living, not only through more appealing programming but also through structural and social supports and by customizing fitness programs to address individual needs, lifestyles, and a more inclusive range of personal and health benefits.

Inducing people to remain active throughout the life span is a hard sell. Many young people simply do not get it. Their bodies stay firm all by themselves, or if they don't have genetically endowed washboard abs, they can figuratively crush the villain who is kicking sand in their faces through the digital manipulation of their video games.

As for adults, most of them say they do not have the time, interest, or energy (Top 10 reasons, 2003). Commuting, family responsibilities, fear of being laid off, rebuilding nest eggs after the burst of the tech bubble—one justification or another keeps most of them off the treadmill and out of fitness centers.

Then there are the seniors. Whether it was fear based in the depression era, the hardships of the war years, or simply the need to work constantly to survive, many seniors spent their youth and adult lives in a world that provided little support for regular sport and fitness participation. Many seniors may first set foot in a fitness facility shortly after they arrive at their retirement homes or communities. They may believe that by then it is too late.

As health fitness professionals, we know how serious the challenge is. We see the symptoms wherever we go. They appear in the form of airline companies charging passengers for two seats when they are unable to fit into one, the popularity of all-you-can-eat buffets, or the January surge in fitness club enrollments followed by the March decline. They can be seen in the dramatic popularity of surgical solutions to middle age or the endless quest for the perfect diet pill. Indeed, even with those who show determination to begin exercising, we witness their looks of frustration when their bodies appear essentially the same after a whole month of training!

But health fitness professionals refuse to quit. They put their collective shoulders to the wheel, they cheer on their clients, they change the choreography to prevent boredom, and they counter client excuses. They make it fun. They divide 30-minute workouts into doable 10-minute chunks. But the rates remain about the same. Force and counterforce.

Adding Value for Active Living

More than 30 years ago, the new field of exercise psychology burst upon the scene of Western science. Within its first decade, researchers proudly proclaimed they had something at least as good as antidepressant medication, an invaluable aid in the management of anxiety, and an organically safe boost to self-esteem and life adjustment (Morgan, 1997; Morgan & Goldston, 1987).

At first, running seemed to be the panacea (Sachs & Buffone, 1984). Of course, it was more than running, but in the 1970s popular magazines put a strong spin on something called the runner's high, and exercise professionals themselves reveled in the potential of running as therapy.

More accurately, Dr. Ken Cooper's (1977) term *aerobics* captured the essence of the new formula for

health and happiness. Biomechanics merged with psychology to demonstrate the merits of aerobic workouts for generating significant psychological payloads (Katzmarzyk, Gledhill, & Shephard, 2002). This idea was clearly adding value to the exercise benefit package.

For better or worse, exercise scientists probing the mechanisms underlying the runner's high promoted images of people training on treadmills or pedaling away on stationary bikes. Indeed, the fitness industry marked its first passage into modernity by moving some of the weight benches off the floor to make room for stationary cycles and treadmills. Shortly thereafter, group fitness studios laid claim to more of the space.

With efficiency in mind, North American scientists searched for the best and quickest ways to guarantee results. Given that physical rather than psychological agendas were more important to most exercise participants, researchers vigorously investigated the calorie-burning, muscle-toning properties of different exercise forms (Montoye, Kemper, Saris, & Washburn, 1996). But as one survey (Flippin, 1987) suggested, the pursuit of physical gains coalesced

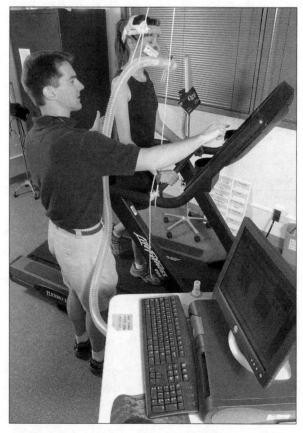

Laboratory studies of exercise influenced options available to exercisers.

with the quest for inner tranquility when exercisers continued beyond their initial year of activity.

In the final quarter of the 20th century, exercise psychologists steadily gained ground, making ever stronger cases for the psychological payoffs of aerobic exercise. A few adventurers offered up to scientific scrutiny activities like yoga and martial arts (Berger & Owen, 1992; Fuller, 1988), but perhaps because of the need to control and replicate research, much of the laboratory look of exercise (stationary cycling, running on treadmills) remained.

As the 21st century commenced, most health fitness professionals professed with rosy confidence that physical activity was not only essential for bodily health but also provided reliable benefits for psychological functioning (Morgan, 1997).

As most regular exercisers would attest, research documenting mood elevation, anxiety reduction, and self-esteem benefits of exercise did not come as a great surprise. What may have been less expected was the legitimization of physical exercise as a bona fide treatment for psychological difficulties (Greist et al., 1979; Morgan, 1997). Even more intriguing was the question of whether a specific exercise or sport might best address particular psychological conditions or needs (Gavin, 1988, 2003).

Western research focused strongly on frequency, intensity, and duration of exercise as related to psychological payoffs (ACSM 2000; Dishman, 1985; Morgan, 1997). Questions of how long one needed to exercise, at what aerobic intensity, and how frequently per week took precedence over investigations of modalities of exercise and differential benefits (Berger & Owen, 1992; Douillard, 1988; Gavin, 1988, 1992).

Through the study of **sport personology** (Vealey, 1989, 1992), the relevance of exercise modalities and their implications for personal functioning came under the microscope of Western sport science. But the questions explored in research on personality and sport were not always clear. Were researchers looking for evidence about why people choose different sports? Or were they concerned with whether sport participation changed personality? In either case, research results resembled a Tower of Babel. Studies were inconclusive in regard to whether different types of people were better suited to different sports or whether different sports offered different kinds of benefits (Diamant, 1991; Furnham, 1990; Mehrabaian & Bekken, 1986; Melamed & Meir, 1995; Sadella, Linder, & Jenkins, 1988; Sage, 1998; Vealey, 1992).

Nonetheless, some writers offered strong opinions about the mind-body connection in sport and exercise, and even about how different exercises or sports related to personality (Arnot & Gaines, 1984; Diamant, 1991; Douillard, 1988; Furnham, 1990). Although these perspectives often lacked the kind of empirical evidence normally required by Western science, they were sometimes based on decades, if not centuries, of practical application. For instance, Chinese doctors have prescribed movement forms from tai chi for different types of mental and physical problems for centuries, and in India yogis based healing recommendations on a taxonomy of postures dating back five thousand years.

Although scientific research on the person–sport matching theme declined toward the end of the 20th century, popular writers rallied around the argument (Gavin, 2003). Literally hundreds of references advance the possibility that individual needs and styles have bearing on sport and activity preferences. Clearly, more research is needed, yet the potential value would seem apparent. Processes by which individuals currently choose fitness options seem haphazard. If health fitness professionals knew more about clients' backgrounds, styles, and needs and if they understood how those factors related to various programming options, they might well be able to guide clients toward more satisfying and sustained fitness involvements (Griffin, 1998; Ray & Weise-Bjornstal, 1999).

Guidance, however, is not only about integrating broader bases of information about individuals with comprehensive understandings of what individual sport and fitness options have to offer but also about communication and support strategies appropriate to clients who are attempting to change longstanding habits.

Active Living in the Perspective of Lifelong Learning

The idea of individualizing fitness prescriptions brings up some intriguing possibilities. To a degree, such prescriptive processes are already in place in most fitness centers. New clients are assessed, typically on physical parameters, and presented with ideas about exercise programs based on their abilities, expressed interests, and medical considerations. The focus, however, is mostly on maximizing adherence so that clients can achieve their largely physical-change goals (Griffin, 1998; Ray & Weise-Bjornstal, 1999).

But with growing awareness of the psychological payload of exercise benefits, individualized prescriptions have the potential for incorporating factors that extend far beyond the physical realm. In light of the common dictum that sport builds character, we can easily envision character-building and skill-building possibilities that individualized fitness programming might foster (Danish, Nellon, & Owens, 1996; Sage, 1998; Shields & Bredemeier, 1995; Smith, 1999).

The significance of these additional benefits can best be understood in light of the fact that the average person exercising at recommended rates of 3 to 5 hours per week will spend thousands of hours in sport and exercise over the course of a lifetime. If these physical training hours double as personal learning and development time, would health fitness professionals have a wider range of incentives to offer current and potential clients? Would the public come to appreciate sport and fitness as providing multidimensional growth and development opportunities?

We know, for example, that many people engage in exercise to look their best, whereas others express less interest in that agenda. Many people are health conscious and will do whatever it takes to minimize health risks; others live like a cat with nine lives. If we combine the agendas to look good, feel good, and be healthy with a host of new incentives for being active, could we entice perhaps another 20% of the population to engage in exercise regularly? Consider some of these added possibilities for exercise payoffs.

Virtually all of us confront difficulties in life. We crash into walls because of ineffective behavior patterns. We face change through aging and major events like transitions, loss, crisis, or calamity. In this respect, lifelong learning is no longer an option for most people—it is a survival strategy. We change or we stagnate. We move with the trends or we are left behind. How many jobs from the 1950s exist today? How many relationships look like those of your grandparents? How many of your life stresses resemble those of the pioneers?

If learning to learn and adapting to change are the rules of the game, how can we play better? In the context of this discussion, what can we take from the world of sports and fitness to apply to the tasks of life adjustment and lifelong learning?

Playing tennis won't improve your calculus grades or directly result in a job promotion, but perhaps we can learn skills through this game that are useful in life. Or maybe the lessons of tennis are not the ones that you need to learn. Maybe you need to run a marathon.

People are different. Let's say that each of us has a personal style. Who someone is may be reflected in what that person does. This concept applies to the world of fitness and sport as well as to other domains of life. A process of creating individualized fitness prescriptions may mean finding activities that closely match an individual's preferences and style so that adherence becomes second nature. Or it may mean helping a person who has a strongly ingrained exercise habit learn additional skills for life through a conscious strategy of selecting new sport and fitness options to foster particular developmental interests.

Understanding the Evolution of Coaching

General information about exercise and fitness benefits surrounds us. In this respect, effective approaches to motivating and advising people to lead active lives would likely use a guided dialogue to emphasize the personal relevance of all this information.

Health fitness professionals who have worked in one-to-one relationships know the power of interpersonal ties and support. We are social animals, and it is fair to say that social connection is an element that needs to be part of our process of working with clients. As an aspiring or practicing health fitness professional, you need to emphasize not only the way that you connect with clients and the public at large but also the scope of your connections.

If you limit your communications to the operation of machines, biomechanics of movement, and formulas for bodily changes, you will strongly address the needs of a limited number of people and inadequately address the needs of a far larger number of people.

What is called for is a process for addressing wide-ranging needs and for communicating information in ways that are supportive and motivating. This process is referred to as lifestyle fitness coaching.

Take a moment to put together what has been presented thus far: Exercise participation throughout North America is far lower than desired and threatens to become even worse. Although sport scientists have made substantial progress in improving both the means and ends of living actively, we do not have well-defined processes for addressing individual needs and lifestyles, and for channeling people into appropriate, personalized fitness programs. Although we may be approaching information overload with public fitness messages, this information is often presented in either limited messages (focusing on fitness devotees) or overbroad messages (generic "do it or else!") that have questionable effect. Recognizing that people need people, can we develop personal processes of communicating with clients that assess and acknowledge their unique needs and lifestyles and that align them with active-living experiences to support their uniqueness and yield the greatest benefits?

Coaching is a tradition firmly rooted in the world of sport and exercise, yet coaching in the context of this discussion has some distinctly different angles and values. The manner in which a lifestyle fitness coach communicates with clients and the nature of the information encompassed in such interactions represent a significant **paradigm shift** for the world of sport and fitness. No single solution is likely to bring about radical changes in population activity rates. But if we accept the premise that matching the benefit potential of fitness options with individual profiles can be useful, then developing appropriate communication processes between clients and health fitness professionals becomes a significant tool for motivating people toward active lifestyles. Moreover, because coaching is a process rather than an event, the guidance and support that coaches provide through clients' experiences of doubt and confusion can help stabilize patterns of active living rather than reinforce episodic encounters with the world of sport and fitness.

Coaching As a Paradigm Shift in the Fitness World

Toward the end of the 20th century, public watchdog agencies and professional associations of fields such as psychology directed increasing criticism toward the fitness industry for boundary encroachments. These critics judged that some personal trainers were serving in quasi-professional capacities as nutritionists, counselors, marriage advisors, and physiotherapists (Atkins, 2002).

Policing themselves, fitness industry professionals attended workshops, participated in focus groups, generated position statements, and, in general, did their best to clarify lines distinguishing fitness professionals from other types of health services professionals. Yet fundamental human dynamics and societal shifts would inevitably thwart efforts to create pristine professional demarcations.

First, in the world of the 1970s, most fitness instructors worked part-time and taught a few aerobic dance classes per week. By the 21st century, many fitness professionals had full-time careers, and newcomers to the industry would settle for nothing less.

Second, in the gradual blurring of lines between mind and body disciplines that characterized the last half of the 20th century, professions began to trespass on one another. People were not machines. We could not intelligently view a person as a composite of separate elements. Mind was related to body. Drugs were in some cases no better than talk. Touch might heal as well or better than surgery. What you ate could profoundly influence thoughts, feelings, and actions. In essence, one could not always isolate and treat a segment of a person's being or experiences with high expectations for success.

For professional societies to expect personal trainers and their clients to spend 2 or 3 hours together each week without talking about life matters was not reasonable. Similarly, to expect trainers to continue to count off pushups without some personal response to a client's voiced concerns was equally unrealistic. Something had to give.

How Coaching Differs From Counseling

In the 1990s, something called **life coaching** began to show up between the lines of a number of professions. Life coaching was not psychotherapy, or nutritional counseling, or spiritual advising, or marriage counseling—at least not in any formal sense. So, what was it?

A definition of life coaching might begin with the statement that it is only nominally related to athletic coaching, although it shares certain fundamental elements. If you bring to mind your definition of a team coach or athletics coach, you may imagine a benign, paternalistic guide or perhaps an autocratic despot. Whatever your framework for defining coaches, we generally see them as making the big decisions and taking the rap when the team or athletes fail to perform.

Take another profession that might seem closely related, namely, counseling. Although counseling itself is generally associated with the field of psychotherapy, this latter field falls further away from the core of life coaching owing to its agenda of addressing deep psychological problems (Prochaska & Norcross, 2003). Counseling, whether from an educational, religious, or psychological backdrop, aims to assist individuals confronting normal life dilemmas and adjustments and is generally short term and problem focused. Professional counselors usually have at least a master's degree in such fields as pastoral counseling, education and guidance, social work, or counseling psychology. As you do with athletics coaches, you might conjure up images of benevolent, empathic counselors or advisors who analyze your problem and tell you what to do. Like athletics coaches, counselors may have styles ranging from collaborative to directive.

In truth, coaching and counseling overlap significantly, yet life coaching may best be seen as a narrow band within the broader scope of counseling. Some would argue with this characterization of coaching, preferring to define life coaching as a wholly separate and new profession. Ultimately such arguments serve mostly to fuel legal and ethical debates, while the core fact remains essentially indisputable: Coaching derives much of its skill base and its principles from the evolution of counseling and counseling theory throughout the 20th century (Cormier & Nurius, 2003; Ivey & Ivey, 2003; Williams & Davis, 2002).

Nevertheless, people who define their work as life coaching differ significantly in accent or emphasis from those who describe their practice within the realm of counseling. A sampling of differences (Williams & Davis, 2002) suggests that coaches as compared with counselors are more likely to do the following:

- Emphasize the present and future more than the past
- Focus on solutions rather than problems
- Frame issues more for goal setting than for diagnosis
- Direct conversations more toward action than analysis
- Orient conversations and structures more for action planning than for insight and understanding
- Use assignments, practice, and homework to foster movement
- Work on growth agendas rather than deficit agendas
- Foster independence and taking responsibility rather than dependency and justification
- Refer clients to any number of allied professionals while continuing to coach them on actions relevant to their visions

Stripped of titles, coaches and counselors may at times be difficult to distinguish. Yet titles are intended to provide indications about areas of focus, ways of working, clientele, and professional boundaries. Someone functioning under the title of a life coach would be out of bounds in asking for details about childhood issues, suggesting psychotropic medication, or giving nutritional advice, yet if a client voiced complaints about problems arising

from these matters, it would be entirely legitimate for a life coach to assist the client in formulating an action plan to gather data, seek expert advice, and embark on a remedial program.

The creation of the coaching niche in the world of professional services was not random. Coaching grew out of an unfulfilled need for straightforward, uncomplicated, affirming, action-oriented, results-focused professional assistance. It also arose from practical concerns.

Fields of psychotherapy and counseling often operate within constraints about time and location. The 50-minute hour has become part of our cultural awareness of the way in which therapists or counselors function (Covington, 2002). Clients meet therapists in their offices at the appointed hour, typically for 50 minutes, and at a normal rate of once a week. Telephone calls are generally restricted to scheduling matters and emergencies.

Life coaching has become roughly synonymous with telephone and even Internet communications. Life coaches also have their appointed hour, but they may arrange for brief follow-ups, check-ins, and in general have a more flexible way of working. Coaches and clients may use the Internet for chat-room group interactions or for transmission of inspirational messages, documents, or e-mails.

Keeping in mind the preceding differences in emphases, coaching embraced many of the societal changes and needs brought about through technological advances, lifestyle patterns, and scheduling needs in a chronically overscheduled society. Moreover, the sanctity of the 50-minute hour simply did not make sense for many of the issues that clients were bringing to their counselors or therapists.

In a world of growing complexity, people need all kinds of assistance to maneuver through our modern mazes. Health care systems, taxation policies, and legal concerns, among others, lead people to the doors of experts. Getting expert assistance is not only a normal process but a wise one as well. Although visiting a psychotherapist continues to have an archaic stigma attached to it, enlisting the support of a life coach may be more palatable to most clients.

With a century of Freudian-fueled psychological wisdom behind us, most people have some awareness of the roots of their issues and needs. What they have difficulty with is change. As Freud himself indicated, insight is half the battle in bringing about a cure (Freud, 1964). The implication was that this 50% was sufficient, but we now know differently. People may have insight about why they eat, drink, or work to excess, but when it comes to adhering to programs of change, commitment vanishes quickly in the face of poorly structured strategies, inadequate social support, and the press of life and old habits. Ultimately, the coaching paradigm was simply more practical and more useful for many people, even those who had previously relied on the assistance of counselors and therapists.

We can readily make a number of observations when we relate this discussion to the work of health fitness professionals and the agendas of their actual and intended clients:

1. Perhaps because they become physically close with clients, fitness instructors and personal trainers have been challenged to remain within the boundaries of their fitness agendas; they are repeatedly presented with other dimensions of their clients' lives that affect health and happiness. Furthermore, if bodies reflect lifestyles and mental states, then it would be difficult for fitness professionals not to notice, or not to care.

2. If we consider the premise that how you do anything relates to how you do everything (Festinger, 1957; Hoelter, 1985; Willensky, 1960), fitness professionals have extensive information about their clients from observing what they do and how they do it at the gym.

3. If we accept the possibility that a segmented, mechanistic treatment of human beings misses the larger picture, then the practice

of doing muscle tests, body-composition measures, and $\dot{V}O_2$max assessments without determining who people are, what they like, what they need, and what their life visions are seems not only unwise but also ineffective.

Toward a Definition of Lifestyle Fitness Coaching

Let us once again piece this information together. We have considered the need for a special process of communication between health fitness professionals and clients that results in uniquely supportive fitness programming and motivational guidance. We have seen how, in spite of attempts to clearly delimit fitness professionals' roles in the last quarter of the 20th century, societal trends favoring holistic treatments coupled with the nature of fitness professionals' relationships with clients have thwarted efforts at rigid role restrictions. Finally, we have reviewed the recent emergence of a new professional category of life coaching. These considerations point directly toward a process that lies entirely within the legitimate parameters of a health fitness professional's work. The process is called lifestyle fitness coaching (figure 1.1) and is defined as

- an ongoing and guided process of dialogue between a client and a health fitness professional that is

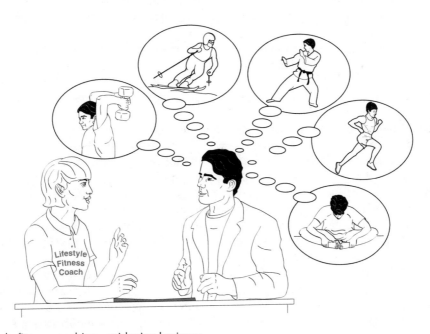

Figure 1.1 Lifestyle fitness coaching—widening horizons.

- informed by comprehensive fitness-related data about client needs, interests, and personal orientations, and

- directed toward broad-based goals of personal and health gains that are

- attained through sustained involvement in physical activities, which are

- adjusted periodically according to the client's evolving life agendas.

Coaching As an Ongoing and Guided Dialogue

In the emerging literature of learning processes, the term *dialogue* (Bohm, 1996; Yankelovich, 1999) occupies a position of great significance. It refers to a special kind of conversation in which learners communicate with one another without preset definitions of the conclusions and without untested assumptions. Learners explore ideas with the intention of discovering answers rather than verifying what they already know or proving their position.

The traditional view of a professional interacting with a client is a kind of "one down" power relationship. One person, the professional, is the expert with all the answers, whereas the other, the client, is unknowledgeable and dependent on the expert's advice. This circumstance, sometimes known as the medical model (Williams & Davis, 2002), has been strongly criticized for the passivity it induces in clients, for the unrealistic knowledge base attributed to practitioners, and for the assignment of responsibility for outcomes to the person who often has the least influence over them, namely, the professional.

In some cases, this traditional view can be appropriate. Fitness experts, for example, need to instruct novice exercisers in the basics of program design, posture, and technique. Even so, the effectiveness of experts' communications will depend on how well they engage clients in a back-and-forth interaction so that they can determine whether clients are understanding, whether they need to account for additional factors in offering prescriptions, or whether they can impart information in ways that will motivate clients better. These subtle differences move us closer to dialogue.

The notion of an ongoing and guided dialogue is not only one of discovery but also one of continuing communication over time. It is not a one-time, fix-it-all-now process. As a lifestyle

fitness coach, the health fitness professional offers a process of communication in which he or she exchanges information in a nonhierarchical manner so that all the relevant data can be made public and validated from both perspectives before action is considered. Each party has different sources of expertise and information that he or she will share in a collaborative fashion. If a power dynamic is present in the dialogue, the less powerful participant may act out of fear or ego or defensiveness and thereby diminish the quality and quantity of relevant information produced in the conversation.

Necessity for Comprehensive Fitness-Related Data in Lifestyle Fitness Coaching

The frame that we need to draw around lifestyle fitness coaching is formed by concerns about how the client will engage the world of active living, which includes but is not limited to sport and exercise. The purpose of gathering data is to inform activity-related intentions and behaviors. This frame is generally broader than the normal one because of the scope of outcomes of fitness involvements that are to be considered. We know that participation in physical activities will affect not only the body but also mental and psychological functioning. Moreover, participation never occurs in a vacuum. Social implications result from all the hours spent exercising, including how a person interacts and with whom.

The scope is framed in the words *lifestyle fitness*. How can we organize fitness programming so that what people need to do best accommodates their lifestyles? In this perspective, all kinds of information that we might not normally consider come into play.

Traditionally, data pertinent to the physical being of the client have been carefully assessed as the primary guides to programming. Although this information is necessary for lifestyle fitness coaching, it may not be sufficient. We can perhaps understand an emphasis on nonphysical parameters in the following light: About 80% of the population needs to exercise more than they do. The 20% of committed athletes, near athletes, and recreational exercisers may indeed have different interests, needs, and personal histories than the 80% group. Motives for the insufficiently active to commit to regular exercise might encompass a different set of incentives than those that we normally encounter in fitness centers. The broader the information bases about actual and potential participants, the greater the chances of finding links to their drives and dreams.

Nature of Goals in Lifestyle Fitness Coaching

Some outcomes of sport and exercise participation have been thoroughly researched and widely publicized; others remain in the realm of discovery, either through systematic research or through the process of dialogue between coach and client.

Lifestyle fitness coaching relies on dialogue to discover what a person hopes to achieve, what he or she is willing to invest, to which paths the person is most likely to commit, and what creativity can be applied to generating nontraditional exercise outcomes that may be part of the person's wish list. This last point may require explanation.

Health fitness professionals are accustomed to hearing such agendas as the desire to lose 20 pounds (9 kilograms) in one month with an investment of 3 hours per week, and they are well versed in presenting the sad facts that such goals are unrealistic. If the health fitness professional can reframe sport and exercise as learning opportunities based in thousands of hours of activity over a lifetime, what else might be possible? What could a person learn? What skills could one develop? What dreams could one fulfill?

If we limit conversations to the set of outcomes documented in research, we will have wonderful things to offer those who exercise regularly, but will these outcomes be sufficient? Will general conclusions from normative studies speak to the distinctive nature and needs of particular clients? Other outcomes are possible, and their identification may emerge through innovative thinking and client-centered programming. Moreover, the attainment of these unique outcomes may require that the person exercise consciously, that is, with his or her personally designed goals in mind.

If this method appears to be offering individuals a menu of undocumented exercise outcomes from which to choose, then consider this perspective of the proposed agenda. If we interpret benefits in the broadest manner possible, we could imagine a client who, as a life agenda, wants to develop greater comfort in social settings. What information do we have that would suggest that this client could achieve her agenda through a strate-

gic approach to exercise participation? To begin, research supports the outcome of anxiety reduction from even short bouts (10 minutes) of aerobic activity (Hansen, Stevens, & Coast, 2001). Furthermore, clinical psychology research documents the validity of "systematic desensitization" procedures whereby individuals are gradually exposed to anxiety-provoking situations under conditions in which they are feeling relatively relaxed before the exposure (Jacobson, 1938). Putting these research-based processes together in a creative program design might result in the following scenario: The person schedules training to begin about 25 minutes before a particular group exercise class commences. She might start her workout with a warm-up and then work out for 15 minutes on a cardio machine such as a treadmill, stair climber, or elliptical trainer. Research tells us that this activity should lower physiological anxiety levels. Then, the individual would join the class. Over time, we would predict that the lowered anxiety level that the person experienced before class would help her in walking into the class, and that the exposure to the anxiety-provoking group situation under conditions of lowered anxiety (sustained by the continuation of aerobic activity) would help to desensitize her to group encounters. As the client progresses, more interactive styles of sport and exercise might be considered. Clearly, this kind of programming requires a certain type of relationship between the coach and the person, as well as coaching expertise and client consciousness.

You are probably aware that in this example we have just leapfrogged over the normal prescription process offered within fitness centers or gyms. With this new kind of advising, we are fully in the domain of lifestyle fitness coaching rather than in traditional practices of fitness advisors.

Domain of Prescriptions for Lifestyle Fitness Coaching

What contains this process within the legitimate framework of fitness is the prescription of sport and physical activity. Although it may be true that psychologists have documented the psychological payload of exercise, it would not be accurate to say that psychologists, or for that matter most other professionals, should be the ones to prescribe exercise programming. The task of aligning individuals with appropriate sport and fitness activities is best left in the hands of health fitness professionals.

Health fitness professionals need to be certified, and although this requirement is relatively new, its demands will deepen in years to come (Lidane, 2003). Fitness advisors and trainers will be held increasingly accountable for knowing anatomy, physiology, biomechanics, and programming requirements for special populations, such as pregnant women, clients with osteoarthritis, people with diabetes, or people with various forms of cardiovascular disease (Cotton & Andersen, 1999). Organizations like IDEA Health and Fitness Association already demarcate treatment issues appropriate for fitness professionals as compared with other allied health professionals (Benefits, 2001). In many instances, team approaches are advocated, and in this regard, the recommended working style of a coach is entirely compatible with team-treatment approaches (Walker, 2001).

In the context of a normal population, in which adults are responsible for their actions and exchange information through dialogue rather than prescriptive mandates, a mature individual chooses to engage in conversations with a lifestyle fitness coach about personal concerns, lifestyle goals, aspirations, intentions, and a whole panoply of human needs and interests with the intention of determining the best programming options for growth and development, at all levels of being. Coaches listen to such information for cues to program design and adherence, not to fix or solve or prescribe psychological, nutritional, or medical remedies.

Of course, many life problems have solutions that lie well beyond the reach of activity **interventions.** Clients may present matters to coaches that might have only a fraction of relevance for activity programming; the remainder of the clients' issues might be referred to appropriate professionals for further diagnosis and intervention or simply considered as general information without need for action. Even so, the fraction of information that may pertain to fitness could help guide scheduling, social contexts, or other supportive structures.

To summarize this point, health fitness professionals seem to have a clear edge on the application of knowledge bases about different sports and physical activities. Certification requirements are becoming more demanding, thereby ensuring adequate competency levels for those responsible for advising clients about programs. Although physical status data concerning clients are necessary for programming, they are frequently insufficient. For those clients who choose to explore the potential that sport and exercise hold as transformative

life interventions, a dialogue between coach and client can be wide ranging in content so long as its primary purpose is the design and motivation of sustained involvement in appropriate physical activities.

Need for Periodic Reviews in the Coaching Process

Change. A behavior pattern that fosters success for a man in his 20s may prove to be a detriment in his 30s. Something that interests him today may lose its appeal next year. What he urgently desires as a single man may become irrelevant when he is a father of three. If we expect change to characterize different quarters of our lives, would we not want to account for program adjustments in how individuals approach exercise over the life span? Your probable answer is yes, and perhaps one of the first concerns you might have would be about the person's physical capacities and needs. In this light, cross-training has been the rubric under which fitness professionals have proffered all sorts of advice to fitness participants. The runner who ignores stretching or who is accustomed to a "10K a day to keep the doctor away" may be in a losing game, unless he incorporates supplementary activities.

Beyond the physical plane, life changes may be more subtle but nonetheless significant. Ages and stages of life bring with them different demands and corresponding needs for new skills and styles of functioning. The hard-charging junior executive may need to learn team-building and mentoring styles as a senior executive. The isolated technician may need to develop social competencies when promoted to workgroup leader. Survival skills for singles are different from survival skills for parents. When good looks fade, a person may need to nurture charm and charisma.

Ruts. We are prone to them. Whether we call it the comfort zone or some other term that characterizes our desire for familiar turf, known venues, or well-traveled roads, as human beings we tend to stick with the known far beyond the point at which its utility begins to decline (McWilliams, 1991).

Managing change in the fitness world is about more than buying new equipment or making sure that centers have the latest programming fad; it is also about helping clients adjust their programs based on personal evolution. Of course, you may be aware of clients who are continuously "adjusting" by trying out the newest techniques or classes with regularity. This sort of behavior is not the same thing. Lifestyle fitness coaching is a process of periodically discussing with clients how their programs are working for them, what benefits they are experiencing, what downsides they are encountering, and what personal and physical needs are emerging in their lives. Through dialogue, coaches help clients reflect and consciously plan for current or anticipated changes in life patterns, interests, and capabilities.

Getting From Here to There!

In many fitness clubs and centers, initiation into membership has a common form. A new client is offered an advisement session with an instructor that serves as a baseline screening process and introduction to the options available at the facility. For example, the instructor may conduct a general interview and administer a broad medical screening questionnaire. After identifying evident training limitations, the instructor may show the client how to use equipment or may even help the member develop a specific weight workout. The conclusion of the session may include general advice about program guidelines (frequency, intensity, and duration) and some motivational strategies. In a general sense, the goal is to help the client get the most from the offerings of the facility. The process is depicted in figure 1.2.

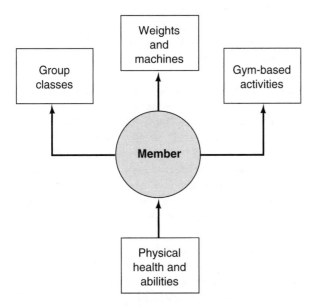

Figure 1.2 A model of elements in traditional fitness advising.

Various goals and resources guide the role of lifestyle fitness coach. Lifestyle fitness coaches meet with clients to review their medical and physical history, their training goals, and their personal styles and preferences. Coaches explore not only clients' fitness goals but also other expectations they have of their exercise involvement. Through dialogue with clients, lifestyle fitness coaches assist clients in determining which sports and physical activities best suit their current patterns and which activities might help them develop skills and abilities that would facilitate desired lifestyle changes. Lifestyle fitness coaches consider a range of activities that extends far beyond the walls of the facility (see figure 1.3). With a framework of active living and lifelong learning in mind, the lifestyle fitness coach most likely regards options available at a fitness center as means to ends rather than as ends in themselves.

What about all the skills that fitness instructors previously applied in work with clients? The simple answer is that they continue to be essential and highly relevant. But lifestyle fitness coaches need additional skills to achieve more balanced and advantageous programming for their clients. Consider this example: Through dialogue with a lifestyle fitness coach, a client decides that she would benefit personally by taking up rock climbing and white-water kayaking. In all likelihood, the client will have decided to do other things in her training, but imagine that these activities are identified through the dialogue as having high congruence with personal and lifestyle goals for this person. Focusing strictly on the activities (and not, for example, on the myriad of personal goals set by the client), you might ask, "How does the fitness center enter this picture?"

We can reframe most fitness center programs as means by which people can develop strength, flexibility, and endurance so that they can easily and safely pursue active lifestyles throughout the year. Lifestyle fitness coaches attempt to understand the active living choices of clients (end goals) and then help clients achieve these goals through fitness programming available at their facilities. In this example, a person who is going to do rock climbing and white-water kayaking will need to develop certain types of strength, flexibility, and endurance. The lifestyle fitness coach will be the client's guide to this kind of development, rather than being the climbing or kayaking instructor. The lifestyle fitness coach collaborates with the member to create a road map to active living and then may serve as a technical fitness expert in the weight room

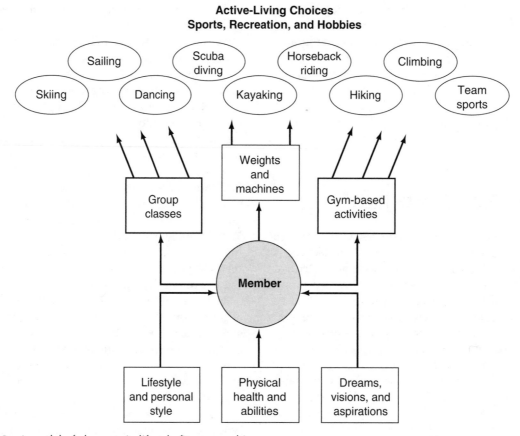

Active-Living Choices
Sports, Recreation, and Hobbies

Sailing · Scuba diving · Horseback riding · Climbing

Skiing · Dancing · Kayaking · Hiking · Team sports

Group classes · Weights and machines · Gym-based activities

Member

Lifestyle and personal style · Physical health and abilities · Dreams, visions, and aspirations

Figure 1.3 A model of elements in lifestyle fitness coaching.

or in other club venues appropriate to the coach's competencies.

As noted earlier, this approach represents a significant paradigm shift within the fitness world. This alteration is important, and it is where we are collectively going. The world of fitness is rapidly evolving. We can quickly identify the emerging career paths of health fitness professionals. In the 1980s one needed to learn how to be a good group fitness instructor. By the 1990s personal training had taken the lead with its individualized, one-to-one crafting of fitness programs. At the turn of the century we began to see scores of personal trainers enrolling in life coaching programs at specialized distance education centers.

Why have all these changes occurred? The answer is simple. People are different, their motivations are multilayered, and they want to reach for the stars. Although it may make good biomechanical sense to have someone sit on a stationary bicycle and pedal for 30 minutes a day at 60% to 80% of their maximum capacity, most people won't do it. As Morgan (2001) remarks, "People give all sorts of reasons for not wanting to exercise. . . . but I think the

real reason is that they don't want to do pointless, nonpurposeful things like running on a treadmill." For each person, different reasons may explain why sound biomechanical prescriptions don't take (see figure 1.4). Learning activity 1.1 might be a useful way to further your understanding of some of the issues presented in this chapter.

With the advent of personal training, custom-tailored programs were coupled with emotional and technical support. Yet even this solution lacked critical elements. Human beings are purposive, goal-seeking creatures. They come to health and fitness centers with a wide range of needs and interests. They arrive with their whole selves. As health fitness professionals gain greater competency in uncovering of the needs, backgrounds, and goals of individual clients, they will be more able to guide and support them in achieving imagined and unimagined results.

So, how do you get from here to there? How can you develop the skill set essential to success—for you and for your clients? How do you make the transition from being a technical fitness advisor to being a lifestyle fitness coach?

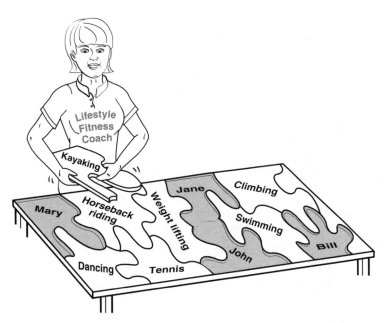

Figure 1.4 Pieces of the puzzle.

Reading this book and mastering its knowledge base form part of the answer. The rest comes with practice, ongoing reflection, and formal and informal coaching from others who have embarked on a similar path. One thing seems certain: By embarking on the path of becoming a lifestyle fitness coach, you will open the door to exciting new career opportunities, complement skill sets you have already developed, and serve your clients in a more holistic manner.

Learning Activity 1.1

Practice Interviews to Understand Exercise Motivations

In your family and friendship network, you are likely to know people who have played sports and exercised most of their lives and some who have rarely participated in physical activities. Ask a few of them if they would be willing to talk to you about their thoughts and feelings regarding sports and physical activities.

Try to find two people who have been active for many years. Ask them the following questions:

1. What have you been doing over the years in relation to sport and physical activity?

2. What has kept you involved for all this time? What kinds of benefits have you experienced? (Look for ways to categorize their answers into such classes as physical, psychological, social, and so forth.)

3. Can you tell me why you do the specific activities that you do?

4. Are there sports or activities that you would not do? Can you tell me why?

5. Do you think you have changed at all because of doing your sports and physical activities? If so, would you tell me how? (Look for ways to categorize their answers.)

6. Is there anything else you can tell me that would help me understand your continued connection to physical activity?

(continued)

Learning Activity 1.1 *(continued)*

Then find two people who have been mostly inactive over their lives, or at least in recent years. Ask them the following questions:

1. Can you tell me what you have been doing over the past few years in relation to sport and physical activity?

2. Do you have any thoughts that you would be willing to share with me about the reasons that you are not more active physically?

3. Can you tell me, in general or specifically, what your attitudes and feelings are about doing physical exercise and sports on a regular (at least three times a week) basis every week for the rest of your life?

4. Are there any sports or activities that you feel particularly attracted to? Can you tell me what attracts you to these activities?

5. Are there any sports or activities that you feel strongly averse to doing? Can you tell me why?

6. What would it take for you to become more physically active in a way that you believe you would enjoy and could sustain?

7. Is there anything else you can tell me that would help me understand your thoughts and feelings about sport and physical activity?

With the results of these interviews in mind, you may wish to reread this chapter to determine whether any of the issues uncovered in these conversations relate to the material presented.

two

Coaching and Active Living

A Formula for Change

*"Whatever the mind is doing,
the body must do also;
whatever the body is doing,
the mind must do also."*

John Douillard

The field of coaching has been defined in such a way that it encompasses vast domains of human behavior. Reflecting this agenda, the International Coach Federation (www.coach federation.org) describes life coaching as "an ongoing relationship, which focuses on clients taking action toward the realization of their visions, goals, or desires." Another well-known center for training life coaches, Life Coach Training (www.lifecoach training.com), states, "Coaching entails working with people who already have a measure of 'success' in their lives, but who want to bridge the gap between where they are and where they want to be in their profession and their personal life. . . . Coaches help their clients design the life they want, bring out their clients' own brilliance and resources so that they can achieve excellence and create purposeful, extraordinary lives." Many people who want support and structures for attaining such goals as changing careers, learning new skills, writing a book, or developing business networks look to life coaches for assistance.

The notion that clients have already demonstrated success in their lives implies that coaching emphasizes development far more than rehabilitation. In Martin's (2001) popular book, coaching is defined as "a holistic process that has the power to balance and harmonise life." Larsen (2002, p. 46) considers coaching "a collaborative relationship which forwards action or deepens understanding, based on trust and integrity. Coaching focuses on the goals, development and dreams of the person being coached, with specific expectations for growth."

In the literature of life coaching, some accepted principles include the belief that agendas must come from clients and that the primary purpose of the coaching relationship is solely to help clients achieve results they desire (Martin, 2001). A long-standing text on life coaching, originating from one of the first coaching schools, identifies three core agendas for coaching—fulfillment, balance, and process (Whitworth, Kimsey-House, & Sandahl, 1998). Each of these is seen to originate within the client.

Whitworth and colleagues (1998) believe that clients enter coaching with a "hunger for fulfillment" (p. 115). Clients are motivated to work with coaches based on a kind of gap analysis, that is, an assessment of the discrepancy between what they have and what they want. Coaches assist clients in working through layers of definitions of fulfillment, generally progressing from external, tangible definitions, such as a new house or a new job to deeper value-laden desires, such as needs for learning and spirituality. Ultimately, coaching philosophy posits that fulfillment is not a matter of having, but rather a way of being.

Another core agenda that Whitworth and colleagues (1998) believe that clients have is achieving balance across the multiple domains of life. With modern-day pressure to perform and achieve in many areas, clients are seen as experiencing a lack of harmony, a sense of being happy with some dimensions but unfulfilled in others. Coaches help clients identify satisfactions with careers, health, financial position, relationships, family, physical environment, personal growth, and recreation. Areas of dissatisfaction are the focus of coaching to bring clients' lives more into balance.

The third and final core agenda identified by Whitworth and colleagues (1998) seems almost paradoxical within the coaching context. With so much of the coaching literature emphasizing action directed toward goal achievement, the process agenda relates more to "being"—to blending with life rather than always trying to make something happen. In focusing on process, coaches guide clients to stay with the moment, to notice what is happening now, and to answer the question of how they want to be rather than what they want to be.

With this general overview of life coaching agendas, you may wonder how it is possible to have sufficient expertise to guide clients through such vast ranges of interests, needs, and issues. Indeed, most professions struggle with such concerns and generally resolve them through the development of specializations.

To work as a health fitness professional, one needs to have achieved certain levels of understanding and education. Moreover, certification examinations in the fitness industry attempt to ensure that professionals manifest a high degree of skill and knowledge in core areas. When this more technical base is aligned with life coaching skills, a reasonable portion of the full range of coaching interventions can be identified.

The domain of sport and physical activity frames lifestyle fitness coaching. Either as a means

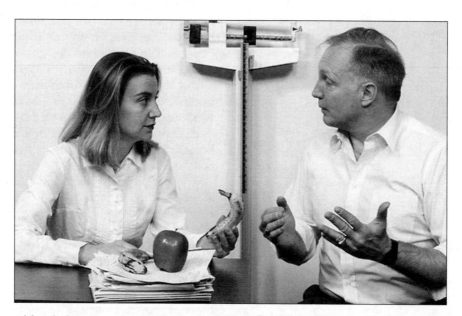

A lifestyle fitness coach with an advanced degree in a discipline such as nutrition or psychology can expand the domain of her practice.

to an end or as an end in itself, active living engagements frame the prescriptive agenda that lifestyle fitness coaches employ. Although coaches may help clients achieve a range of interests in fulfillment, balance, and process, a boundary is drawn around the work of a lifestyle fitness coach. With high levels of interest, skill, and knowledge in sport and physical activity, lifestyle fitness coaches are best able to embrace the wholeness of their clients within a most important dimension of their lives, namely, active living. Lifestyle fitness coaches who want to expand their repertoire to include additional domains of expertise, such as nutrition, will find that the principles emphasized in this book will apply equally well to a more encompassing agenda.

It is difficult to delineate all the reasons why people choose to be clients in lifestyle fitness coaching. What you are personally able to offer clients will partly depend on your specific credentials and education. Some health fitness professionals have advanced degrees in psychology, nutrition, physiotherapy, kinesiology, business, and other disciplines. How your unique constellation of talents combines with the skill set of coaching will serve to orient your practice. Trained health fitness professionals may apply lifestyle fitness coaching in several ways:

- Assisting clients with adherence to health fitness programs
- Supporting clients in their pursuit of more holistic approaches to sport and activity commitments
- Helping clients develop competencies in addressing the challenges of change through the successful completion of a cycle of change related to active living
- Enabling clients with self-esteem and body-esteem issues to engage the world of sport and fitness as a means of overcoming self-limiting beliefs and behavioral patterns
- Codesigning programs with clients in support of personal or lifestyle changes that the client can reinforce through reliable participation in physical activities
- Helping clients generate new perspectives about self and life through active-living engagements
- Providing support and guidance for people who, because of illness or injury, have experienced insurmountable obstacles to active living

- Assisting clients who are pursuing typical agendas of weight management, health enhancement, performance improvement, or stress reduction by providing well-rounded guidance, emotional support, goal setting, action planning, and implementation skills in the service of autonomous action
- Supporting activity-based change processes, while cocreating action strategies for clients to address correlated health and lifestyle change issues
- Collaborating with mental health professionals in team approaches to help clients develop healthy and functional living patterns
- Educating individuals and groups about the multidimensional benefits of active lifestyles

Having drawn boundaries around the nature of lifestyle fitness coaching, we can take a reasonable next step by considering the meaning of exercise and a rationale for its role as a powerful agent of personal transformation.

Understanding the Modern-Day Exercise Mandate

Why do people exercise? Moreover, why do they do what they do when they exercise? If you reflect on your own answers to these questions, you might realize that your response could differ from day to day, and you may be aware of change over different periods of your life. The meaning and shape of one's relation to exercise evolves over a lifetime. As a health fitness professional you may seek to motivate and support people in their commitments to exercise, yet there are few roadmaps to promoting lifelong fitness in the 21st century. Rapidly changing lifestyles have opened up uncharted territory that necessitates imaginative and individualized fitness programming (Dallek & Kravitz, 2002; Green, 1986).

In truth, we have never before had a population with so little need to be physically active. Yes, people have to get out of bed, make breakfast, do house chores, go shopping, and travel to and from work, but few have to do manual labor for 8 or more hours a day (Solomon, 1984; Stamford & Shimer, 1990). This trend toward effortless work and labor-free lifestyles will most likely accelerate in coming decades. The implications of these changes for human exercise needs and the evolving roles of health fitness professionals are profound.

In surveys of the inactive population, respondents offered several reasons for not exercising (Top 10 reasons, 2003): no time, no energy, lack of discipline, expense, tedium of exercise, embarrassment, apathy, and lack of understanding of exercise benefits. Even when people finally overcome their resistance or obstacles to exercise, they stand a 50% chance of dropping out within the first 6 months (Dishman, 1988).

Fashion Trends in the World of Fitness

One way to appreciate current meanings attached to the concept of exercise is to take a historical look at fitness and the industry that surrounds it. Even if you have only recently become involved professionally, you are likely to realize the exponential growth of this industry in the past century. Growth and change have been so pervasive that they sometimes create an image of fitness as trendy and faddish. By examining developments over time, we can see what lies beneath these superficial changes. Starting from the rather narrow base of the "physical culture" movement in the early 1900s, a growing sophistication about human physiology and a deepening attention to human diversity can be identified in the myriad exercise programs of the 20th century (Dalleck & Kravitz, 2002; Green, 1986).

Some of you may recall the Charles Atlas ads that served as the icon for fitness in the 1950s. The appeal was one of being strong ("a real man") so that no one would ever "kick sand in your face!" By the mid-1960s other motives were linked to exercise. Fear of heart disease fueled the early growth of running, an activity that soon became the cultural equivalent of what it meant to exercise. Within a few years, however, the runner's high had to make room for the aerobics revolution, which derived some of its momentum from the Me Generation's obsession with youth and beauty. Motives for following trends in fitness were packaged and marketed, using appeals that ranged from self-protection to health promotion and on to beauty. The greater the number of motives offered up for public consumption, the greater the rates of participation—up to a point! As noted previously, in spite of all the scientific data supporting the need to exercise, historically only about 20% of the adult population have been serious enough about exercise to commit to it three or more times a week (Dishman, 1988; Dishman & Buckworth, 1997; Centers for Disease Control and Prevention, 2003).

Fitness, as we know it today, may be seen as a by-product of the postindustrial age. People have only recently confronted a medically mandated exercise agenda that they have to account for in their daily programming (ACSM, 2000; Blair & Brodney, 2000; Chodzko-Zajko, 2000; Pate et al., 1995). With a population of wide-ranging interests, temperaments, and physical capabilities, the fitness industry has focused its creative energy on the development of diverse exercise options to motivate and maintain involvement. Although we may know the biomechanical requirements for maintaining strength, flexibility, and cardiorespiratory functioning, most people will require something more than the promises of health, vitality, or physical change to sustain engagement in activities that they often see as time consuming, difficult, repetitious, or unattractive (Morgan, 2001; Taylor, 1994).

Chapters of the Fitness Story

If we think of modern fitness as a story with many chapters, we might view the first chapter, which roughly covers the period 1964 to 1990, as focusing on the determination of training parameters—intensity, duration, and frequency of exercise—along with fine-tuning biomechanical knowledge. The second chapter, which is currently well under way, would then be more about creativity—designing new forms of exercise to address the panorama of psychological and physiological needs of different sectors of society, including the young and the old, the firm and the infirm, the skilled and the unskilled, the willing and the unwilling. Although research continues to extend the frontiers of biomechanical knowledge, particularly as it relates to previously excluded segments of the population (e.g., the aged and those with chronic medical conditions), the creation of new fitness options seems to have a momentum driven as much by entrepreneurial interests as by market forces.

A third chapter may now be beginning. Building on foundations of exercise requirements, physical and psychological benefits, and programming options, processes that are more personalized seem to be emerging whereby fitness professionals can evaluate people in ways that permit the structuring and support of programs specifically adapted to the clients' needs and lifestyles (Gavin, 2003; Griffin, 1998; Ray & Weise-Bjorstal, 1999). Although options for active living are extensive, what means do we currently have for appreciating the interests and agendas addressed by different exercise forms? To some degree new fitness forms appear in the market place for reasons that are at least unstated, if not unidentified. Think, for instance, of the recent explosion of interest in yoga and classes based on martial arts. A decade ago, it was rare that fitness centers offered either of these activities, yet now they are omnipresent. Why? What needs do they address? What agendas do they fulfill? To whom do they appeal? What cultural changes do they reflect? Advancing knowledge concerning these questions will move us from a randomly creative stage of fitness evolution to one more focused on matching specific, identified needs within the population.

Being Clear About What Clients Need

What will it take to meet the lifelong needs of people who have to search continually for the time, energy, and motivation to incorporate physical activity into their daily schedules? As a health fitness professional you may intuitively sense what programs appeal to different people. You may observe that more men than women use the weight room, that more women than men take dance-style fitness classes, or that yoga classes generally appeal to older rather than younger participants. Novelty sometimes drives participation in activities. At other times, the personality of an instructor may make a class popular.

Programming has typically been about catering to the needs of different people. Health fitness professionals regularly attend conventions, obtain training in new types of classes, and bring these skills back to their clubs, often with great success, at least for a while. An instructor's enthusiasm for a new training method can be contagious, but even that wanes over time. What may be missing in this picture is an understanding of individual clients and what they need for sustained connection to active living. Offering dozens of types of classes per week at a fitness center makes good sense. With an underlying logic of providing something for everybody, a fitness center can be successful by having more options than the club across town does.

Yet, the assumption seems to be that the best way to grow the fitness industry is to offer more diversified fitness options. With this logic, fitness participation is thereby limited to fitness facilities. Most of the population at large rarely, if ever, set foot in a fitness center, and those who do often have to organize their days around their training. Working out at a fitness center is not just a matter of hopping on a treadmill or joining a class. This form of fitness experience involves getting there, changing, and sometimes waiting until equipment becomes available or the class begins. Then, the

participant must reverse the process—showering, changing back into street clothes, and commuting to the next part of the day's agenda.

Another assumption is that a fitness center is more about doing than it is about learning. In spite of the fact that personal training has been a staple of the fitness industry for decades, the concept of education within most fitness facilities is foreign. One might not expect group fitness instructors to spend time during classes educating participants about different aspects of exercise, but it would seem normal that the work of most personal trainers would contain an educational component. Yet personal trainers are paid for training, not talking. Or, at least while they are talking, the normal expectation is that their clients are exercising.

One motivation for health fitness professionals to enroll in courses in life coaching may relate to the idea of being paid for talking to clients. Based on their experiences, health fitness professionals are aware that clients' adherence to exercise, their ability to address challenges to commitment, and their feelings of accomplishment are based on the professionals' understanding of clients' unique needs, interests, values, orientations, and lifestyles.

One can certainly imagine a client whose agenda for hiring a personal trainer is to increase muscle strength and tone or to decrease percentage of body fat. Moreover, it may be possible that this client is so motivated that all he wants to do is to receive guidance, instruction, and support in doing specific exercises necessary to achieve his goal. That is, this fictional client has no interest in talking to the trainer or in discussing extraneous (nontraining) subjects. If this client adheres entirely to the prescribed training regimen, there may be no further issues to consider—other than the curious fact that this client continues to hire a trainer with whom to exercise, probably long after he has learned how to perform the exercises.

More likely scenarios manifest greater complexity. Clients have difficulty adhering to the regimen. They express feelings of boredom. Progress doesn't come fast enough. They eat too much at night and counteract the desired effects of training. Or life happens, and they bring their outside-the-gym experiences into their training, in terms of either energy level or commitment or the need to talk.

In these more complex relationships, the role of the health fitness professional has added dimensions. The professional is not just a technician or an instructor but also a motivator, a supporter, a listener, and sometimes a counselor or coach. If we do not acknowledge these added dimensions as legitimate aspects of the professional's role, then we would have to frame them outside the working relationship of professional and client.

Aligning Health Fitness Professionals' Roles With Clients' Needs

Health fitness professionals often operate with **implicit personality theories** (Spinath et al., 2003) based on how clients show up and the kinds of sport and fitness programs they choose. An experienced professional can usually sense when someone is likely to gravitate toward the weight room, focus only on the step machine, or be the first to sign up for kickboxing. Understanding clients' personal styles and preferences can be a deciding factor in professional success.

Maybe you know people who define themselves by the activities they do: "I'm a swimmer," they say, or "I'm a bodybuilder." You may know others who run with the crowd, who take stability ball classes because it is trendy. Novices may take their cue from what their neighbors do, what they see on TV, or what will embarrass them least. Although choice should always remain in the hands of the consumer, what role might health fitness professionals play in coaching people about the wide world of fitness?

Consider this possibility. You have a 25-year-old client for whom you put together an ideal 5-day-a-week program based on the latest biomechanical and medical information. Would you expect this client to be doing exactly the same program 20 years later? If this client continues to exercise over those 20 years, what factors do you imagine could influence her decisions to modify her training?

Variety is the spice of life! Yet why and how we vary our choices and behaviors may relate to values, interests, needs, and other factors that we can probably articulate. Random change can be risky. Following the fads as a trial-and-error approach to finding one's fitness niche has a low success rate. Staying with the same program year after year can also have a downside. Overuse injuries, changing life conditions, or other factors can potentially compromise adherence to one's preferred practices. Ideally, individuals should have access to information and guidance that advance comprehension of their unique needs and interests, especially as they change throughout the life span.

As we complete the second chapter of the fitness revolution and move toward the opening of the third chapter, we need to offer people more than strength, health, beauty, and longevity. One reason that we need to is that we can. A more potent reason is that doing so will satisfy a wider range of human needs and thus engage a greater proportion of the population.

Dreams and Visions for the Future of Fitness

Most of us have hopes for how we would like people to relate to their bodies and their involvement in physical activity. But the daily reality that we confront may seem worlds away from where we would like it to be. Consider this vision a way of focusing on the potential that lies ahead.

Imagine yourself as a lifestyle fitness coach whose goal is to cocreate with clients positive connections with physical activity throughout the life span. In working toward this goal, your task will include educating, guiding, motivating, supporting, and instructing clients concerning the needs of their bodies, the physical and psychological parameters relevant to participation in different activities, the risks and benefits related to their activities, and the specific processes of activities they choose. This agenda may be far broader than what you typically address in your current role. Remember that you are facing a world where people have a good chance of living into their 80s and 90s, where medical innovations will keep us functioning longer, and where self-sufficiency and autonomy will be key criteria for both individual happiness and societal prosperity.

In this future vision, guidance concerning the body and physical activity would begin at an early age in school curricula and in community-based programs as well as in the home. Children would learn about their bodies in positive ways rather than in ways that induce guilt, shame, and embarrassment. They would discover that their bodies are unique and require special care and handling if they are to be sources of competency, joy, and fulfillment for as long as possible. They would come to understand human anatomy and learn that muscles must be strong and that joints must be supple. They would find what suits them best by exploring their personal styles and preferences. They would realize that no single approach to fitness works for all people, that different sports have different "personalities," just as they do. They would come to appreciate the requirements for a successfully aging body so that their childhood investments do not jeopardize their future happiness.

As these children enter early adulthood, their needs may change, and with these changes will come new orientations to physical activity. Depending on the paths they choose, they may need to learn new social skills or psychological approaches to problems, and they will find trustworthy allies in specific sports and physical activities recommended to them by knowledgeable health fitness professionals. Rather than relying on designer drugs to alter their psychological realities, they can adjust their sports and fitness programs to give them a natural boost in the directions they desire. If they need to counterbalance the stress of advanced studies or an aggressive career path, their lifestyle fitness coaches will be there to recommend sports and activities that complement their lifestyles. Or perhaps as they enter early adulthood, the physical requirements of doing their work or studies will suggest specific physical exercises of stretching or muscle strengthening to offset the effects of, for example, sitting in front of a computer monitor for 8 to 12 hours a day.

With the onset of middle age, lifestyles may evolve again, interests may change, and the body may express different preferences and tolerances. Addressing the social and psychological changes of midlife, lifestyle fitness coaches will guide people toward activities that can reawaken creativity, widen horizons, or take them in new, yet unexplored directions that had long been their souls' yearning. In this positive vision, the now middle-aged adults will know about their bodily needs and will easily recognize the necessity of engaging in strengthening programs for continuing their active lifestyles. They will also have learned to optimize the myriad daily opportunities for physical activity inherent in the ordinary rituals of maintaining their lives, commuting to work, and going about their business.

As these individuals move into the period of redirection, formerly known as retirement, they will have developed competence and skills in a variety of sports and physical activities, so they will have the benefits of choice and control at this stage of life. They will be able to choose from a menu of activities that they have practiced and enjoyed at earlier stages in life to rekindle their spirits, provide new perspectives, or give them exactly the kind of energy they need for the task at hand. Their bodies will be in good condition, barring the unforeseen misfortunes of disease and accident, and even then, their bodies will be the best they can be. They will not be limited to what we currently define as options for the aged. They will indeed be vigorous and continue to access the full potential of mind and body with the aid of physically active lifestyles.

Perhaps you know an octogenarian who represents the fulfillment of such a lifelong vision. More likely, you know many more who do not resemble this optimistic portrait of aging (Chodzko-Zajko, 2000). As noted earlier, advances in medicine and surgical intervention will keep most of us living longer, yet the core issue is quality of life, not quantity of life. As a lifestyle fitness coach you can be a key contributor to this positive vision.

Learning how to access the kinds of information implied in the foregoing descriptions so that you can help clients is what this book is about. Upcoming chapters will help you develop methods for conversing with clients in ways that inform you of their needs and visions and that allow you to influence them based on the expertise that you have gained as a health fitness professional.

Guiding Human Development

Most high school students are given opportunities to consult with guidance counselors for advice concerning careers and further education. In helping students understand their options and how personal interest patterns correlate with career possibilities, guidance counselors use tests and interest inventories to create profiles for each student so that they can match these profiles with corresponding career options and educational programs (Holland, 1985).

What if you could offer novice exercisers access to information and dialogue that would guide them toward activities that matched their life orientations, their personalities, and even their agendas for personal development? Just as people with different physical makeups are suited to different exercise programs (Arnot & Gaines, 1984), so too are people's lifestyles and personalities more or less appropriate to sustained involvement in different sports and fitness pursuits.

Human beings are creatures of habit. We become what we do. The more we engage in a behavior, the more natural it becomes, the more it represents our way of being. The adage "Sport builds character" suggests that participation in a sport or a regular exercise program influences our personalities. If personality appears in habits of behavior or patterns of relating to the world, can we change these? Evidence produced during a century of psychological study answers with a cautious yes (Seligman, 1995). Caution arises from research telling us that change is not a simple matter—that it takes time, effort, and clear guidance.

Consider this: A 20-year-old who exercises daily will invest over 3,000 hours in this process each decade. If she lives to the ripe age of 90, she will have spent close to 21,000 hours exercising. Someone who exercises three or four times per week will accumulate fewer hours but will nonetheless invest approximately 10,000 hours over a lifetime.

Returning to the concept of habit, we recognize that people usually form behavior patterns through repetition over time. If you knew that different sports or fitness programs reinforced particular behavior habits, might you then be able to guide people toward choices that could augment their effectiveness in the world? With all the hours that people spend exercising, could you design programs to sharpen their skills for living and help them develop psychosocial competencies that might enhance their effectiveness and well-being?

What a person chooses to do over a long period of time conditions not only the body but also the mind. Even when a sport or exercise program seems simple from a biomechanical perspective, it can have subtle complexities at a psychological level. Consider, for instance, an activity like running on a treadmill. If one's body is physically capable, the activity may not seem complex. By contrast, playing basketball or completing a lengthy dance choreography appears to be more intricate.

Delving beneath the surface, however, we might ask such questions as these: What keeps someone running on a treadmill? What determines the pace that he sets? And will he come back tomorrow? As simple as running appears to be, we know that more people are capable of training for a 26.2-mile (42.2-kilometer) marathon than actually ever do. So, even for seemingly simple activities, we must ask several questions: What habits and characteristics do they rely on and thereby reinforce? How does this habit development differ from that of the dancer or basketball player? More fundamentally, we might ask why someone becomes a marathoner whereas someone else only wants to dance.

Appreciating the Determinants of Choice

What do we know about the reasons that people do what they do, especially in the exercise realm? Considering the obvious, here are some of the factors that play into our choices:

- Physical characteristics, including height, weight, and physical condition
- Medical history, including injuries and illnesses
- Family history and values
- Interests and predispositions

- Culture and environments
- Behavior shaping through school programs
- Prior experiences with physical activities
- Relationships with peers and significant others
- Socioeconomic status
- Personality
- Accidents of fate

Research provides some knowledge about who is likely to exercise and who is not, which factors reinforce participation and which ones discourage it, and even how sedentary people can be motivated to exercise (Dishman, 1988; Gavin & Spitzer, 2002; LeUnes & Nation, 2002). Whenever you meet a client who has never exercised, has a yo-yo relation to exercise, or has persisted in only one activity despite accumulating problems of overuse injuries, you are likely to be dealing with a stacked deck.

Clients come to you with lengthy histories that shape and support their behavior patterns. In the best circumstance, these patterns have worked in their favor. Recognize, however, that many fitness participants seek your counsel because something is not working well for them. They may struggle with consistency or be amidst a major life transition. Clients' motivations for exercising can be simple or intricate. Their reasoning for choices can be clear or cloudy. Whatever their dynamics, you can be certain of this at least—years of life conditioning will have resulted in deeply set patterns of thinking, feeling, and acting.

Although we may believe in free will, in our ability to make rational choices based on values, needs, and aspirations, paradoxically many of our choices seem predetermined. As noted earlier, we are creatures of habit. For better or worse, we form some habits before the "age of reason" (approximately 7 years of age) or in response to situations that no longer exist. Precisely for these reasons, the work of a lifestyle fitness coach is to help people examine how well their habits or behavioral patterns serve them now.

Someone may come to you with a desire to lose weight, tone up, or reduce the risk of heart disease. If you are able to take into account this person's patterns and lifestyle, your chances of success will increase. Moreover, if in addition to their negative reasons for exercising (fear of death, dissatisfaction with body proportions, and so on), you can add such positive motivations as taking charge of one's life, developing new social skills, or nurturing latent talents, you will provide your clients with further incentives to actualize all their potential.

The Nature of Change

Why change? For some people, life is fine just the way it is. Ultimately, the question of change reduces to whether we currently have what it takes to cope effectively with the life demands of today and tomorrow. Typically, life moves along in a more or less comfortable way until something happens to make current patterns outdated, ineffective, or unsatisfying. Rather than continue with this state of affairs, the rational choice is to change, and even when we try to avoid change, life sometimes pushes us into it.

Now comes the paradox. As creatures of habit, we have many automatic behaviors. Typically, when we are under stress, these habits are more evident than ever (Schultz & Searleman, 2002). By definition, any change, even positive change, is stressful (Jones & Bright, 2001). So when life switches its agenda for us, we usually have to drop old habits and behave differently. Yet, the stress of change causes us to rely on habitual behaviors even more! Imagine someone who charges ahead in all life situations. In a high-stress situation, this behavior is even more likely to emerge. What will happen if this straight-ahead charge is directly into the face of danger or into some other form of self-defeating reactivity?

If skills or behavioral habits are inadequate for situations that the individual is currently confronting, how can this person develop new patterns that are more effective? In a preventative mode, can she develop new habit patterns and bank them for the future? In a metaphor of sport, can someone who is a runner learn to swim in preparation for the possibility that someday she may reach land's end? If the scope of your work is to help people get the greatest range of benefits from the thousands of hours that they will invest in physical activity over their lifetimes, can you offer them all the physical benefits that normally accrue and add to this a host of personal development possibilities that will serve their desires to be all they can be?

How we adapt to reality may be indicative of our level of mental health. Continuing to apply the same solutions to the problems of life even though they repeatedly bring failure and dissatisfaction is neither wise nor health promoting. On a physical plane, the bodybuilder who continues to train despite crippling injuries and chronic pain is not befriending his body. The smoker who continues to light up despite a chronic, hacking cough is not choosing wisely. The student who habitually puts studies aside until the night before final exams is not ensuring success.

People cannot leave the choice of physical activity to habit alone. Habit may persist in the face of overwhelming evidence of its inappropriateness or detrimental effects. Sport and exercise programs are unique bundles of learning challenges. To engage in any sport and achieve at least a modicum of success, an individual must confront particular situations, deal with various emotional reactions, learn new moves, build specific musculature, and eventually form new habits.

The game of tennis, for instance, is not just a matter of learning to hit a ball over a net. Tennis involves intricate mental and emotional processes including strategic thinking, remaining calm under fire, focusing in the moment, being flexible in response, dealing with feelings of winning and losing, and managing or retraining some habits of mind and body. Unlike a computer that responds unemotionally to certain cues and stimuli, human beings think and feel and hope and wonder. We react to competition. We may feel socially awkward when surrounded by cheering spectators. We may even have behavioral habits of diving headfirst into action but rarely stepping backward. We may strike the ball with too much or too little force, or with inadequate follow-through. We may move too quickly or too heavily, or we may not be flexible enough in our choices of where to move next. If you consider these physical actions as metaphors for how people live their lives, imagine the potential for personal transformation that lies within the coaching process that you can offer individuals in your areas of expertise.

Take this analysis one step further. Why might a person choose a step aerobics class over an hour on a step machine? No single answer has certitude because hundreds of explanations may be valid. Irrespective of the reasons for choosing one activity over another, put yourself in this situation and do an imaginary before-and-after study: Consider doing an hour on a step machine one day and taking a step aerobics class the next day. What do you think would be the difference between how you feel during and at the end of each experience? From a physiological perspective, you may have achieved similar levels of energy expenditure, yet your social and psychological experiences would be different. Project this one-hour experience into a year or more of training either on the step machine or in the step class. What experiences might you have had? What habits might you have formed? What attributes would you have reinforced?

Conditioning and Core Change

Lifelong fitness needs to be seen in light of core changes that individuals can create in physical, psychological, social, and even spiritual well-being. Sport and other forms of physical activity can serve as pathways to personal growth, especially when programs are consciously designed with lifestyle and personal development as part of the agenda.

From your personal experience and from your professional training, you know that exercise elevates moods, that it temporarily relieves feelings of stress and anxiety, and that it contributes substantially to feelings of personal well-being (Gavin, 2003; Morgan, 1997; Hays, 1999). Add to these benefits the potential for exercise to serve as a safe training ground for developing personal traits and behavioral patterns that foster success and happiness (Shields & Bredemeier, 1995; Danish, Nellon, & Owens, 1996; Smith, 1999). Doing the "right" sport or fitness programs can make it possible for your clients to learn new ways of coping, more effective strategies for action, new ways of relating, and a more integrated approach to living.

As a lifestyle fitness coach you may not always advise clients to do a new sport, but you may ask them to do what they are currently doing differently. How someone plays the game or participates in an activity can be as important in fostering personal development as the activity itself. Ultimately, what works best is a combination of the right exercise or sport program and the right way of engaging in that activity. The word *right* refers to what is right for clients—at this juncture in life, based on what they currently need most to support their desired directions for change. Your role as lifestyle fitness coach is to help clients bring together all the relevant information about their lives to formulate plans of action to which they can and will commit. In time, your role will be to help them reflect on this plan and revise it as needed.

However many hours you invest in training and conditioning your body will double as time directed toward mental change. Conditioning as described by fitness experts may conjure up images of physical actions like performing push-ups dozens of times to strengthen particular muscles. When psychologists talk about conditioning, you are likely to hear descriptions of behavioral control techniques aimed at helping people deal with such symptoms as anxiety or depression. The word *conditioning* in these two instances appears to have different meanings, but consider how these two types of conditioning are essentially alike and how both support personal change.

From your school days, you know that mental learning is, in part, a function of repetition. Experiencing something repeatedly allows you to move

experience from short-term to long-term memory and from a superficial awareness to an imprinted way of knowing. At subtler or even unconscious levels, you may have repeated experiences that condition you to think and act in predictable ways. This kind of learning or conditioning eventually adds up to what we may call your personality.

Martin Seligman's (Peterson, Maier, & Seligman, 1993) work on "learned helplessness" illustrates this kind of conditioning. His studies show that some forms of depression—or, as he labels it, learned helplessness—result from early life conditioning. Seligman also found that the trait of optimism may result from psychological conditioning.

Here is one way it might work. Imagine that from your earliest days, you were surrounded by positive, affirming people and, therefore, developed a strong belief in yourself and your capabilities. Now, imagine the opposite, that you met rejection and criticism throughout your childhood and, as a result, developed a fearful, self-doubting personality. In both cases your mind was conditioned to certain attitudes and beliefs based on frequent repetitions of verbal and nonverbal behaviors directed toward you. In the end, you learned to believe that you were either able or unable to manage and control your life.

Now examine the seemingly different experience of physical conditioning. When you practice a physical action repeatedly, you develop strength and competence in related functions of the body. A child who learns to swim and has frequent opportunities to practice swimming develops a body conditioned to the movements and coordinated actions of this sport. In contrast, a child who never practices swimming is at great risk in open waters because the necessary musculature and coordination for swimming is lacking.

The examples of learning emotional reactions and psychological beliefs represent conditioning the mind; the example of learning to swim reflects conditioning the body.

This contrast of mental and physical conditioning is, to a large degree, an artificial distinction. The conditioned swimmer will have developed not only a body-based competency through training but also a set of beliefs about his abilities in the water. So, too, the learned optimist will not only have incorporated the belief that she can take charge but also have demonstrated this belief in action. For the most part, the mind does not encounter life without a behavioral counterpart, nor does the body engage in action without some type of mental activity. Personal reality is highly integrated. Living requires both sides of the mind–body equation. A person who has learned to be optimistic will still be at risk in deep waters if she doesn't know how to swim, and even our swimmer may sink if he has learned to feel helpless in stressful situations.

Conditioning as a process of repeated thoughts or actions affects your mind and body because you function as a more or less integrated whole. The important news in this for lifestyle fitness coaches is that people can engage in processes of self-development through methods of mental or physical "calisthenics" because body and mind constitute flip sides of personal reality.

Can You Really Change Who You Are?

You can build bigger biceps, increase your running speed, or learn to play tennis effectively, but can you change personality traits or other mental characteristics? Although genetics plays a significant role in behavior, life experience exerts strong influence on personality and other individual qualities. You may not be able to change all your personal characteristics, but there is clear evidence that you can change some personal traits through consciously directed efforts (Seligman, 1995).

Personality represents characteristic ways in which you behave, especially in relationships with other people (Cashdan, 1988; Sullivan, 1953). Personality also shows itself in your habitual emotional responses to life. Personality traits that distinguish people include how self-confident they feel, how extroverted or introverted they are, whether they tend to be optimistic or pessimistic, how they respond to stress, whether they react impulsively or deliberately, and how much personal drive and ambition they have.

What portion of personality is determined by genetics and what is the result of life experience may not be as critical a question as how much room there is for change over the life span. Although there are limits to change, there is little doubt that personality can be influenced through a variety of activities.

Whether it results from in-depth psychotherapy, education, psychological skills training, or simply life experience, a vast body of evidence tells us that profound changes occur in adult life. In fact, they are commonplace. Some people are able to bring about change through self-help programs that, when followed carefully, produce significant improvements in how they feel about themselves, how they validate and affirm themselves, and how they function in the world.

For others, self-help guides are not as effective as face-to-face conversations with counselors, coaches, or therapists that enable them to get in touch with core dilemmas and needs. Whether it happens through psychotherapy, peer support, or some other form of helping relationship, these interpersonal approaches work by providing constructive feedback, challenging faulty beliefs or irrational thinking, and creating new experiences of social relationship that are healing (Prochaska & Norcross, 2003).

Activities like meditation, self-reflection, or positive affirmations are also highly respected strategies for producing behavior change (Benson & Stuart, 1992). Meditation programs can help people feel less anxious and more in control through a process of sitting quietly for 30 to 60 minutes a day and observing their breathing or repeating a mind-centering mantra. Alternatively, change may occur through repeating such affirmations as "I am whole and healthy" or "I am successful and happy" in support of the mind's desire to create positive realities.

These proven methods for personal change rely on a fundamental mechanism that is at the heart of sport and fitness. In a word, it is called practice. Through repetition and committed action over time, we learn to think differently and eventually to behave in ways that are more effective. Because the world of sport is typically associated with themes of competition, performance, and winning, you may believe that the concept of practice has distinctly different objectives for health fitness professionals than it does for therapists. What this book will demonstrate throughout is how you can use the practice dimension of any sport or fitness program to enhance personal development and achieve such personal changes as becoming more assertive, being more spontaneous, living more adventurously, developing greater self-reliance, and creating more satisfying social interactions.

Another connection that **mind methods** have to sport and exercise pursuits derives from the fact that, to be effective, personal growth programs require an arena in which practice can reliably and safely take place. In successful change efforts, practicing new behaviors occurs most effectively when conditions are controlled to protect and foster growth (Hubble, Duncan, & Miller, 1999). Like a young flower that needs specific nutrients, weather, and moisture, people in transition require conditions that maximally support their intentions to grow. Moreover, people eventually express in actions the changes fostered by therapy or personal growth programs. Through consciously designed fitness programs, the action components of personal growth agendas may find safe venues that support and reinforce growth.

An example may clarify these points. Someone who struggles with irrational fears and anxieties can benefit by talking to a therapist and trying to understand himself better, yet the person eventually needs to deal with the physical dimension of these emotions in a way that the body can understand. To be free of fear and anxiety, words alone may be insufficient. The person may need to channel these emotions on a physical level, whether that happens through massage, yoga, tennis, or deep-breathing exercises. Psychology finds expression through the body, and to effect change, physical experiences need to be repatterned just as much as thought processes have to be revised.

This point deserves repeating. If you are feeling anger or rage, it is unlikely that you can just talk yourself out of these feelings or simply count to 10 and expect your feelings to disappear entirely. Emotions have a physical reality. You harbor emotions in your body, and your body needs avenues for dealing with them (Prestera & Kurz, 1976; Reich, 1949). If you do not have healthy outlets for your emotions, you might end up converting these feelings into physical symptoms such as headaches, hypertension, colitis, or even cancer (Zautra, 2003). The mind never works alone. It has its constant companion, the body, which we must embrace in any program of healing or change.

Working on a body level to energize and direct personal transformation can be extremely powerful (Frank, 2001; Murray, 1951; Smith, 1985). At the same time, this approach does not equate to doing things to your body while your mind passively awaits transformation. Through the conscious use of sport and exercise for change, the body becomes as valid a starting place as the mind for personal development work. The idea of conscious exercise means that after initiating a process of personal change through the body, a person must form a partnership with the mind. The mind is likely to resist change when it is treated as a reluctant or irrelevant passenger.

An In-Depth Analysis of the Psychosocial Structure of Sport and Fitness

Each fitness activity or sport is a complex set of mind–body demands. Most often we tend to look at the physical requirements for participation; less

often do we explore the embedded social and psychological agendas.

Let us take a **psychosocial** tour of a kickboxing class. You need not have taken any kind of kickboxing class to profit from this tour. On the other hand, if you have been in too many classes to count, you may want to set aside your prior experiences as you take on new eyes to see what may occur beneath the surface.

First, you may want to try on a new identity. You are an overweight and slightly out-of-shape 40-year-old. Next, you need to situate yourself in time and space. Imagine that you have just finished work. It is 5:30 on a weekday evening, and you are walking into a sprawling, new, multilevel fitness center. A friend recommended that you visit this center to try out a killer kickboxing class that begins at 6:00 p.m.

In your new identity, you may sense an energy shift as you enter this building for the first time. Mobs of people are coming and going, mostly at a fast pace. Some are alone, like you, and others in company. Your energy level may increase a notch as you become aware of the strangeness of the environment and as you anticipate the killer class that you are about to attempt.

You go through the routine of registering at the front desk, paying for the class, and signing a waiver that releases the center from responsibility should you injure yourself. The notion of injury may cause a momentary spike in your anxiety. As you complete your sign-in, you find yourself discretely examining people at the center and drawing comparisons to yourself.

Minutes later, you are in a modern and attractive locker room. There doesn't seem to be a whole lot of privacy when you change into your workout clothes, and in the back of your mind, you may hear a voice evaluating the outfit that you brought for class.

The studio is on the other side of a large area that contains scores of stationary bikes, treadmills, stair climbers, elliptical trainers, rowing machines, and other workout equipment that you may not have seen before. Digital displays catch your eyes as your ears fill with the whirring, beeping, buzzing cacophony of a modern fitness center.

At this moment, you find yourself peering through the glass door of the studio. You pause before entering. About 20 people are already in the room. Some are wearing baggy shorts and T-shirts, whereas others are wearing revealing, skintight outfits. Although there doesn't seem to be a set dress code for this class, you are nonetheless tempted to reassess the outfit that you are wearing.

A group of people rushing to occupy their favorite spots sweeps your body into the room and derails your momentary hesitation. You gravitate toward the rear corner near the door, but someone is already there. You end up in the middle of the class surrounded by strangers.

Time for an attitude check. How are you feeling? Class hasn't even started, yet you have already had a bit of an adventure. Are you at ease, or are you just trying to look cool? You notice that no one seems to be paying any particular attention to you, and although this circumstance allows you some breathing space, it might cause you to feel alone.

You distract yourself from introspection by looking around the room. You catch reflections of about 50 people in the mirrored walls of the studio. If you were inclined to hide, being in this room would make doing so extremely difficult. You see someone who you think is the instructor. He is adjusting the sound system and seems to be preparing equipment for class. He looks to be about 6-foot-3 (190 centimeters), not much more than 25 years old, and extremely muscular. Again, you mentally assess whether you are up to this experience.

The class starts. The instructor welcomes everybody in a pleasant voice. He seems friendly, and any anxiety you might have decreases slightly. He invites participants to take care of themselves, even if that means slowing down or stopping. His permission lets you know that this will not be an ultraendurance contest.

He starts with gentle warm-ups that enable you to gain confidence. Yes, you can do this exercise. You have done it before or at least something like it. He encourages everyone to breathe fully through the warm-ups. Your joints begin to loosen, your muscles relax, and you may even notice that your mind is unwinding.

The pace quickens. Without awareness of the transition, you are hopping from side to side, back and forth, punching and kicking the air. The action is a little intimidating. Most of the movements are new, and you don't have eyes in the back of your head. As you kick your leg to the side, you pray it doesn't connect with someone's body.

At the half-hour mark, you notice that a couple people have stopped moving. The instructor's face glistens with sweat as he continues to call out directions. For a moment, the class moves in unison. You become part of this pulsating organism.

A sudden stop and a call to check your pulse. Given the opportunity, you take another attitude check. Where are you? How are you feeling? Bottom

line? You probably answer, "Good!" Something about the movements, the spirited instructor, and the harmony of the group in motion have eased your mind and your feelings—and strangely, you feel as if you are beginning to grow eyes at the back of your head. You are more aware of all your body parts, not just your front, but your sides and back, neck and head, shoulders and feet. You certainly have lost that awkward self-consciousness you felt just before class began.

After another flurry of kicks, punches, dives, and dodges, the cool-down begins. You do a dozen variations of the standard sit-up, innumerable push-ups, some completely new exercises, and then the final stretches begin. You notice that the floor around you resembles a small wading pool. You furtively mop your sweat with a towel.

You know that the end is coming. Movements are slower. Sensual stretches and deep breathing release the last wisps of tension in your body. The instructor compliments you all on your effort, and, in turn, loud clapping tells him that he has done a great job.

Not much talking occurred during class, but now more of a social atmosphere prevails. You feel a bit closer to these strangers. You shared an eventful hour, and found it worthwhile.

Now that class is over, let us examine its psychosocial nature. A good way to begin is by realizing that all sports and physical activities have rules and demands. If you want to play the game, you need to abide by the rules. Rules govern not only required physical actions but also your personal psychology. In analyzing the rules of group fitness and, more particularly, a kickboxing class, you may gain insight into how the underlying structure of an activity can support personal development. We can see this structure from three different yet integrated perspectives:

1. Psychosocial demands, or the emotional, social, and behavioral requirements for participation
2. Anatomical demands on the muscles and joints used in the activity
3. Movement demands pertaining to the types of movement required by the activity

Psychosocial Demands for Activity Participation

In analyzing a kickboxing class, let us begin with simple observations. Our first observation may be that all fitness classes are group activities, yet they do not require participants to interact. Think of a team sport like basketball for contrast. In basketball, active verbal and nonverbal exchanges occur between players throughout the game. In group fitness classes, the only one likely to be speaking is the instructor, and his communications are mostly commands or words of encouragement. Participants may communicate through eye contact, facial expressions, or unintentional body contact, but the "game" does not require such interaction.

Next, you might observe that kickboxing is a leader-centered activity. Participants follow the instructor and make few decisions other than to stay and to follow. In this regard, long-term participation does not foster leadership skills, decision-making abilities, or even self-reliance. In the extreme, it can feed dependency by reinforcing a person's belief that he can't exercise unless he takes a class in which someone shows him what to do.

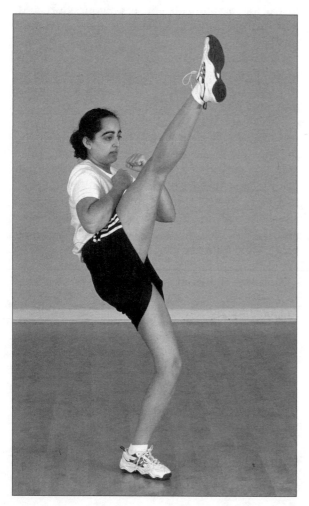

Even though a kickboxing class is a group activity, participants will generally not be interacting with each other. Such a class requires only a moderate level of sociability.

Group fitness classes are mostly noncompetitive in nature. No prizes go to those who kick the highest, groan the loudest, or sweat the most. This fact does not mean that everyone behaves noncompetitively. Participants take their personalities to class. If they are competitive, they will find opportunities in this or any other encounter to transform the experience into a contest. Although kickboxing classes aren't intentionally competitive, the imagery that instructors use during the class may encourage participants to think of pitting themselves against imaginary foes. Nonetheless, staying in the class requires a level of cooperation with the instructor and with one's classmates.

In what ways does a kickboxing class involve you mentally? For beginners and before routines become predictable, it requires a moderate degree of mental focus. You need to concentrate! Movements change frequently, so participants must pay attention to the instructor. As time goes on, the class may become more predictable, so you will be able to engage your body with less mental effort.

Why is mental focus important? If you are preoccupied or worried at the beginning of class, a focused activity like kickboxing encourages your mind to switch tracks and come into the present moment. As a result, both your mind and your body experience a release from energy-sapping tensions.

The next dimension is more complex. Kickboxing classes are a mixture of spontaneity and control. Unlike weight training, for example, in which movements are highly controlled, a kickboxing class includes an element of surprise. Unless an instructor is so predictable that you can anticipate each change in command, your body needs to be ready to shift from movement to movement at a moment's notice. The mental set that prepares you for these sudden shifts in movement and direction develops inner qualities of flexibility that you may apply in other life encounters.

Generally, group fitness classes are not aggressive in style or content. With such a wide variety of classes in fitness centers, however, you need to consider the content of a class before assessing whether or not it encourages aggressive actions. Think of a stretch-and-flex class. None of its movements or instructions would encourage aggressive thoughts or behaviors. Most step classes would also have low aggressive content. Kickboxing, on the other hand, involves strong actions and the imagery of defense and attack. Bear in mind that we are not using the term aggressive in a negative manner. Rather, the term implies forceful movements of the body in overcoming resistance or counterforce (real or imagined). Over time, such training may increase participants' comfort level with strong, assertive actions and makes the likelihood of such behaviors higher in other arenas of life (Gavin, 1988; Gill, 2000).

A beginning student may experience kickboxing as a moderately risky activity because of its challenging movements and the possibility of injury. On an emotional level, some risk of social embarrassment may be present in a class in which you don't know the moves, the implicit rules, or your classmates. What would be an example of a safe activity? Pedaling your stationary bicycle at home while watching TV sounds safe. You can go at your own rate and stop at any point without risk of embarrassment. In addition, the movements of stationary cycling are contained and repetitive, and unlikely to put your body in jeopardy.

A kickboxing class, like most other group fitness classes, falls into the category of other-directed or externally motivated activities. To understand this concept, think of a marathon runner who rises at 5:00 a.m. 7 days a week to run 8 to 10 miles, alone, through all kinds of weather—no matter what. This activity requires a high degree of self-discipline, whereas ongoing attendance at kickboxing classes has more external support. A class has a fixed schedule, an inspiring instructor, peer support, motivating music, and a controlled and encouraging environment. Marathon runners must generate most if not all of their motivation from within, whereas group fitness participants can rely on external structures and interpersonal support to make commitment happen.

To summarize, a kickboxing class shows up in this psychosocial analysis as an activity that emphasizes the following qualities:

- dependency on a leader,
- a moderate level of sociability,
- a non-competitive process,
- high levels of concentration or mental focus (at least for the first few classes),
- some physical and psychological risk taking,
- reliance on others and external motivations,
- moderately aggressive actions, and
- a balance of spontaneity and control.

In the long term, a commitment to kickboxing classes will serve to reinforce these qualities in people who consistently choose this as their fitness program.

Psychological Significance of the Anatomical Demands of an Activity

Understanding the potential of exercise for changing your personality comes not only from knowing whether the activity requires aggressive, social, or competitive actions but also from understanding how it affects the structure of your body. For example, what muscles do you use in a kickboxing class? The answer partly depends on the instructor and the level of the class. Generally, however, kickboxing classes are intended as an overall muscle strengthening experience, as well as a cardiorespiratory conditioning program. Your arms and torso come into play in punching, swinging, and bending motions, as well as in the push-up and sit-up routines that may constitute part of the cool-down. Moreover, kickboxing involves a lot of legwork, so these classes should develop strong leg muscles.

What might strong leg muscles have to do with your personality (Dychtwald, 1977; Gavin, 1988, 2000; Kurz & Prestera, 1976; Reich, 1949; Smith, 1985)? To appreciate the psychological relevance of leg muscles, picture two rather extreme body types: The first one has strong legs but a relatively weaker upper body (arms, torso). The second has powerful arms, shoulders, back, and abdomen but relatively less developed legs. Imagine these two pitted against each other in a series of contests. Mr. Legs would probably win all the foot races and would be able to hold his ground in any standoff, but Mr. Arms would likely be the victor in contests like arm wrestling, bench pressing, and other types of manual control.

In psychological terms, the upper body has been related to social control and manipulation, whereas the lower body is thought to influence movement and emotional stability (Dychtwald, 1977). Through participation in kickboxing classes, participants can develop high potential to mobilize themselves, move into action, or firmly stand their ground when life demands it. Because these classes also emphasize upper-body development, participants' ability to express their needs and control their environments would also be reinforced.

Does lopsided training lead to lopsided personality? In extreme cases, an exercise program that overdevelops your arms, shoulders, and back while only minimally developing your legs may reinforce a psychological imbalance. From a psychological perspective, this kind of program "exercises" your competency in reaching out, taking charge, and controlling your environment, but it may not engender a corresponding sense of emotional security or

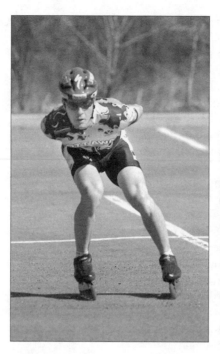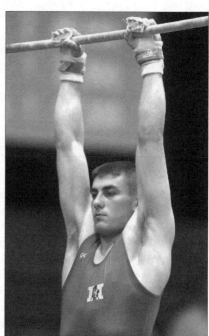

Figure 2.1 Training and extensive practice develops bodies in a specific manner. The lifestyle fitness coach can guide clients to see the relationship of physical development to functional usage.

stability. Conversely, if you overdevelop leg muscles while neglecting upper-body exercise, you may develop a strong sense of emotional grounding and personal security but do little to enhance your ability to manipulate your social–emotional world (Dychtwald, 1977; Gavin, 1988; Smith, 1985).

Much of the thinking about body structure and functioning in relation to personality derives from a subspecialty of clinical and counseling psychology (Krueger, 2002; Smith, 1985). Evidence appears mostly in case studies rather than in large-sample statistical research. For this reason, we must apply caution and common sense to these interpretations. One commonsense framework that health fitness professionals can readily grasp is the relationship of physical development to functional usage. An analogy from the automotive domain may fit here. Driving a Hummer in New York City may impress others, but how well does it function? A Hummer is fuel inefficient, difficult to park, an obstruction to other drivers' range of vision, and perhaps a bit of a menace on the road (e.g., by taking up too much space). By contrast, a Mini Cooper is small, zippy, and fuel efficient but a bit of a sight in a 10-car pile-up.

The fundamental point is that different sports develop bodies in unique ways. Genetics alone does not cause people to look like bodybuilders, swimmers, or dancers. Their identifying muscular development often derives from extensive practice. The massive thighs of the speed skater, the short, firm calves of the long-distance runner, and the

muscular chest and arms of the gymnast are natural outgrowths of training (figure 2.1).

At a biomechanical level, muscular development occurs because each muscle has specific functions. Some muscles extend a limb; others flex it. Some move the limb away from the body; others move it toward the body. These functions of muscles also have psychological implications. The strength of muscles and the flexibility of joints partly determine your range of behaviors, as well as your social reality as created through physical impressions.

Consider, for instance, how a lack of muscular strength in your abdomen and lower back might affect your self-image (Kurz & Prestera, 1976; Smith, 1985). When the middle of your body looks and feels collapsed because of weak muscles, your sense of pride and self-esteem may diminish. Knowing where you are strong and flexible tells you not only what exercises you need in your quest for physical health but also where you most need to work to foster personal development.

Psychological Implications of Movement Patterns in Activity

How might kickboxing movements affect your mind or emotions? Kickboxing classes obviously require different movements than weight lifting does. What might not be as evident is that daily kickboxing practice may support personality change quite different from that conditioned by a regular routine of bodybuilding.

To appreciate the psychology of movement (Gavin, 1997; Lamb & Watson, 1994; North, 1972), you might recall someone saying to you, "I knew it was you by your walk." What did your walk reveal? What characteristics of mood or energy did your steps convey? Your walk is like your signature, that is, a set pattern of movements that reveals deeper aspects of your nature. Your individuality appears not only in your footsteps but also in your rhythms, gestures, and ways of using the space around you. Some people seem to fill a room, whereas others recede into the walls. Some people always run, some saunter, and others dance through life. Each movement quality can be correlated with aspects of personality.

The link between personality and movement is based on the fact that different exercises or sports promote different styles of movement (Santana, 2002). An individual who has had 15 years of classical ballet training will express this conditioning in everyday movements. Likewise, someone who has studied yoga for years will manifest this training in life. Extensive involvement in particular sports and exercise changes your movements in a more or less predictable manner. As your movement patterns change through exercise, so too might your personality undergo change.

To illustrate the power of movement to influence internal feelings and states of mind, consider the following statement from a dedicated runner (Kepner, 1993):

> One day last spring I was having an exceptionally good run. . . . I was around the 14-mile point and I was preparing to cross a one-lane bridge when all of a sudden a large cement mixer turned the corner. . . . I never thought for a second about stopping and letting the truck pass. I simply continued and said to myself, "Come on you son-of-a-gun and I'll split you right down the middle—there will be concrete all over this road!" The driver slammed on the brakes and swerved to the right as I sailed by. That was really scary afterward, but at the time I really felt good. I have felt equally strong and indestructible many times since then, but I have never taken on a cement truck again.

This story underscores the importance of practicing movement patterns that are most beneficial for your personality. People diagnosed as having a coronary-prone, or type A, personality usually show a preference for fast, forceful movements, and if left to their inclinations would choose sports that foster this aggressive and potentially self-destructive pattern (Friedman, 1996). Similarly, rigid or compulsive individuals might feel more comfortable in a daily routine of stationary cycling, yet they might do well to stay away from such exercises because the inherent movement pattern could reinforce these psychological traits instead of "exercising" other qualities. But we must realize that people don't always have to change what they are doing; they may have intuitively chosen what is right for them. The hard-charging executive may recognize her need for something like yoga to reduce stress. Or a person may like to run because it gives him precisely the kind of mental and physical release he requires. If we consider the explosive, forceful, multidirectional movements of a kickboxing class, we might begin to appreciate the psychological qualities that long-term participation might promote. One does not throw a punch in the same way that you sculpt the air in a ballet class. A kick or a punch calls for a powerful explosion of energy directed at a point in space. Moving with intention and control as you duck, dodge, kick, and punch reinforces movement potential that may readily transfer to everyday life.

A vast literature dating back to the beginning of the 20th century addresses the use of movement training for affecting personal change (Lamb & Watson, 1994; North, 1972). With an understanding of movements normally required for participation in different sports and fitness programs, we can gain insight into the personality patterns that these different activities might reinforce. In working with clients, we can engage them in a dialogue about the potential of movement for actualizing their personal growth agendas.

Extensions and Limitations of Activity Analysis

This brief analysis of one type of fitness experience—kickboxing—is founded on three diverse fields of study: sport and exercise psychology, clinical and counseling psychology as related to body dynamics, and dance and movement therapy. The illustration of one activity can help you understand extensions to all other active-living engagements. This analysis has conveyed several fundamental points:

• **Physical activities have psychosocial representations.** Just as you can describe certain biomechanical aspects of physical routines, so too you can identify probable psychosocial characteristics.

• **Long-term participation in an activity conditions not only the body but also the mind.** The analysis of kickboxing—or, for that matter, any activity—becomes relevant in the long term. When someone engages in a specific activity over a period of months or years, its potential to condition new habits of thinking, feeling, and acting increases.

• **Experience will be your teacher.** A great deal of clinical judgment is represented in this analysis. As a lifestyle fitness coach you need to study your field intensely. Remembering that the realm of physical activity, in and out of the gym, forms the boundaries of your legitimate role, you will need to understand the wide world of sport and fitness. If you have primarily spent your time in a weight room and know little about racket sports, group fitness classes, outdoor recreation, or martial arts, exposing yourself to these pursuits will enhance your success as a coach.

• **Nothing is absolute.** The intentions of Western science are to describe, explain, predict, and control behavior. Science seeks formulas in which to insert values of variables and, thereby, to obtain reasonably accurate predictions. Unfortunately, we are a long way from being able to do that with human behavior. In another tradition of science we intensively study an individual and derive the most precise predictions for that individual based on a thorough analysis of all known relevant factors (Dunn, 1994). Perhaps with that approach we can find acceptable levels of confidence and reliability. We can never accurately analyze activities or sports without accounting for a participant's unique nature. Should anything you have read so far imply that if you participate in sport A for X hours, you will develop Y degrees of personality trait R, please erase that impression. Lifestyle fitness coaching is based on a dialogue in which no one has the answer at the outset. The coaching process is one of discovery. As coach and client intensify their inquiry, exploration, and testing of assumptions, they become more likely to arrive at the right answer, where right is defined in relation to this client rather than to people in general.

At this point, I invite you to apply what you have learned in this dissection of kickboxing. No doubt you are intimately familiar with at least one sport or physical activity. Try your hand at analyzing it in a fashion similar to what we did with kickboxing. Learning activity 2.1 will be a useful exercise in developing awareness that you can apply in lifestyle fitness coaching.

Learning Activity 2.1   Psychosocial, Anatomical, and Movement Demands of Sports

The analysis of kickboxing in chapter 2 provides a kind of template for dissecting other sports. Choose a fitness activity (like weight training) or a sport (like soccer) with which you are familiar, likely one in which you have participated extensively. Now, follow these guidelines to analyze its demands.

Psychosocial Demands

• How much social interaction does this activity require?

• Are the physical actions highly repetitive and predictable, or do they vary greatly and require spontaneous changes in response to situational demands or other elements?

• Do social supports or other factors make participation easy for a newcomer to this activity? For instance, having motivating music or the guidance of an instructor can help. Having teammates or classmates can be encouraging. If not, do you see this activity as relying on a high degree of internal motivation to sustain regular participation?

• Is this a gentle or forceful activity? Are the movements or actions demanding and even aggressive? Or are they relaxing and soft?

• Is this a competitive activity? Does it require high levels of collaboration or teamwork? Or is it solitary?

• Must you pay attention every second when you are doing this activity? Every once in a while? Or virtually not at all? Does the activity own your mind while you are engaged, or can you watch TV, listen to your radio, or daydream?

- Is this a dangerous activity or a safe one? What are the risks, if any? Are they social, psychological, or physical? Can you be hurt easily? Could someone feel embarrassed easily if he did poorly at this activity? Would a newcomer's self-esteem be at risk in doing this activity?

Anatomical Demands

- What muscle groups does this activity strongly employ? Does this activity emphasize the growth and development of muscles? If so, which ones? Does it emphasize flexibility, that is, does the activity improve range of movement? If so, which joints are most affected?

- What might this kind of development help a person do in the real world outside the fitness arena? For instance, in a threatening situation, could the person run away faster or defend herself better? Would the activity increase energy flow in the body by helping to unblock areas that the person might hold rigidly? Think through the real-world applications of the physical development that this activity might foster.

Movement Demands

- Are movements required by this activity likely to be fast, slow, or a mixture? If a mixture, what are the approximate percentages?

- Are movements required by this activity likely to be extended or contracted? Does the activity foster reaching and stretching more than it does the forceful contraction of muscle groups (as in weight training)?

- Are movements linear or nonlinear? Does the activity cause the participant to move up and down, side to side, backward and forward, and in circular or zigzag patterns? Or are the movements mostly straight ahead?

- Are movements forceful or soft? How much muscular force must the participant generate to do this activity? Does it vary throughout the course of the activity, or is it relatively constant?

- Are movements precise and controlled or flexible and potentially inexact? For instance, to swim well, movements need to be controlled and relatively precise, whereas free-form movements such those as in improvisational dance can be uncontrolled and imprecise.

- What are the implications of these movement qualities? For instance, when a participant always has to move in a fast, direct (linear), forceful, contracted, and controlled manner to participate in an activity, what psychological qualities might the participant develop? How would these translate into real-world behaviors?

Choice, Commitment, and Change: Essential Ingredients for Coaching

People who exercise regularly enjoy making periodic assessments of progress. These assessments typically take the form of weight or body-composition changes, increases in muscular definition, or gains in cardiorespiratory function. You might add to this list of assessments depending on the goals to which your client commits in the lifestyle fitness coaching process.

You will certainly be able to inform your clients of the probable physical changes that they will experience through regular participation in physical activity, but what psychological or personal changes can

you count on? Will a specific fitness program have the same predictable effect on all your clients? Will 5 miles (8 kilometers) of running increase your clients' self-esteem as much as a routine of weight lifting will? Can a highly competitive game of racquetball reduce feelings of anger as much as a lengthy yoga class will? Just as the required training or even the likelihood of running a sub-30 minute 10K will vary among clients, so too where and how a client enters a relationship with you speaks to the nature and extent of potential change along nonphysical dimensions. What is your client's starting point? What is he willing and able to commit? What other factors will influence change potential?

Personal change through active-living engagements comes slowly, but surely. Just as excess weight gradually melts away through exercise, personal development deepens through practice. By the time clients become cognizant of changes, they may have little conscious awareness of how they behaved before the change. The transition is like the change that occurred when you first learned to ride a bicycle. After you breezed around your neighborhood on your maiden voyage, remembering how it was before you could ride was nearly impossible.

Progress assessments that you make with your client will likely require personal journaling and record keeping (see chapter 10). People might normally step on a weight scale once a week, but rarely do they take their psychic temperature on a weekly basis, or count the number of times that they have asserted themselves with others. If lifestyle fitness coaching is the nature of the relationship that you have with your clients, you will have the opportunity to create ways of monitoring progress that uniquely reflect the contracts that you develop with them. As time goes by, you will have additional victories to celebrate as your clients achieve not only their physical change goals but their more personal ones as well.

Left to their personal wisdom, most people yield to old inclinations, to the path of least resistance. They tend to choose what reinforces their personal habits. Gregarious individuals gravitate toward group-based activities. Aggressive people choose aggressive sports. Adventurous people press the limits in risky sports. As long as people stick to the familiar, change on a personal level will be modest and in line with one's current predispositions.

Your work as a lifestyle fitness coach will invariably involve helping both inactive and active clients move out of their comfort zones (McWilliams, 1991), away from the status quo. For novice exercisers, your coaching may serve to identify activity options that closely match their patterns, whereas for habitually active clients, your work may be to guide and support them as they challenge ingrained styles and habits of action through new activity choices. For instance, with a shy novice, you would look for activities that might protect him from social challenges, whereas for a shy habitue who is working as much on personal as on physical agendas, you may cocreate opportunities for interaction within physical activity. In both cases you must manage degrees of challenge and a process of change.

Fully understanding client agendas, hidden and overt, is a significant part of your work. Once you

have identified these agendas, you will have placed yourself on a kind of map with certain destinations. Moving toward these destinations involves commitment to begin the journey, persistence in the face of unknown challenges, and a willingness to explore the insights and dilemmas that may occur along the way.

The words *choice, change,* and *commitment* summarize the messages of this chapter. We began with a sampling of definitions of life coaching and then identified a specialized focus within this broad field, identified as lifestyle fitness coaching. By framing this specialty within the context of sport, fitness, and other active-living pursuits, we then considered the wide-ranging effects that activities can have on physical, social, and psychological dimensions of a client's life.

Only rarely do people who are completely content with their lives upset their states of equilibrium to pursue the path of change. More typically, crisis, calamity, or other changes provoke people to engage in a process of change (Tedeschi, Park, & Calhoun, 1998).

The Chinese pictogram representing the word *crisis* comprises two symbols, one standing for opportunity and the other for danger. When people ask to be clients in a coaching process, they are likely already experiencing the need or desire to change because of various forces. To ensure that they avoid danger and maximize opportunity, they wisely seek assistance.

Clients working with lifestyle fitness coaches have a choice about whether or not to take action and then about the kinds of actions that they will pursue. With choice comes the likelihood of change. Clients do not consciously choose to work with coaches to remain the same. Although they may unwittingly sabotage change, they consciously wish to change. Finally, when action is defined, commitment is required. Saying that you want to lose 20 pounds (9 kilograms) by exercising five times a week and managing your diet is much easier than consistently committing energy and action to reaching that objective.

Coaches "forward the action" (Martin, 2001) by assisting clients in processes of choosing, changing, and committing. Lifestyle fitness coaches operate within the realm of sport, exercise, and active living as the means to achieving clients' visions, dreams, and goals. Along the paths of clients' journeys, the coach will serve as guide, supporter, wizard, sage, and truth teller.

The Coaching Relationship

L ife is about relationship (Cashdan, 1988). Whether as a professional, friend, family member, or citizen, we are shaped by the nature and extent of our social interactions. To some degree, we know who we are in the reflected impressions we see in others. This chapter delves into important relationship qualities and issues that are core to the work of lifestyle fitness coaches. Because the material reviewed has a strong theoretical flavor, the chapter includes learning activities that will help you derive concrete and practical understanding.

As Miars and Halverson (2001) note, most people are engaged in some form of helping relationship every day. Some kinds of helping may occur informally, whereas other types of helping have a more formal face. Accordingly, expectations of helpers will vary according to whether the helper is considered family, friend, or professional. We expect certain types of support and advice when we share concerns with friends, whereas professional helping often has a different dynamic. In general, professional helpers bear greater responsibility throughout the helping process, and we expect them to be objective, purposeful, and knowledgeable.

In considering how we function in relationships, a recent concept helps frame relevant aspects of personal readiness and ability. Daniel Goleman (1995) popularized the term **emotional intelligence** and, in so doing, broadened our appreciation of human competencies. Critical elements of emotional intelligence include the degree to which an individual has self-awareness, is able to self-regulate personal behaviors, is self-motivating, is capable of experiencing and expressing empathy, and can readily access

"In the beginning was relationship."

Martin Buber

personal resources. Emotional intelligence reflects how much the person is able to establish rapport with others, create an atmosphere of trust, generate interpersonal confidence in relationships, listen effectively, and appropriately influence others. Virtually every writer on the topic of helping relationships has highlighted the first factor noted, self-awareness. Cormier and Nurius (2003), for instance, plainly state that clients and the circumstances of helping will often "push your buttons," because we all have personal histories that affect our perceptions and our reactions. According to these authors, self-awareness has to do with taking responsibility and learning how to manage our sensitivities. As we move deeper into discussions about coaching, we will see how closely this concept of emotional intelligence relates to one's ability to function effectively as a coach.

Clients typically engage professional helpers to resolve some concern or difficulty or to foster personal growth (Miars & Halverson, 2001). Clients agree to work with professional helpers concerning one or more of the following types of goals (Brammer & MacDonald, 1999):

- To cause changes in behavior or lifestyle
- To increase self-awareness, insight, or understanding

- To obtain relief from suffering
- To change thought patterns or self-perceptions

Although it may seem obvious, helping relationships are a process of enabling clients to change and grow in directions chosen by the client. The effective professional helper fosters clients' awareness of possible alternatives and encourages clients to accept responsibility for taking action on one or more of these alternatives (Capuzzi & Gross, 2001).

Although a range of values and ethics inspires professional helping relationships, two values are especially relevant. The first is a belief in the dignity and worth of the individual, and the second is respect for the client's right to self-determination (Shebib, 2003).

You no doubt have experience as a client or patient in a helping relationship. For instance, in visiting a doctor, lawyer, accountant, counselor, or professor while in school, you positioned yourself as someone seeking advice, counsel, or help. Learning activity 3.1 provides an opportunity for you to explore the quality of helpers based on your personal encounters before you consider ideas that are more theoretical.

Learning Activity 3.1 What Really Helps: A Personal Review

Throughout your life you have experienced helping relationships in a variety of forms. Appointments with doctors, lawyers, accountants, teachers, counselors, and others are situations in which you were the person in need of help or guidance. How did you feel in these situations? What did the professionals do that seemed to put you at ease? What might they have done to empower or disempower you? How much trust did you feel in them? What specifically did they do to engender trust?

Take time to reflect on the different experiences you have had and identify qualities or behaviors of the helpers that either fostered or detracted from your sense of trust and confidence in their abilities. What caused you to believe that they could help? What did they do that made you feel whole and respected in the relationship?

Helpful Qualities or Behaviors   ### Unhelpful Qualities or Behaviors

_____   _____

_____   _____

_____   _____

_____   _____

_____   _____

Promoting Growth Through Relationship

Beliefs others have about us carry weight. One of most dramatic illustrations of this fact can be found in studies of the **self-fulfilling prophecy,** wherein one person's expectations of another's behavior, conveyed repeatedly over time, tends to be incorporated by the other and enacted in accordance with expectation (Smale, 1977).

A parent who believes that his daughter will succeed in school is more likely to have a high-performing child than one who thinks that his child will fail. People emerge into adulthood having adapted consciously and unconsciously to the expectations of others. Helping relationships, such as those with coaches and counselors, are thought to hold the potential for correcting some of these early life biases that shaped a client's life.

Carl Rogers (1951, 1961, 1967, 1980), one of the founders of humanistic psychology, wrote extensively on relationships and the qualities of helpers that nourish clients' growth. A central theme of his writing was the belief that people are in the process of becoming, that people can change, and that they are not bound by their past. Rogers' position represented a dramatic shift in beliefs about human nature derived from an earlier Freudian perspective (Freud, 1964). Rather than treating clients as products of their pasts and incapable of altering their behavior, Rogers and his followers urged helpers to view clients as having strength, potential, inner power, and the capacity to change. In Rogers' (1961) view, a helper's attitudes and feelings toward the client were far more important in determining outcomes than were any particular skills or techniques that the helper possessed.

A classic tale of helping that Rogers (1951, p. 69) described was of a man who successfully completed counseling after an unsuccessful prior experience with another counselor. When the second counselor inquired why the client was able to work through his issues so successfully with him, the client responded: "You did about the same things he did, but you seemed really interested in me." Although some of Rogers' (1961) reflections about effective helping relationships have become almost prescriptive, his profound concern for the client and for the quality of the relationship formed by a helper's thoughts, feelings, and actions can be framed in simple questions that helpers might ask themselves in the process of working with clients:

- How can I act so that clients will perceive me as trustworthy?
- Can I permit myself to experience positive attitudes of warmth, caring, liking, interest, and respect toward clients?
- Can I be strong enough as a person to be separate from my clients?
- Am I secure enough to permit clients their separateness?
- Can I allow myself to fully empathize with my clients' feelings and world perspectives without evaluating or judging?

The Latin phrase *sine qua non* (literally translated as "without which nothing") captures the importance of relationship dynamics in helping. The relationship is considered by many to be the principle medium by which clients bring forth significant ideas and feelings to form the working agenda of helping (Brammer et al., 1993). The quality of relationship established by helpers with their clients determines whether in fact anything happens at all. Goldstein and Higginbotham (1991, p. 22) felt that the quality of the relationship serves "as a powerful positive influence on communication, openness, persuasibility, and ultimately, positive change in the client." A number of factors influence the formation of helping relationships, and many of these rely on the helper's awareness, attentiveness, and use of self in relation to his or her client (Cormier & Nurius, 2003).

The Working Alliance

In the coaching literature as well as in the broader literature of helping and counseling, the term **working alliance** has been advanced as a perspective for understanding what needs to happen between coach and client (Bordin, 1979; Greenson, 1967; Sexton & Whiston, 1994). Coaching as a form of helping is defined as a partnership—an agreement to collaborate in working on an agenda defined by the client. Three necessary elements of this alliance appear in the form of (1) agreement on goals, (2) agreement on tasks, and (3) an emotional bond between coach and client.

When a coach attempts to form a working alliance with a client, each party's history in relationships will have bearing on the success of the alliance. Focusing on the coach's behavior, a number of patterns must be considered (Brems, 2001). Coaches may have needs for intimacy that are either excessive or insufficient to form effective alliances with clients. They may have needs for approval that sometimes constitute a reversal of roles between coach and client. A coach may be too transparent in disclosing personal information or may be too private, thereby causing clients to feel objectified. Although an emotional bond must be present between coach and client, the coach's level of emotional expressiveness may be more or less appropriate to the client or the client's agenda. Other issues, such as dependency or trustworthiness, will also influence whether or not a coach can establish the necessary climate for the collaborative alliance required in helping.

Coaches need to be competent within their domains of involvement, yet it will ultimately be the quality of the alliance established between coaches and clients that makes a difference (Rogers, 1961; Sexton, Whiston, Bleuer, & Walz, 1997).

Containment and Holding

Have you ever had an experience in which someone approached you with a perplexing human drama or a need to talk driven by grief or despair? Most of us have been present to friends, family, or sometimes relative strangers who simply needed to talk about their experiences and wanted nothing more than for us to listen. In reflecting on such experiences, you might remember how you wanted to say something, wanted to come up with just the right words to make the person feel better, yet you realized that nothing you could say would achieve this result and, in fact, that there was little that anyone could say to resolve the drama or emotions expressed. So you simply listened—with all your heart and soul. At the end of this process, the person probably thanked you profusely for being there, and you might have felt bewildered, thinking to yourself, "But I really didn't do anything."

To understand the process of helping and, thereby, the function of a coach, one needs to grasp the significance of **containment,** or the creation of a **holding environment** (Winnicott, 1958). Experts like Kohut (1984) and modern-day theorists like Hendrix (2001) offer insight into the healing capacity of the space that we create for others to express their realities. In a world of action and doing, it is profoundly important to understand the role of simply being—without the compulsion to do something. Just as day makes sense in relation to night, doing gains significance in its connection to being. When someone comes to us for help, our immediate thought is often about doing: "What can I do that will make this person feel better?"

As we will see in upcoming chapters, the process of helping begins with understanding the client's story. If a threatening person is interrogating someone, the story that the person tells may be replete with distortions, deletions, and misinformation. The kind of relationship that a coach wants to create with a client would clearly be one of support and should be nonthreatening in nature. For a client to tell the complete story, a coach needs to create a safe environment where the client's thoughts, feelings, and behaviors can be contained without judgment and with respect. Creating such an environment is not always easy.

To contain another's story is to be fully present, to open oneself to that person's felt meanings, and to allow oneself to experience what it might be like to have lived her story. This task requires not only a readiness to listen but also competency in conveying to the other a sense of boundaries and security. Often, people tell deeply meaningful stories to others in confidence, and certainly in professional helping relationships, confidentiality is a requirement.

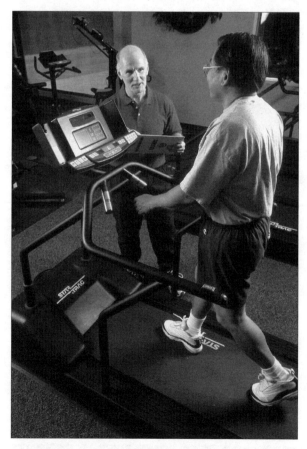

A successful lifestyle fitness coach must aim to form a working alliance with his client.

Learning Activity 3.2   Why Do You Want to Be a Coach?

What motivates you to learn about coaching and to consider this highly rewarding yet challenging career path? Please take a few minutes now to write down your motivations.

- What are your primary motivations for becoming a coach?
- What do you feel would be your unique contributions as a coach?
- What skill set that you believe you possess would most help you in your work as a coach?
- What life experiences have you had that support your decision to move into coaching as a career?
- What kind of feedback from friends, family members, or clients helps you understand your interpersonal skills related to the coaching profession?

Although these may seem normal and acceptable bases for such career decisions, it is nonetheless important to remain personally vigilant concerning the hidden needs embedded in such agendas. For instance, the desire to give others what one has personally received and clearly valued may result in an insistence that clients accept the coach's obviously useful guidance. The quest to do for others what someone has done for you may translate into a personal crusade to ensure that someone has the benefit of what you once received from another. Similarly, when insights and awareness come flooding to mind, the desire to ensure that another person has the advantages of your knowledge can become a form of tyranny. In summarizing the risks of such motives for helping, Cormier and Nurius (2003, p. 17) suggest that well-intentioned coaches driven by their personal stories can behave toward clients with "pride rather than humility, insistence rather than invitation, telling rather than listening, 'expert-ing' rather than collaborating, and making or coercing rather than assisting."

What Does It Take to Really Help?

As a coach you will continually experience opportunities to explore your relation to three themes related to working in a helping context with clients: competence, power, and intimacy (Cormier & Nurius, 2003):

Competence

No matter how many degrees you have or how many certifications you pursue, an exploding knowledge base in the health fitness professions places you on a never-ending journey of learning. Ironically, what

you know now may serve as an impediment to the acquisition of new learning, especially when what is new represents a paradigmatic shift in knowledge or understanding. Developing technically based competencies may be comforting at times. Being able to enlist the aid of machines or formulas in determining answers helps reduce ambiguity about the solutions that we derive. Blood lab analyses, $\dot{V}O_2$max assessments, or formulas for body composition offer some degree of concreteness and allow professionals to feel expert in their judgments. Yet as you move away from technical analysis into the soft sciences surrounding lifestyle fitness coaching, certainty diminishes and the quest for knowledge to reduce ambiguity or increase precision multiplies. The more deeply you work with clients, the more likely you are to encounter questions and certain imponderables. But coaching is an action-generating process, so you need to conclude analyses and make decisions. Invariably, you will experience doubt and second-guessing. Should you have done something differently? Was your choice the wisest?

Understanding your personal sense of competency and your history of success experiences will provide clues concerning your vulnerability to doubt, negative self-beliefs, or tendencies to be self-critical. In the chaos created by self-negation or denigration of your competencies following a perceived failure, a number of courses of action are likely. Some of these can be productive, whereas others may be dangerous or even harmful. Trying to bolster self-confidence by asserting the correctness of your actions or the client's ineffectual style will not work. Nor will it be helpful to turn to clients for reassurance, that is, to ask the client to take care of you in moments of doubt. On the other hand, seeking counsel, talking with colleagues, working with a supervisor, researching the literature, or simply owning your feelings can reverse the downward spiral of self-doubt.

Effective coaches make contingency plans for occasions when things do not go as they had hoped, rather than hoping that things never go wrong. It is normal to question and even to doubt. How you manage these predictable episodes in a helping career ultimately determines whether you survive and how well you help.

Power

Knowledge is power, and coaching roles themselves come packaged with client expectations that convey to one's title as lifestyle fitness coach a patina of power. Some coaches attempt to deny possession of any differential levels of power in relationships with clients. A feeling of discomfort in being perceived as powerful may cause a coach to minimize influence attempts and perhaps to fail to intervene when such action can help.

At the other extreme, a coach can misuse power through the conviction that because he has the knowledge, he necessarily has the power, that because he has the position, he needs to be obeyed. Coaches who assume that they know what is right for their clients are likely to misuse power based in their role and expertise. With some clients, this pattern can continue indefinitely, in a dysfunctional way. A client who is highly dependent or needy may be willing to submerge personal opinions or even values in return for the coach's approval. Indeed, the client may collude to such a degree as to convey to the coach impressions of success. The client may lose weight, gain muscle, act more assertively, or develop apparent confidence, so long as client and coach implicitly agree to this power dynamic. But if the client objects or the coach steps too far over the line, the whole system quickly falls apart to reveal the underlying reality.

The **lifestyle converter** is a form of power abuse described by Cormier and Nurius (2003). A coach who is personally committed to certain ways of living or personal practices may use communication techniques in a conscious or unconscious manner to manipulate clients into adopting her preferences. Coaching then turns into a cult exercise in which one either becomes a true believer or is banished from the relationship.

Intimacy

The term *intimacy* in the context of professional relationships may seem misplaced, yet to work effectively with clients, coaches need to ask questions and discuss information that goes deeper than merely personal. A normal human response to revealing such information is to feel vulnerable, and to reduce client discomfort, coaches are often advised to engage in certain limited self-disclosures as a way of leveling the field. As Jourard (1958, 1964, 1968) indicated long ago, however, self-disclosure begets more self-disclosure, so clients who feel somewhat relieved that they are not the only ones who have issues are encouraged to talk more deeply about themselves. Inevitably, a feeling of intimate connection between coach and client develops. In fact, this emotional bond becomes one of the necessary conditions for discussing and resolving client issues.

Coaches can abuse intimacy or, conversely, engage it inadequately. A coach may have strong needs for intimacy and, as a result, may decide to probe deeper than necessary to attempt to bond with clients at a level inappropriate to the contracted working alliance. When a coach feels emotionally insecure and needs to experience intimacy with clients, she may behave in a manner that prevents the client from talking about necessary topics. For example, to avoid feeling rejected, the coach may prevent the client from experiencing emotions like anger or irritation.

Fears of intimacy or strong emotionality represent another potential liability in coaching relationships. A coach who needs to remain objective, professional, and aloof may dampen clients' emotional expressions or their willingness to experience vulnerability through opening up to the coach.

Most people have issues surrounding competency, power, and intimacy. Effective coaches are unlikely to have worked through all there is to resolve in these areas, but they devote themselves to becoming aware of their personal dynamics around these themes, and they do whatever is necessary to ensure that their personal dynamics are appropriate and productive to their client relationships.

Consider this example. A coach probes deeper than necessary to gain understanding of a client's history and agenda related to active living. The client, feeling somewhat exposed, looks embarrassed. In response, the coach decides to self-disclose to ease the client's tension. Subsequently, the client opens up more, and the coach, thinking his self-disclosure was productive, reveals even more personal information. Soon, coach and client are exchanging intimate details of their lives with comfort. At the end of the session, the coach senses that he went too far and feels rather exposed. Moreover, he wonders how the client feels and what her expectations will be for the next session. Clearly, the coach went too far in this case and will need to work with awareness to bring the relationship back to a more appropriate level of sharing related to the client's legitimate agenda. The coach could probably benefit from supervision in this situation, both to bring the relationship back on track and to explore the personal dynamics that propelled him to move so strongly toward intimacy.

The Coach's Power to Influence

The term *manipulation* has negative connotations in Western society, yet social scientists (D. Johnson, 2003) readily acknowledge that most communication is about influence. We manipulate one another with words, actions, and nonverbal communications. Where one person's attempt to change your behavior fails, another's succeeds. Indeed, some people influence us more easily than others do. What elements of character, presence, or relationship make one person more powerful than another? If a particular person can influence you, does that mean that she will be equally influential with others?

The agenda for coaching derives from the client (Martin, 2001; Whitworth et al., 1998). On this point, most practitioners and writers seem to agree. Furthermore, the means to the ends desired by clients should ideally come from the client, or at a minimum, the client should wholly agree with them. So where does influence come in?

Clients may be motivated to change or to pursue some goal, but typically they need help unearthing the reasons, values, needs, and personal dynamics that pertain to their wishes. Then they may require assistance in formulating plans that are robust and realistic. Once engaged in action, clients typically need support, and although the coach should not be their sole source of support, coaches can provide invaluable aid by assisting clients in structuring systems of support.

We could argue that if clients could do all these things on their own, they would not need coaches. Yet those in the coaching world normally identify the client as someone who is reasonably well functioning, has manifested sufficient levels of success in life, and is motivated to pursue identified goals and change processes. From this perspective, influence should be rather straightforward and uncomplicated, and, in fact, many times it is. Nonetheless, the coach is in a position of influence and should do far more than be a passive listener to a client's musings.

Most textbooks on counseling (Ivey & Ivey, 2003) devote major sections to two classes of skills, defining one roughly as attending and the other as influencing. The interweaving of attending and influencing skills in interviews and counseling processes is based on the notion that the counselor first obtains the client's story (through attending) and then works toward influencing change. This flow from attending to influencing characterizes even more objectively based change processes. For example, although blood-lab reports, CAT scans, and MRIs aid diagnosis of problems, physicians will nonetheless augment their objective data by using such attending skills as asking questions before they attempt to influence a patient to change a behavior or to subscribe to a form of treatment.

In coaching as in counseling, the relationship between the coach's attending behaviors and her use of influencing skills should be based on client feedback. An important determinant of the timeliness of employing influencing skills is whether the coach has established sufficient rapport with the client to attempt to direct change. A common recommendation is that the coach continue to build rapport through use of attending skills until two conditions have been met. The first is that the coach has sufficient information to begin the process of influencing the client, and the second is that the coach has an adequate basis of rapport with the client, that is, that the **core relationship conditions** have been sufficiently established.

The importance of a coach's ability to influence client thoughts, feelings, and behaviors can be traced back through the history of coaching or even further back through the literature on counseling. Perhaps the first significant contribution to understanding the dynamics of influence in coaching and counseling relations appeared in 1968 when Strong published his landmark article on counseling as a process of social influence. Strong reflected on the difficulties that clients have in successfully pursuing valued change processes. He suggested that the awareness that a client has of current behaviors as contrasted with some preferred or more beneficial pattern creates a sense of dissonance, or internal discomfort. One way to reduce this discomfort is to discredit the person who has raised the client's awareness of the discrepancy, namely, the counselor or, in our perspective, the coach.

This reasoning led Strong (1968) to hypothesize certain variables that would decrease the chances that clients would resist helpers' influence attempts and, thereby, increase the probability of successful change. Strong (1968) identified three helper characteristics thought to make the relationship more positive and to enable clients to be more receptive to helpers' influence attempts. These were expertness, attractiveness, and trustworthiness. Goldstein and Higginbotham (1991) called these factors relationship enhancers because of their capacity to positively affect the working alliance. In his initial model Strong believed that the optimization of a helper's ability to influence occurred in two distinct phases.

In the first phase the helper deliberately engages in actions or manipulates the environment in ways that convey to the client a sense of the helper's expertness, attractiveness, and trustworthiness. According to Strong (1968) the helper uses whatever sources of power are available to establish influence potential with the client.

Based on how effectively the helper has presented herself as attractive, expert, and trustworthy, the second phase revolves around the client's world. No matter what a coach thinks she is communicating, only through the client's interpretation do these communications take on meaning. In this phase the client must come to a place of regarding the coach as influential, almost independent of whether the coach merits such regard.

In a more recent rendition of this model of influence, Strong and colleagues (Strong, Welsh, Corcoran, & Hoyt, 1992) added a third component to this social influence model, which they described as follows: "Client responsiveness to the ideas and recommendations presented by counselors is a function of their dependence on counselors. Dependence is a motivational factor that gets generated through the helping relationship" (p. 7). What is critical to note here is that for a coach's influence to reach its greatest level, the client must experience a form of dependency on the coach. Although the notion of dependency carries with it certain harmful connotations, one reality of the coach–client relationship is that the client hires the coach because of a perception that he needs help to achieve his goals. Implicitly, the client initiates the relationship with the intention of being dependent on the coach, yet for this intention to be actualized, the coach must behave in ways that create safety around client dependency and vulnerability (phase one) and the client must perceive that this is so (phase two). When the client proceeds through these two phases in the desired manner, then the success of the helper's influence attempts will be contingent on the degree to which the client allows himself to experience dependent feelings with the coach.

Expertness

We have already considered aspects of expertness, as discussed by Strong (1968), in earlier remarks about competency. However, a review of how coaches can appropriately help clients perceive their expertise will be useful here.

Being perceived by clients as an expert does not depend on years of experience (Heppner & Heesacker, 1982). Clients do not necessarily perceive experienced practitioners as more expert than novice practitioners. Competencies in verbal and nonverbal communications are more likely to influence client perceptions of coaching competence (Barak, Patkin, & Dell, 1982). Of course, in initial contacts with clients, a coach's reputation and such external trappings as degrees, certifications, and awards will create transient impressions of expertise (Cormier & Nurius, 2003). These, however, will only allow the coach sufficient time to build more substantive manifestations of expertness through actual demonstration of coaching skills. If the coach does not demonstrate competency in behavioral interventions with clients in initial meetings, clients will be more likely to terminate their relationships before progressing toward their goals.

The coach's versatility in dealing with client differences is a critical consideration in establishing expertness with clients. What may seem appropriate professional behavior in a North American context could be perceived negatively by clients from different backgrounds. A coach may be highly accomplished in the health fitness field, but if he commits certain psycho-socio-cultural gaffes, technical expertise or professional accomplishments will count for little.

Cormier and Nurius (2003) list particular nonverbal behaviors associated with clients' perceptions of helpers' expertness, including the appropriateness and quality of eye contact, a forward lean of the body when communicating from a seated position, and the fluency of the helper's speech. Verbal behaviors relevant to perceptions of expertness include (1) the relevance of questions asked by the helper, (2) verbal indications of attentiveness, coupled with a lack of interrupting behaviors, and (3) the degree of directness and confidence evidenced in verbal communications.

Attractiveness

Attractiveness may seem an odd dimension to consider, yet it is so central in most of our other relationships that it would seem odder if it were omitted.

The adage "Beauty is in the eye of the beholder" offers clues about the nature of attractiveness in coaching relationships. Attractiveness is a matter of perception, and it is also the case that we like being around people who make us feel good about ourselves; this is another way of understanding the dynamics of attraction. So we are not just talking about physical appearance, although in many cultures people who are perceived as physically attractive have more power than those who are not (Robinson & Howard-Hamilton, 2000). Strong (1968), among others, considered attractiveness a mix of the helper's degree of similarity to the client, his friendliness, and the client's perception of how likeable he is. Physical attractiveness per se probably figures into the equation earlier in the relationship (Cormier & Nurius, 2003) but gradually diminishes in importance. What begins to take precedence over physical appeal is the helper's interpersonal attractiveness, which relates more to skills in working with clients. How well the helper attends to the client, how responsive he is to a client's signals, and even the degree to which the helper is willing to engage in appropriate levels of self-disclosure with clients (Edwards & Murdock, 1994) tend to increase perceptions of attractiveness and, therefore, interpersonal influence. As always, versatility comes into play in understanding how clients of diverse backgrounds will perceive behaviors intended as overtures of friendliness or what actions they will find likeable.

Trustworthiness

The development of trust with clients hinges on many factors. People vary in their willingness to trust others (D. Johnson, 2003), and although trust may eventually develop after a long series of trials and tests, one mistrustful act can easily destroy it. Such helper characteristics as genuineness, congruence, respect, versatility, and empathy will help establish trust, yet the challenge of creating trust will be larger or smaller depending on clients' personal histories with other helpers and the degree to which the helper is thought to possess certain characteristics that might be culturally defined as meriting trust, for example, age, sex, or similarity in ethnicity. As D. Johnson (2003) indicates, it is appropriate that people earn trust in relationships rather than receive it automatically. In this light, coaches should prepare themselves to be tested and should not react defensively when clients are unwilling to trust them unconditionally, irrespective of how trustworthy they have proved to be in past

relationships. In fact, Zastrow (1999) argues that distrust is more likely than trust in relationships of cross-cultural helping.

Understanding the Relational Underworld: Transference

When people are in intense, intimate relationships over a period of time, some predictable dynamics begin to occur. Patterns and a unique language begin to evolve, and each person's identity may become connected with others with whom the parties have had relationships. Traditionally, this dynamic has been labeled **transference**. Although this technical term has its origins in psychoanalytic literature, its relevance to coaching relationships is unmistakable.

An experience that most of us have had is meeting someone new who reminds us of another person in our lives. From the outset of this new relationship, we may need to be conscious about how our previous relationship may affect the development of the current one. Appearances, mannerisms, or some other aspect of the person triggers in us an association to the previous relationship. Recognizing physical similarities is easier than identifying a resemblance that occurs at a psychological level.

An earlier discussion about intimacy noted that people have different preferences for levels of intimacy and even different reactions to the experience of intimacy in a relationship. For instance, someone who seems quite grounded in a friendship relationship may begin acting strangely once the relationship turns a corner toward more intimate connections. Common wisdom would suggest that perhaps this person is reacting to prior experiences. For instance, someone who has experienced pain and loss in intimate relations may begin to distance himself when signs of closeness increase in frequency. This circumstance represents another face of transference.

Corey and colleagues (2003) identify transference in a helping context as the "unreal relationship." As seen in coaching, transference would be a process whereby a client projects onto the coach thoughts, feelings, or attributes that they had experienced in relation to other significant people in their lives. As these authors note, "Transference typically has its origins in early childhood and constitutes a repetition of past repressed material. Through this process, clients' unfinished business produces a distortion in the way they perceive and react to the [coach]. The feelings clients experience in transference may include love, hate, anger, ambivalence, and dependency" (p. 46).

Perhaps a more practical way of looking at transference is that the client focuses more on the helper than on himself (Young, 2001). In so doing, the client avoids the necessary work of the coaching relationship. Watkins (1986) discussed five patterns of transference that seem common to helping relationships; these have been framed within the work of lifestyle fitness coaching:

1. **Coach as ideal role model.** The client emulates the coach's behavior, including modes of dress and manners of speech. He is exceptionally complimentary of anything the coach does or says. Although flattery and imitation may be ego gratifying, the coach may eventually feel some irritation with the client's adoration. In addition, the coach may begin to worry about the excessive influence he has on the client's attitudes and behaviors.

2. **Coach as wizard.** The client sees the coach as having all the answers, as being all knowing and flawless in judgment. Conversely, the client acts in a self-denigrating manner, criticizing his own judgment and knowledge. When coaches receive such high praise, they may begin to focus on the potential of falling. They may begin to worry about making mistakes and, ironically, begin to doubt themselves. Self-aware coaches usually can feel the setup in such overblown feedback.

3. **Coach as ultimate caregiver.** The client sees the coach as a loving and nurturing person with whom the client feels totally safe and secure. The coaching relationship becomes a private haven where the client can open himself to all feelings; however, the client confides that this all-embracing nurturance only happens with the coach. This kind of response from a client may encourage the coach to give excessively out of a desire to help. Over time, however, the coach will begin to feel depleted, experiencing an energy drain occasioned by this client's extreme need.

4. **Coach as resister.** The client acts as if the coach is standing in the way of his progress, either through questioning or through requests for concrete planning. He frequently tests the coach and acts defensive and mistrustful with him. The coach can easily become caught in a kind of self-fulfilling prophecy in which the more the client mistrusts, the more uneasy and cautious the coach becomes. Invariably, this exacting awareness may cause the coach to trip, thereby proving to the client how untrustworthy he is.

5. **Coach as irrelevancy.** The client uses the time with the coach in an aimless, goalless, and unmotivated manner. Although physically present for sessions, the client blocks progress by diverting the coach's efforts to focus or direct discussions. Because the coach is being paid, he may begin to feel rather useless and come to doubt his own competency. Feelings of resentment and annoyance toward the client may also build as the client continues to thwart the coach's efforts toward progress.

Countertransference

Of course, relationships are two-way streets, so coaches may also project attitudes, feelings, or thoughts onto their clients. This phenomenon bears the label **countertransference**. Corey and colleagues (2003) describe it as any projections coming from the helper toward the client that can potentially get in the way of helping the client. See learning activity 3.3 for sample cases of both transference and countertransference.

All this may seem foreign to what health fitness professionals normally consider when they work with clients. In transitory, short-term, and technically oriented relationships, it is nonetheless probable that transference and countertransference are operating. In these relationships, however, these dynamics are unlikely to have much bearing on the outcome. If a client comes to a fitness center to have his body composition assessed or to obtain estimates of cardiorespiratory functioning, he may project feelings of resentment onto an advisor based on earlier life experiences in which he had to undergo painful assessment processes, but his results will be largely unaffected and he will continue in his life largely unchanged by the experience.

Oddly, in relationships such as coaching in which the helper is doing his utmost to promote safety and support, the likelihood of transference projections seems to increase (Kohut, 1984). The belief is that the safety created by the helper eases the client's expressions of long withheld emotions. In this regard, we might refer back to our earlier consideration of the holding environment.

The phenomena of transference and countertransference are often seen as mystifying elements of relationships that should be studied only by people training to be psychological counselors, social workers, psychotherapists, or psychoanalysts. This kind of thinking is fundamentally flawed and probably arises from a mistaken assumption that these dynamics are necessarily

Learning Activity 3.3   Examples of the "Relational Underworld"

To gain awareness of transference and countertransference, read the following case histories and consider the questions that follow each case:

The Case of Henry

Your client, Henry, has been working with you for over a year. Although you have made great progress with him in terms of his attainment of both physical and psychological change goals, you are aware that Henry is nowhere near being ready to work independently. In fact, the more progress he makes in your work together, the more questions he brings to you and the higher he sets the mark for achievement. Although he is respectful in scheduling appointments and telephone check-ins, he seems to save all his decision making for times when he can talk with you. He says, "You have such good advice . . . You're a genius. Without your input, I simply wouldn't know what to do."

- What do you think is going on with Henry? How do you understand his behavior?
- How might you discuss his behavior with him?
- If you had a number of clients with similar patterns, what might this imply about your style?

The Case of Carla

Your client, Carla, has become increasingly critical of your work. She implies that you are sloppy and disorganized, and that you act like a robot with her. You have thought about her feedback and asked some of your colleagues for their opinions about your work. So far, Carla's remarks seem baseless. You are beginning to dread your meetings with her.

- What do you imagine might be going on with Carla?
- Do you think it would be appropriate to talk to her about her remarks and your feelings?
- If so, what exactly would you do and say?

The Case of Ben

Your client, Ben, is successful in his work and seems to have a wonderful family. He is so good at what he does that you often wonder why he needs you as a coach. You find yourself judging Ben's success sometimes, attributing his accomplishments to his wealthy family or sheer luck. When you are coaching him, you are aware of looking for flaws in his plans, emphasizing what isn't working for him, or simply not congratulating him when he does something well. In your own family, you always defined yourself as the underachiever, especially compared with an older sibling.

- What do you think might be happening in your relationship with Ben?
- What do you believe an appropriate plan of action might be?
- Do you think it would be appropriate to talk to Ben? Do you think it would be helpful for you to talk to someone else?

negative or even pathological in nature. In the previous chapter, we considered the fact that human habits arise from experience, often repeated experience. In this chapter, we began with the thought that human life is essentially social. So, the habits we form are often embedded in a social context. That is, we behave similarly in social situations.

Taking this one step further, the more similar the situation, the more likely that habitual responses will appear.

When we meet someone, we enter into the relationship with the fullness of our personal histories. For many, this history is exactly what allows us to be trusting and open, until otherwise indicated by the responses that we receive. This dynamic is a form of transference.

The gift afforded coaches by understanding transference comes in the knowledge that the clearer we are about ourselves, the more we will have worked through our own filters and biases, and the more receptive and supportive we can be toward clients. The better able we are to intercept client projections for exactly what they are, the more effectively we can use them in enabling clients to reach their goals.

If you believe that you carry no conscious bias toward a client, if you have behaved compassionately and supportively, and if you have lived up to your end of agreements, then complaints about your behavior, your effectiveness, the results achieved, or other matters may be unmasked as unresolved issues emanating from your client's past. Then, with some of the skills that we will review in upcoming chapters, you can caringly discuss these matters, always with the client's agenda in mind. To say this differently, you need not confront all transference projections. You can simply receive them as information and deal with them according to the contract you have with your client.

The flip side of this situation occurs when you as a coach struggle desperately to make sense of all your client's complaints about your behavior because you have failed to recognize that your client is reacting from the "unreal relationship" (Corey et al., 2003). This is not to deny that you will sometimes make mistakes or that on occasion your biases will bypass your professionalism. Not every complaint is evidence of transference; not every feeling is a projection. We do form new relationships. We do like some people a lot and have difficulty with others, simply because of our experiences with them.

We receive yet another set of gifts by understanding these matters, and it comes from our examinations of transference and countertransference. The nature of intimate helping relationships (Cashdan, 1988) is that our basic dynamics play out at levels of which we may have only vague awareness. For instance, you may work with a client who is conscientious about her program, who is never tardy, who always takes your advice without resistance, yet for whom you have a niggling feeling of irritation. A common way to deal with this feeling is to attribute it to some personal issue of yours or to override its messages in your interactions with her. You certainly don't want to show this excellent client that you feel irritated with her! Yet this inner voice is sending you a message. If you have behaved clearly, professionally, and compassionately, an irritation that keeps

surfacing is a signal that something deeper may be occurring. Because you have no axe to grind with this client and because you have done your best to create a safe holding environment, some aspect of your client's behavior may be at root. Indeed, she may commonly elicit irritation from others even though she constantly works at being the very best employee, the most solicitous friend, the most determined client, and so forth. Certainly, the irritation could be all yours, yet through reflection, with supervision, and after careful observation, you could discover that this client is blind to the edginess of what may be her perfectionist ways.

The bottom line here is that when you have done your personal work to be a clear receiver and thoroughly professional, your deep awareness of clients may be based on the ability to tune into a different frequency of their communications. So, before you toss out the data, spend a little more time exploring its potential messages about your client.

A Strategy for Dealing With Transference

Although it may never be entirely clear whether a client's strong emotional reactions to a coach represent transference or honest and appropriate responses to perceptions of the coach's behavior, coaches can use the following strategy to increase the likelihood of positive outcomes. Young (2001) proposes steps for dealing with transference, and these have been reconfigured to address potential issues in the coaching relationship:

Step 1: Express Acceptance of the Client and Her Communications Without Retaliation

When transference is operating, clients may eventually erupt with strong negative feelings toward the coach. Especially when these expressions are unwarranted, the coach needs to communicate empathy for the client and a genuine appreciation for the reality of feelings that the client is experiencing.

Client: "This is a total waste of my time and money. Where are we going with all this? I think your ideas are pointless and stupid."

Coach: "I really hear how upset you are with me, and at the same time I'm glad you're willing to let me know how you feel. Now that you've brought it up, I can't think of anything more important for us to do than to spend time trying to understand what's happening. Would this be okay with you?"

Step 2: Explore the Client's Thoughts and Feelings

In the face of the coach's accepting attitude and behavior, the likelihood that the client will retreat into feelings of shame, hurt, or fear of retaliation will decrease. The coach's role at this point will be to encourage further expression and clarification of the sources of the emotions.

Client: "I simply don't think this is working out. I keep coming here and get the feeling that my lack of progress is all my fault."

Coach: "Thanks for telling me this. Are you aware of any messages coming from me that sound blaming or that make it look like it's all your fault?"

Step 3: Work With the Client to Find New Patterns for Expressing Feelings and Getting Needs Met

By maintaining a reassuring, accepting attitude toward the client throughout the dialogue, the client is likely to feel an increased sense of safety in expressing emotions and working through complaints, without having to wait until the emotional buildup has reached uncontrollable proportions. Even when the client has legitimate issues with the coach's behavior, her manner of expression can be the focus of new learning. If the coach at any point turns to self-justification or efforts to prove his effectiveness, this learning opportunity will likely be lost.

Client: "No, I think it's me feeling like I'm not doing enough, and I guess I took it out on you."

Coach: "That sounds like an important awareness. No matter how it came out, I'm glad we've gotten to this point of understanding. So, there are two things we might discuss now: The first is why you feel you're not doing enough, and the second is about how to more comfortably express your feelings about our work in the future. Does this sound right to you?"

Gaining Wisdom

Becoming a coach and understanding the unique relational emphasis of coaching take more than time. Depending on your level of experience and your professional training, undertaking certain tasks can facilitate your learning. Kottler's (2000) book *Nuts*

and Bolts of Helping offers some practical guidance for promoting skill acquisition and wisdom. The following suggestions rely on Kottler's writings but are conceptualized for the role of lifestyle fitness coach:

- **Talk to practicing coaches.** Through either the Internet or your personal relationship network, identify a few people who are working as coaches. Ask them about their experiences. Learn from their practices and then translate what they are telling you into the world of sports and fitness.

- **Become a client in a coaching relationship.** After you have talked with a few coaches, you might find someone whose style seems to work for you. Arrange a time-limited coaching experience. We all have areas in which we can benefit from a solid helping relationship. Some examples of issues that you may wish to address include time management, dealing with conflict, promoting your business, and planning a career shift, among others. Because contracting is an important part of the coaching relationship, draw lines around the area where you can profit the most and try it out.

- **Practice coaching in a small learning group.** Find a couple of colleagues who are on a similar learning journey. Arrange to work in pairs, so that the third person is available as a more objective observer. Person A coaches B, B coaches C, and C coaches A. You can arrange to have your coaching sessions privately and then get together as a triad for debriefing.

- **Videotape or tape-record your sessions.** Camcorders are reasonably available and will provide surprising feedback when used in your practice coaching. If you don't have a camcorder, a tape recorder will be sufficient. No matter how much you know or how well you are able to recite principles for effective communication, your personal habits will continue to permeate your practice until you are able to identify them and work strategically to change them. This piece of advice, if followed, will be one of the most powerful learning tools at your disposal.

- **Read and discuss.** Form a support system, perhaps with your triad or with others as well. Agree to read particular books or articles on the topic of coaching and meet weekly or biweekly to discuss what you read. Learning about coaching and relationship issues comes alive through interaction. Although you may come across useful techniques or principles in books, it is mostly through the exploration of these materials and through practice that you begin to own them for yourself.

• **Engage in continuing education.** If this is to become your career path, you will find it helpful to organize your time and other resources around a 5- or 10-year plan for learning. Of course, learning does not stop at that point, but setting an initial objective at, say, 5 years gives you enough room to reach a new plateau, where you may further refine your direction. Indeed, dozens of professional conferences occur each year on the topic of coaching, but they may take place far from your home and therefore uncomfortably stretch a limited budget. The good news is that continuing education opportunities are as close as your computer or your local college or university. Coaching groups offer chat rooms that you can join. Colleges and universities offer classes on psychology, counseling, theories of personality, human motivation, helping relationships, interpersonal communication, and a myriad of other relevant subjects. You don't have to go into debt attending national conferences. If your goal is to learn how to help people envision their futures and reach their goals through your work in the health fitness world, unlimited opportunities for learning how to improve your skills are available in your local area.

Goals, Boundaries, and Ethics in Coaching

"If I keep from meddling with people, they take care of themselves, If I keep from commanding people, they behave themselves, If I keep from preaching at people, they improve themselves, If I keep from imposing on people, they become themselves."

Lao-tse, 2300 B.C.

A deceptive simplicity characterizes the agenda of coaching. Kottler (2000) captured it in three questions a coach might discuss with a client: Where are you going? How will you get there? How will you know when you arrive?

Yet all one needs to do is search the Internet or library for books on coaching or helping professions to discover how complex this agenda can become and how much a coach needs to be prepared for ways in which clients may answer these questions.

Of a client's many interests and needs, lifestyle fitness coaches can legitimately address only a subset. As Kottler (2000) notes, we have to know where clients desire to go, and in this regard, we need to know whether and how we are able to assist clients in their quest.

This chapter addresses three interrelated themes: goals, boundaries, and ethics. Games and sports are likely to have goals, and usually they include rules for participation and for the attainment of goals. Coaching clients typically arrive with a more or less articulated agenda, and they will have chosen you as a coach because they believe that you have the training and qualifications to assist them in realizing their vision. Through dialogue, coach and client will translate the client's agenda into some type of contract indicating the boundaries of the agreement relating to the working alliance. What unfolds after initial discussions may reveal new dimensions and previously unexpressed goals, and revisions to the contract may be in order. As coaching progresses, client needs and interests may diverge not only from original intentions but perhaps also from the realm of coaching competencies. At this point, the rules come into play. Broader perspectives of the boundaries of coaching relationships lead directly to consideration of ethics.

Goals

In the literature of sport and exercise, goals and goal setting are major themes (Buckworth & Dishman, 2002; Gill, 2000; LeUnes & Nation, 2002). Goals may be framed in terms of outcomes, performance, or processes (Weinberg & Gould, 2003), although it is readily acknowledged that all three play important roles in directing behavior change (Filby, Maynard, & Graydon, 1999). **Outcome goals** typically focus on the result or end of some engagement, such as a contest or a quest to lose weight. One client may aim to win a race, and another intends to lose 10 pounds (5 kilograms). Both are outcome goals. **Performance goals** are the achievement of standards of behavior or performance, irrespective of others' actions. An athlete may have a performance goal of achieving a personal best, whereas a coaching client may have a performance goal of training daily at a particular level of intensity for a minimum of 30 minutes. Finally, **process goals** emphasize the actions or even qualities that one wishes to characterize behavior. A runner may have a process goal of focusing on her breathing and extending her stride, and a coaching client may have a process goal of enjoying what she is doing while she is training.

Coaching and counseling literatures also emphasize the importance of goals and goal setting (Cormier & Nurius, 2003; Ivey & Ivey, 2003; Reynolds Welfel & Patterson, 2005; Shebib, 2003; Whitworth et al., 1998). Fulfillment, balance, and process, three types of coaching goals identified by Whitworth and colleagues, may be seen as parallels of the outcome, performance, and process goals referred to in the context of exercise and sport. Shebib (2003) identifies only two types of goals: outcome and process. Within the context of coaching, these would concern what a client wants as a result of the coaching relationship (outcome) and what means a client is willing to commit to in order to attain these results (process). Process goals refer not only to the actions agreed on by coach and client but also to the coaching process itself. How often will coach and client meet? What are the terms of the relationship? What responsibilities do clients and coaches bear for activities between sessions?

Clear goals are essential in coaching. A distinction that might be made between coaching and counseling (or psychotherapy) clients is that the former will likely have specific intentions for the coaching process that represent forward movement (movement toward), growth, and development, whereas the latter may have vague and diffuse objectives often representing a desire to move away from negative states of being or patterns of behavior (Bandura, 1969).

Goals provide direction (Shebib, 2003) and thereby serve to guide clients' actions. Goal statements also help clarify the boundaries of the coaching relationship—what can or cannot be accomplished. In this regard, Cormier and Nurius (2003) indicate that another function of goals is that they permit helpers to assess whether they have the skills, experiences, and credentials to address clients' agendas effectively. Having goals also directs coaches to use different strategies and interventions appropriate to assisting clients' goal attainment. Finally, goals provide frameworks for evaluation and assessment of progress (Bandura, 1969; Shebib, 2003), and interim goal statements can help clients experience success and reenergize action commitments.

Qualities of Effective Goals

How should goals be formulated to serve client needs best? Thirty years of research on goal formulation and goal setting has advanced our understanding of the essential elements of effective goals. Locke's research (1968; Locke et al., 1981; Locke & Latham, 1985; Locke & Latham, 1990), in particular, has consistently shown that goal setting has a powerful effect on behavior. Some of the more germane implications of Locke's research can be summarized as follows:

- Goals should be stated at levels of moderate difficulty, rather than being either too easily attained or too difficult to reach.
- The more specific the goal statement, the better it is.
- Feedback about progress is critical along the path to goal attainment.
- Goals that are imposed will not be as effective as those that involve or originate from clients.
- When goals are publicly acknowledged, they are more likely to be attained.
- Having both short- and long-term goals is beneficial.

Principles of Goal Setting

Lifestyle fitness coaches should emphasize goals and goal setting not only in the beginning of coaching but throughout the process. Goals are not static; they evolve with increasing levels of knowledge and experience. As clients learn more about themselves and as they engage the realities of their commitments, goals may be further refined and shaped. The following principles of goal setting drawn from the sport and fitness literature (Weinberg & Gould, 2003) may be seen as building on Locke's (1968) conclusions:

- Goals need to be specific.
- Goals should be set at moderate levels of difficulty.
- Short- and long-term goals should be established.
- Goal setting should include the three types of goals—outcome, performance, and process.
- Strategies for achieving goals should take into account a client's personality and motivation.
- Goal-setting structures should include feedback and evaluation processes.
- Goals need to be recorded and progress systematically assessed.

The SMART goals approach is a popular model for framing client goals (Smith, 1994). The letters stand for the words *specific, measurable, action-oriented, realistic,* and *timely* (see figure 4.1). Using this model for the different types of goals (outcome, performance, and process) that clients have will facilitate success.

Boundaries

All relationships function implicitly or explicitly within the framework of boundaries or contracts and agreements. How these dynamics play out in coaching relationships has major implications for personal well-being, satisfaction, and individual and collective outcomes.

Lifestyle Fitness Coaching and the Concept of Boundaries

What do we mean by the term *boundaries*? A tennis court has boundaries. So do football fields, basketball courts, and swimming pools. You clearly know

when the football goes between the goal posts, when a swimmer is in the right lane, or when a basketball player is out of bounds. As a lifestyle fitness coach you will rely on boundaries in the same way that you do on a playing field. They serve as guides for making calls regarding what is within limits and what is out of bounds, and in this respect the discussion of boundaries is often picked up in the context of professional ethics.

In sport as in life, the rules of the game are intended to be clear. For example, the race begins only when the gun is fired. Yet, an element of interpretation may come into play, as when referees make "judgment calls" about whether actions were intentional or accidental.

Subjective elements related to boundaries can be problematic. The more effort you invest in clarifying role and relational boundaries, the more readily you can identify out-of-bounds behaviors.

Professional boundaries stem from definitions of your role, job skills, and responsibilities (Gavin & Gavin, 1995). The longer a profession has been in existence, the more likely it is that professional associations will govern it and delimit actions considered fair or foul. Even so, most professions have some equivalent of an ethical review board to debate the inevitable gray areas that emerge in practice. Professions are not static entities but dynamic, evolving systems that must continually examine and monitor the frontiers of practice. Professional boundaries evolving in the coaching field will help guide your actions in a wide array of situations, but they can never cover all events that you are likely to encounter in your professional career (Williams & Davis, 2002). We will consider this matter further in the section on ethics.

Boundary Crossings and Violations

In discussions of boundaries, a useful distinction has been made between a **boundary crossing** and a **boundary violation** (Corey, Corey, & Callanan, 2003). Certain professional behaviors have the potential for creating the conditions for eventual misconduct, yet they are not inherently wrong. Examples of such behaviors include accepting a token gift from a client, giving a client a hug after a victorious experience, accepting an invitation to a large social gathering sponsored by your client, or regularly attending meetings of community organizations in which your client is also a member.

Some writers (Smith & Fitzpatrick, 1995) argue that such actions pave the way to boundary violations and to serious breaches in ethical conduct. Behaviors identified as boundary crossings

SMART goals capture essential elements of effective goal setting as demonstrated in research. Depending on the type of goal under consideration (outcome, performance, or process), what each of the five elements of SMART represents will vary. An illustration of a SMART outcome goal follows, along with identification of the five elements of SMART.

SMART	Example
S = specific	My goal is to lose 20 pounds (9 kilograms) in 20 weeks starting Monday, January 5 and ending Monday, May 24. In so doing, a related goal is to reduce my percentage of body fat from 27% to 22%.
M = measurable	I will measure my progress in the following ways: 1. I will weigh myself each Monday morning starting January 5 and ending Monday, May 24, and I will record my weight. 2. I had my body fat estimated by my coach using skinfold calipers on January 3. I will have another measurement of body fat using the same method during the week of March 15 and again during the week of May 24. 3. I will keep a detailed record of my caloric intake each day, recording the number of calories that I consume each day starting January 5 and ending May 24. 4. I will record each of my training sessions in terms of frequency, duration, and estimated caloric expenditure in a weekly training log beginning January 5 and ending May 24.
A = action oriented	My action plan is as follows: 1. I currently consume approximately 3,200 calories per day. By keeping track of my caloric intake, I will monitor my food consumption to maintain or slightly decrease this level of intake over the next 20 weeks. 2. I will increase my activity level for the next 20 weeks by engaging in cardiovascular exercises five times a week for 60 minutes each time with an estimated increase in caloric burn of 800 calories each time. 3. Specifically, I will use the treadmill or step machine twice a week for 60 minutes and on the other 3 days will take an hour-long spinning class or an equivalent class experience (e.g., circuit training).
R = realistic	My goal is realistic for the following reasons: 1. A pound of fat (0.45 kilograms) contains approximately 4,000 calories. Twenty pounds (9 kilograms) of fat contain approximately 80,000 calories. I currently eat approximately 3,200 calories per day. By maintaining my food intake and increasing my activity level, I will burn 4,000 extra calories per week. Over the 20-week period, this will translate into a weight loss of 20 pounds (9 kilograms). 2. My coach has estimated that with an increase in activity and with the estimated weight loss, the percentage of decrease in body fat is realistic. 3. I have scheduled my training periods for the next month without problem. If alterations occur in my work schedule that might affect my training, I will work with my coach to create alternative exercise strategies. 4. I have the support of my coach. 5. In the past I exercised regularly. Although the initial weeks may be challenging, I am committed to achieving this goal and know that I was able to train at similar levels in the past.
T = timely	I will begin my program on January 5 and continue until May 24. At that point I will reevaluate based on experiences and results. In the interim I will evaluate my progress biweekly with my coach. I will assess changes in my weight weekly and changes in my percentage of body fat after 10 and 20 weeks.

Figure 4.1 An illustration of SMART goals.

represent "a departure from commonly accepted practices that could potentially benefit clients" (Corey, Corey, & Callanan, 2003, p. 250). The more serious matter, boundary violations, has been defined as "a serious breach that results in harm to clients" (Corey, Corey, & Callanan, 2003, p. 250). Boundary crossings are considered problematic because they tend to blur professional boundaries. Moreover, when matters of diversity and cultural difference become part of the equation, what may seem to be a completely innocent expression on the part of the coach may assume meaning of far greater proportion by the client. Although these discussions are more often found in the literature of counseling and psychotherapy, the dynamics of coaching in the physically intimate realm of sport and exercise may be more similar than dissimilar to those of intentionally deeper encounters.

Guiding Boundary Formation: Role, Resources, and the Situation

If you think of boundaries as limitations to thought, action, or even the expression of feeling, what might guide the establishment of limits?

- **Your role.** As a lifestyle fitness coach you will have a particular domain in which it is legitimate for you to work. Your training, contracts with clients, and personal characteristics and limitations will help to define your scope of work. Moreover, although you may be competent to administer a certain service, legal limitations imposed on professional groups may restrict the activities of members of this profession. For instance, you may be an insightful, skilled communicator with an undergraduate degree in psychology and extensive knowledge of psychological issues, yet it would be illegitimate for you to switch into a psychotherapeutic role with a coaching client even though you might be able to do it well.

- **Your resources.** Even with all these demarcations of professional action, at times you will have to make a judgment call. When your personal resources are at low ebb, you may better serve yourself and your client by not taking on a particular activity. An example might be a client request for an additional session when you are tightly booked and need time to address your own needs.

- **The situation.** In another respect, situational dynamics may supersede normal boundary limitations and require intervention. Most rules have exceptions that apply in unusual circumstances. Imagine that a client breaks down and cries uncon-

trollably in the midst of a session because she has just had a miscarriage. This issue may not be part of your contractual relationship, but because of the severity of the matter, it would be appropriate to listen to your client with great empathy. But if you find yourself making so many exceptions that rule enforcement becomes the exception, you may want to examine your criteria for exceptional circumstances—or what kind of situation you are in (Gavin & Gavin, 1995).

To explore your sense of professional boundaries as a coach, take time to complete learning activity 4.1, which will help you integrate this discussion of boundaries on a personal level.

Coaching Agreements and Contracts

As D. Johnson (2003) remarks, whenever we interact with others we will find some interests in common and others in conflict. Managing the mix of shared and opposing interests to reach agreements takes both wisdom and skill. We can define an agreement as a mutually determined understanding of a commitment to action. Although the terms *agreement* and *contract* are often used interchangeably, some important distinctions will be noted later in this discussion.

Critical elements of agreements and contracts have been summarized here in the context of lifestyle fitness coaching, based on D. Johnson's (2003, pp. 271–272) perspectives:

1. The coaching agreement (or contract) must meet the legitimate needs of coach and client, and both parties must perceive it as fair. The agreement should detail rights and responsibilities of both coach and client in implementing the agreement. These should include but are not necessarily restricted to the following:

    a. Who will do what when, where, and how? This item includes the specification of the beginning and end of the agreement, as well as other timed events (e.g., length of sessions).

    b. Concrete and descriptive statements of behavioral expectations.

    c. Arrangements for reviews of how the agreement is working, and renegotiation of terms and conditions, if and when necessary.

    d. Explicit stipulation of exchanges of resources, materials, fees, and other matters.

Learning Activity 4.1   Identifying Your Perspectives About Professional Boundaries

Complete the following sentence stems and consider what you might learn about the boundaries that you expect to have in coaching relationships.

- "As a lifestyle fitness coach you should always . . ."

- "As a lifestyle fitness coach you should never . . ."

- "I think the limits of my professional role are determined by . . ."

- "In working with my clients, it is my business to . . ."

- "In working with my clients, it is none of my business to . . ."

- "Some good rules to follow in ensuring that I don't encourage or allow clients to step over my professional boundaries are . . ."

What do these notes tell you about your professional boundaries? What do you think is unique to you, and what pertains generally to the profession of coaching? Did you experience any uncertainties, conflicts, or inconsistencies in completing this exercise? What might you do to resolve these matters?

2. The coaching agreement (or contract) should be based on objectively justifiable principles. For example, fees, meeting schedules, terms of working together, and limits of the working relationship should be based on principles of professional expertise, normative patterns in the industry, mutual respect, or scientific merit.

3. The process of reaching agreement should be part of the pattern of strengthening the ability of the coach and client to work cooperatively and to come to an amicable resolution of any differences that might arise in the course of the relationship.

The fewer the assumptions embedded in an agreement or contract, the better off both parties will be. Even when the parties are operating in good faith, they may have different assumptions about the agreement. Let's look at a few situations in which assumed agreements may develop:

- Imagine a coaching relationship in which the coach serves coffee at the first three meetings. The client may assume that part of the working arrangement is that the coach always provides coffee.

- If a client repeatedly shows up 5 to 10 minutes late for appointments, but the coach always give him the contracted 45-minute session, the client may reasonably assume based on the coach's behavior that he is entitled to the full session whenever he shows up.

- What happens if a client answers cell phone calls during sessions without comment from the coach? Even if sessions end at the agreed-on time, the implied agreement is that telephone calls during the session take precedence over the coaching agenda.

- If the location of meetings between coach and client varies greatly during the first month of the relationship (e.g., coffee shops, offices, public fitness areas), what assumptions might emerge about both the nature of the meetings and the options for meeting venues?

All these situations have one thing in common: People observe behavior patterns and infer the rules or agreements. Regardless of what you state as the agreement, actions speak louder than words. Each time a variation to the agreement occurs without comment or discussion, it holds the possibility for altering the agreement. Over time, both coach and client may come to assume that their agreement

is something different from what was originally stated (Gavin & Gavin, 1995). This is not to say that agreements should remain fixed, rather that the parties need to acknowledge variations or changes explicitly and either define them as exceptions or incorporate them into a revised agreement.

Psychological Contracts

Assumed agreements make up part of what is known as the psychological contract (Levinson, 1976). Based on your personal history, you develop expectations of others' behaviors. On your birthday you assume that everyone will make a fuss. When you go to work at a new club, you expect that your old work habits will have the same results. You enter a new relationship and assume that because you are committed, the other person will be also. You make doctors' appointments and expect to be kept waiting. You hire an employee and expect the person to do as told.

Maybe these aren't your expectations, but whatever your experience, you have expectations! As a lifestyle fitness coach you will have expectations of the people with whom you work—and they will have expectations of you. You may know what you expect of yourself but have less complete information about what others expect from you. Or you may mistakenly assume that you know what is expected of you—and operate on those assumptions.

Being successful in coaching involves initiating conversations to make explicit the expectations that others have of you, as well as the expectations that you have of them. In this way, you will know exactly where to direct your energy and what areas you are accountable for.

Distinguishing Contracts and Agreement

If an agreement is a mutually determined understanding of a commitment to action, a contract may be thought of as a more binding agreement, typically with legal implications if the contract is broken. Contracts, therefore, are more likely to be formal and signed by both coach and client, whereas agreements tend to be ratified verbally and through handshake (Gavin & Gavin, 1995). As coaching relationships take shape, the parties should agree on the terms and conditions of the work as early as possible (Brammer & MacDonald, 1999). As Gladding (2000) suggests, written contracting helps clarify the coach–client relationship by giving it direction, through protecting the rights, roles, and obligations of both parties, and thereby ensuring the likely success of the relationship.

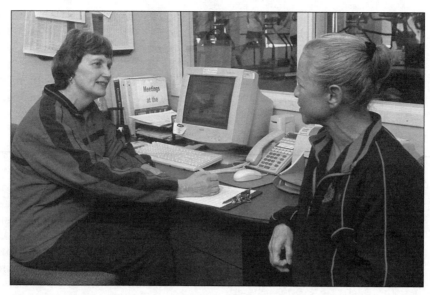

Written contracts help clarify the coach–client relationship.

Detailing elements of an agreement in writing gives it added weight and significance. Shebib (2003) thinks of a contract as a road map that provides general directions about how to get from one point to another and confirms that both coach and client have explicit intentions to move in the same direction. An important function of contracting noted by Shebib is the increased ownership that clients feel about agreed-on objectives when contracting has been thoroughly engaged. An often overlooked aspect of contracting is the specification of terms and conditions for ending the relationship. Coaching relationships, in particular, might best be framed as time limited rather than open ended. The goal-directed, action-focused orientations of coaching enable both client and coach to gauge progress and to identify probable points of termination or renegotiation.

Exploring the Who, What, When, Where, How, and Why of Agreements and Contacts

As noted earlier, an important framework for understanding the elements of coaching agreements and contracts can be found in the questions who, what, when, where, how, and why (Gavin & Gavin, 1995).

Who?   Who is involved? It may be just you and the client, although you could be involved in a team approach in which a medical doctor, nutritionist, personal trainer, or other allied health professional works in collaboration.

What?   What is involved, or what are you contracting for? What is your goal for the relationship? What is the client's goal? Exactly what services are you providing? What are you expected to do to achieve these goals? What is your client expected to do? Are some expectations so obvious that you assume them instead of making them explicit?

When?   When will this happen? You should know not only when certain things are expected to happen but also for how long or over what period. If a client hires you for 2 hours a week, you might want to stipulate not only the exact hours of meeting but also the minimal duration of your contract, for example, 6 weeks. Another critical aspect of this question concerns when terms of your relationship might not apply. Your clients may approach you during unscheduled periods to discuss their issues. Is this acceptable? How often and at what times are you willing to accept telephone calls?

Where?   Where does this happen, and where doesn't this happen? Do you meet your clients only in an office? Do you visit clients' homes? Do they come to your home?

How?   How do you do this? What does the working relationship look like? Traditionally, health fitness professionals enact their responsibilities in a hands-on manner rather than a style of sitting and talking. What methods will you use? What training and certification do you have to warrant your use of these approaches?

Why?   This last question is really the first that you need to answer, but it appears last because the why of a relationship is often hard to answer immediately. Through the rapport-building process of detailing a client's interest in achieving certain personal growth goals or physical improvement objectives, coaches can begin to understand the reasons behind intended actions. Why is this goal so important that the client is willing to devote time, money, and effort toward its accomplishment? Too often, we assume the why. An overweight client asking for guidance and support in maintaining an exercise program to shed excess weight may hardly have to be asked why, yet the value in doing so can be substantial. Is the motivation coming from the client or from others? Does a larger issue need to be addressed while the client is undertaking a specific lifestyle change?

Figure 4.2 provides an illustration of a detailed coaching contract. You may wish to reflect on elements that you deem important to include in a coaching contract.

Problematic Nature of Informal Agreements

Entering informal agreements may be tantamount to agreeing to follow conditions only so long as it suits one or the other party because, in these types of agreements, consequences for failing to meet conditions are vague and nonspecific (Gavin & Gavin, 1995). Informal agreements give both sides excuses to back out. A coach and client informally agree to work together whenever they can, until one of them fails to show. A client informally agrees to try out a recommended exercise program for a while to see what happens. How long is a while? What needs to happen for the client to move beyond the trial stage?

Referring to something as an informal agreement may have to do with fear and doubt—fear that something more formal would be too binding and doubt that you or your client will live up to the terms of a real agreement. Informal agreements may be a way of sitting on the fence. Although this may accurately reflect where you are, if it doesn't you will need to work toward a formal agreement or contract.

A formal agreement is one in which you take the time necessary to be explicit about all the expectations and all the answers to who, what, when, where, how, and why. Even when you are uncertain about things, you can still have a formal agreement about what you and the other party need (who, what, when, where, and how) to come to terms that are more definite.

A mistaken notion is that agreements are informal until they are written. You can have a formal agreement that is oral. Of course, oral agreements are more likely to be problematic because of memory lapses, semantics, or trustworthiness. You may

forget. Or your idea of what it means to pay at the beginning of the month may mean before the 15th. Or you may have no intention of living up to the agreement because as Bart Simpson says, "I didn't do it! Nobody saw me! You can't prove a thing!"

Ethics

The prevailing sense of professional ethics is one of benevolent wisdom reflecting fundamental values and morals with which few would disagree. Ethical guidebooks may resemble recitations of the Ten Commandments or other religious precepts. Of course, one should not kill. Obviously, one should not steal. Then comes the question, "Why should I read this stuff? It is all too evident." If that is your reaction, then at least the first step of appreciating ethical principles and boundary considerations will be easy—your question reflects a fundamental agreement with core values of the profession.

The second step, however, may not be as easy. Such matters as restricting friendships with clients usually arise in discussions with novice coaches and helpers. Why can't we be friends? Or, when the coaching relationship ends, why prohibit friendship then? Exceptions to the rules always come to mind, and the debate begins.

Some professions like psychology have become increasingly restrictive over the decades concerning the limitations on relationships between professionals and their clients. Certainly, some of this tightening of rules derives from experience and clear intentions to protect clients' welfare. A sexual relationship between a professional and client always provokes dramatic discussion and virtually unanimous agreement concerning its prohibition. Seemingly innocuous ethical matters, however, are more likely to trip us up. We might make an innocent assumption that a new client should automatically understand the rules by which we work. We might slip a little too far into self-disclosure in an attempt to help a client grow through the lessons of our own lives. We might feel quite competent to do something although we have not completed formal training in that area.

These instances highlight the need for deeper reflection about ethical codes. What does it mean when a code says that the professional must be competent? Of course, this is the case, yet how does one document competence? What experiences must one have had to be considered qualified? Or what does it mean that a coach is responsible for a client? How responsible and for what exactly?

Lifestyle Fitness Coaching Contract

Claudette Demers

BS (kinesiology), ACE personal trainer, YMCA LFC certification (master coach)

Date: September 15, 2005

Parties to the Agreement

Coach: Claudette Demers

Client: Charles Grovner

1. In general terms, what am I agreeing to do?

Coach	Client
1. Meet with you for 1 hour a week face-to-face for 10 consecutive weeks at a mutually agreed-on time at the rate of $___ per hour.	1. Show up for scheduled meetings on time for 10 weekly sessions, starting today.
2. Be available by phone or e-mail for agreed-on check-ins up to three times a week.	2. Commit myself to the coaching process and to the goals that we agree on.
3. Work with you through dialogue to help you determine the best program for your objectives and to provide ongoing support for your goal-directed activities.	3. Phone or e-mail you about my progress or issues that come up, within the limits that we have set.
4. Inform you about issues that arise that affect our working relationship and your progress.	4. Be willing to talk to you about any issues that pertain to my progress or how we are working together.
	5. Pay you each session at the agreed-on rate of $___ per hour.
	6. Pay for any sessions cancelled without 48 hours of notice.
	7. Pay for any extra telephone calls at the rate of $___ for 10 minutes.

2. In general terms, what am I expecting you to do?

Coach	Client
1. Attend all scheduled sessions.	1. Help me with the design of my program and with clarification of my goals.
2. Follow the program that we develop.	2. Provide me with support for my program and my goals.
3. Provide me with all necessary information relevant to the coaching process.	3. Give me feedback about things that I need to know and do.
4. Keep me informed about any new issues or factors that may impede your progress or require program adjustments.	4. Be available to me by phone or e-mail as arranged in our sessions.
5. Pay for all sessions and extra phone calls on time.	5. Keep all our discussions private.

3. When and where will these things take place?

   We will meet at my office at the Sport Center on Wednesdays from 5 to 6 P.M. for the next 10 weeks. Telephone calls will take place as agreed on in our sessions.

(continued)

Figure 4.2 A sample contract between a lifestyle fitness coach and client.

4. What is the duration of this agreement?

   From September 15, 2005, to November 24, 2005

5. What are the client's goals and objectives?

Client
Stated in SMART terms
To be completed in our September 22, 2005, meeting:
First goal
S
M
A
R
T
Second goal
S
M
A
R
T
Add for other goals

6. What costs are involved?

   $___ per hour for weekly sessions

   $___ for each 10-minute period (or part) of each telephone call beyond agreed-on weekly check-ins

7. When and how will the client pay these costs?

   The client will pay in cash or by check at the beginning of each weekly meeting.

8. What conditions or actions would make this agreement invalid?

Coach	Client
1. Failure to attend two consecutive meetings without notice.	1. Failure to keep to scheduled meetings.
2. Not living up to program agreements for a period of 2 weeks, unless extenuating circumstances exist.	2. Failure to respond to e-mails or be available for agreed-on calls.
3. Nonpayment.	3. Not being helpful in ways that we have agreed to in our meetings.
4. Behavior inappropriate to our professional relationship.	4. Giving me advice or information that is wrong or jeopardizes me in some way.

Signatures

_____   _____

Coach   Client

Figure 4.2 *(continued)*

This discussion appears here, before the presentation of the skills or tools of lifestyle fitness coaching, to set the stage for the work that you will do. If you choose to move quickly through this material, either make an appointment with yourself at a later date to sit in quiet reflection with some of the examples offered or create time to discuss with colleagues their opinions and interpretations of these ideas. You can more easily appreciate the palpable nature of boundary issues and ethical matters through dialogue and reflection on your practice. Reading alone will inform but not necessarily educate.

Distinguishing Ethics, Values, and Morals

Most of us carry with us a definition of the term *ethics*. Occasionally, our definitions may blend with other terms, and we may not fully understand the implications of ethical violations.

Corey, Corey, and Callanan (2003) provide a thorough review and consideration of ethical concerns within the helping professions. As a lifestyle fitness coach, you might find it helpful to understand some distinctions these authors make between ethics and related concepts.

Corey et al. (2003) distinguish among the terms *values*, *ethics*, and *morality* in the following manner:

Values pertain to beliefs and attitudes that provide direction to everyday living, whereas ethics pertain to the beliefs we hold about what

constitutes right conduct. Ethics are moral principles adopted by an individual or group to provide rules for right conduct. Morality is concerned with perspectives of right and proper conduct and involves an evaluation of actions on the basis of some broader cultural context or religious standard. (p. 11)

Values

Values are personal and not necessarily about right or wrong. They are individually held beliefs and attitudes that guide action. According to Ivey and Ivey (2003), parents, religious upbringing, or traumas (such as accidents, wars, personal violations) that people have experienced usually shape deeply held values. You might want to reflect about experiences in your life that shaped your attitudes and beliefs by completing learning activity 4.2. What life events were most significant in forming your values? Can you relate experiences that you have had to the values that guide your daily actions?

Victor Frankl (1969), a prominent psychiatrist who wrote about his experiences as an inmate in a Nazi concentration camp, argued that human behavior constantly raises issues of values. People make choices in life. As they exercise these choices, their values become evident. Values are learned to such an extent that some believe that one can make a child value virtually anything if that child is raised

Learning Activity 4.2   Identifying Experiences That Shaped Your Values

Below, describe one or two pivotal events in your life that you believe shaped your character in some way. After you have done this, attempt to identify the specific values, attitudes, or beliefs that these experiences may have influenced.

Events and experiences

_____

_____

Values (attitudes and beliefs)

_____

_____

_____

_____

_____

and reinforced in particular ways (Gladding, 2000; Hackney, 2000).

Our decisions are related to our values, and when our choices do not result in the reinforcement of our values, we will normally feel unhappy (Brown & Srebalus, 2003). Values influence our outlook on life. If you place a high value on money, you may direct most of your efforts to obtaining money. The goal of getting money may justify any means for obtaining it. In this respect, a value does not imply good or bad, right or wrong. Of course, when we ask people what they value, they may recite words like wisdom, friendship, freedom, happiness, equality, or world peace (Parrott, 2003). Yet, as guides to action, a good diagnostic indicator of a person's values appears in the things that she chooses, in the ways that she acts, or in her behavior toward others.

As a lifestyle fitness coach, can you act in ways with clients that are value-free? The simple answer is no. The fact that you exercise regularly is an expression of values, as are most other choices that you make in life. How is it possible to be authentic and open with clients without revealing your values? A coach's values are part of his work with clients (Coonerty, 1991). As Okun (1982, p. 229) suggests, "In an interpersonal relationship, whether or not it is a helping relationship, values are transmitted either covertly or overtly between the participants."

Another perspective on values is that they form an integral part of personality (Parrott, 2003) and therefore are inseparable from who the coach is and how he approaches the tasks of coaching. What this implies, of course, is that clients tend to seek out coaches with similar values or with values congruent with goals that clients are seeking.

If values are part of who the coach is, attempts to come across as value-free in the coaching process are doomed from the outset. But having values does not mean that one needs to impose these values on clients. Ideally, the values that a coach has about people and life in general are ones that reflect positively on his character and approach to helping. Because values derive from experience, a reflective coach (Schon, 1983) would devote time and effort to understanding and changing those values that seem contrary to effective human relationships and the promotion of well-being. A coach who drinks excessively or who has a habit of smoking would not be the best role model for clients working on health behaviors.

A few summary points concerning values deserve emphasis. First, values are not, by definition, positive. We can value things that are, in society's perspective, bad. Second, we cannot hide our values. They are evident in all we do. Any attempt to mask our value orientations from clients would be futile. Third, having values does not mean imposing values. Finally, values change through experience and awareness. The first step in this process may be to know fully what your values are and to evaluate how well they reflect the way you want to be in the world as a person and as a coach.

Ethical Codes

The core of ethical responsibility is that the professional "do nothing that will harm the client or society" (Ivey, Ivey, & Simek-Morgan, 1997). The burden of responsibility for ethical practice rests on the coach's shoulders. Clients who come for help may be vulnerable and susceptible to undue influence by helpers. Another perspective of ethical practice is that it is grounded more on who coaches are rather than on what they do (Parrott, 2003). The cornerstone of ethical practice in this regard is virtue (Gelso & Fretz, 1992). Virtue is defined as "a habit, disposition, or trait that a person may possess or aspire to possess. A moral virtue is an acquired habit or disposition to do what is morally right or praiseworthy" (Beauchamp & Childress, 1983, p. 261). According to Parrott (2003), "Virtue is nourished by deep roots anchored in the bedrock of the self, yet the virtuous helper does not acquire ethical behavior merely through good intentions. A helper with solid character begins by becoming legally and ethically competent, and this incorporates a solid understanding of the law and of client rights."

A code of ethics can be defined as "the values of a profession translated into standards of conduct for the membership" (Gibson & Mitchell, 2003, p. 431). Legality is certainly relevant to ethical behavior, yet as Corey et al. (2003) point out, laws define the minimum standards that society will tolerate. Ethical codes speak more to ideal standards, to the maximum aspirations of a professional group for relationships with clients and the conduct of its members.

Although it is implied, all codes of ethics require practitioners to act in accordance with relevant governmental statutes and regulations. Occasionally, ethics and the law may be in conflict. For instance, what occurs in helping relationships is most often bound by a client's right to confidentiality, yet some circumstances—such as when working with minors—may require a professional to breach this ethical principle. Whenever such conflicts are identifiable, ethical guidelines require professionals to inform clients of conditions under which rights of confidentiality do not apply.

Ethical codes guide practitioners and help them make ethical decisions in their work. Moreover, such codes also serve to regulate the behavior of professionals and therefore have practical implications with punitive consequences for noncompliance. A professional may face charges of having violated the ethical code of a profession without having necessarily violated the law.

Morality

As you consider these initial thoughts about ethics, you might realize that such discussions cannot take place without some mention of morality. As Corey et al. (2003) note, morality has to do with perspectives of "right and proper conduct" based on some evaluation of actions emanating from a cultural or religious standard. Morality, then, is necessarily embedded in community and cultural values. Yet, as Brown and Srebalus (2003) observe, the ethical codes one finds in most North American professional societies (psychology, law, medicine) are remarkably similar in their reflection of moral standards for right and proper conduct.

Before we review common elements found in numerous codes of ethics, let us first consider the core matter of moral principles that are generally reflected in these codes. Meara, Schmidt, and Day (1996) identify six moral principles that form the foundation for professional behavior: autonomy, nonmaleficence, beneficence, justice, fidelity, and veracity. Applying these principles to the actions of lifestyle fitness coaches is an ongoing process of learning and striving for excellence in practice. Here is what each of these principles might imply for your work with clients:

• Autonomy means that as a coach you would work to promote the independence and self-determination of clients relating to what you do together. You would encourage them to be self-directing rather than dependent. Paradoxically, dependency may be an important component of the coaching relationship in the beginning phases, yet as the relationship develops, coaches would promote greater self-sufficiency.

• Nonmaleficence essentially means that coaches will do no harm to their clients and will avoid the identifiable risks of harmful actions. Responsibility for awareness rests with the coach. Clients may not be cognizant of the potential effects of certain training processes, and they may not

know about the kinds of issues that could emerge in discussions of goals and objectives. Although a coach cannot foresee all possibilities, many issues surrounding the dynamics of helping relationships have been identified and therefore constitute part of the coach's responsibility in avoiding potential harm to clients.

• Beneficence is the principle of promoting good for clients. Coaches intend to help their clients through the working alliance, yet at times it becomes evident either that a coach cannot help a particular client or that the work a client intends will not be helpful. This principle places responsibility on coaches to ensure, to the best of their abilities, that their actions with clients will be beneficial.

• Justice refers to the fact that coaches strive to provide equal treatment to all clients. This concept does not mean that coaches have to be equally skilled in working with all types of clients or in all issues that clients might bring them, but rather that within the range of their expertise, coaches treat all clients fairly, without discrimination, and with sensitivity to their unique backgrounds and issues. Where feasible, this principle also carries with it an expectation that coaches will adapt approaches and processes to the needs of clients whom they deem themselves capable of helping.

• Fidelity is about making honest promises and honoring commitments to clients. This principle asserts that coaches will be trustworthy in all their actions with clients. To do so, coaches need to be proactive by informing clients of dimensions of the working alliance of which clients may not be fully cognizant. Making an honest promise is about truth in advertising, or marketing themselves accurately in what they are trained to do, areas of competence, expectations of clients in order to profit from the relationship, and responsibilities of the coach in the relationship.

• Veracity is closely related to fidelity. It means that the coach will always be truthful. A concept in helping relationships known as informed consent requires coaches to tell clients in advance about such items as fees, cancellation policies, and limitations to the relationship. A coach is neither wise nor moral if his announcement of policies after the fact surprises clients.

The majority of helping professionals have integrated these moral principles into their styles of working and living. None of these principles is likely to come either as a surprise or as a stimulus for significant change in behavior. In spite of good intentions, however, on occasion we simply do not see ourselves accurately or we make assumptions about another person's knowledge or understanding. The coach who assumes that a new client should know that the session ends, no matter what, after 60 minutes, likely does not have an immoral intention, yet the behavior can be immoral.

Communality of Ethical Codes

A list of different associations or professional groups whose work is conceptually and structurally aligned with that of lifestyle fitness coaching appears in "Associations With Ethical Codes Relevant to Coaching" below. The ethical codes of these associations have significant overlap and communality (Koocher & Kieth-Spiegel, 1998) as expressed in the following nine principles (Brown & Srebalus, 2003):

1. Professional action shall bring no harm to clients.
2. Clients have the right to choose their own directions.
3. Be faithful to your clients, your profession, your organizations, and ultimately to yourself.
4. Be just and fair to all your clients, thereby ensuring nondiscriminatory professional actions.
5. Be of benefit to your clients by promoting their welfare.
6. Treat all clients with dignity and respect.
7. Be fully accountable to your clients.
8. Care deeply for those you accept as your clients.
9. Maintain clear and unwavering professional boundaries.

Again, this list of nine principles, which builds on the six moral principles, is unlikely to contain surprises. If you read professional codes of ethics, you will quickly discover all the fine print, along with details about the implications of these statements. Coaching organizations, such as the International Coach Federation (cf. Williams & Davis, 2002), largely mirror more established entities such as the American Psychological Association (2002) in their ethical codes.

Several practical implications might be important to explore in relation to the role of lifestyle fitness coach:

• **Proper training and ongoing education.** To be of benefit to clients and to ensure the absence of harmful interventions, coaches must not only be properly trained but also continue to pursue learning and educational opportunities.

• **Client rights.** If clients are to be self-determining, they must fully understand the parameters of the coach–client relationship. One would not want a client to self-determine an exercise program without expert guidance. Yet coaches need to be vigilant for indications that clients are complying unwillingly with programs because they believe

Associations With Ethical Codes Relevant to Coaching

Although professional qualifications in the life coaching field (Martin, 2001) are difficult to specify, organizations like the International Coach Federation have made significant efforts to formalize certification processes required for membership. Moreover, a number of organizations that certify life coaches, as well as more established associations in the helping professions, have detailed ethical principles. The following organizations or associations may provide useful guidance.

• International Coach Federation: www.coachfederation.org
• American Counseling Association: www.counseling.org
• American Psychological Association: www.apa.org
• American Association for Marriage and Family Therapy: www.aamft.org
• Association for Counselor Education and Supervision: www.acesonline.net
• National Board for Certified Counselors: www.nbcc.org
• Life Coaching—United Kingdom: www.uklifecoaching.org
• Executive Coaching Network: www.execcoach.net

they have no choice or because they think that the consequences for noncompliance would be significant and negative. Certainly, coaches need to assure clients of their rights to privacy and the confidential nature of the coaching relationship. In this lies a responsibility for coaches to inform clients fully of all matters pertaining to their agreements, actions, and aspirations.

• **Exceptions to rules of confidentiality.** Common sense tells us that in a life-and-death emergency or in the event that a coach has information that might save a client's life, the coach would have a reason to breach confidentiality agreements. This principle extends to such unlikely situations as a client's revealing to his coach that he is intending to end his life or that he plans to harm someone else. Similarly, if the coach has clear evidence that the client is abusing or neglecting minors or elderly or disabled individuals, the coach might breach confidentiality agreements. Legal statutes will also stipulate other conditions under which a coach must make records and conversations with clients available to the courts.

• **Boundaries of caring.** Caring more for another than for oneself may be a choice, but doing so is rarely an ethical obligation. Moreover, at times caring may slip into more intimate feelings and concerns, from the perspective of either client or coach. Caring is always viewed in relation to the contract and nature of work occurring between coach and client. A coach may become concerned about a client's health or well-being, especially if he sees the client intentionally putting herself at risk. Yet to intervene in such cases, a coach will always need to frame his actions within the legitimate bounds of his profession and the contractual nature of the relationship.

• **Referrals.** Coaches may refer clients to other professionals or for other services. Two forms of referral can be seen in instances where the coach effectively turns over all connections with the client to other professionals versus instances in which the coach retains an overseeing or facilitative role in referrals while maintaining a primary connection with the client. For example, a coach may deem it inappropriate or ineffective to continue working with a client and therefore may suggest to the client that she consider working with another professional or in another fashion on her own or with a group. The coaching relationship then officially ends, even though the client may not have reached the intended objectives. In the second type of referral, the coach may discuss with the client certain ancillary activities, perhaps through work with other people. These may be allied health professionals, or they could

be other service providers, for example, lawyers, realtors, or financial planners. Of course, the way in which a coach makes any referral would incorporate principles of free and informed choice. In practice, this might mean giving the client a list of service providers, describing what one knows about each, and offering suggestions for how the client might obtain independent assessment of these professionals' competencies. Implicit in the concept of referral is the notion that even when a coaching relationship is not viable or when the coach is unable to provide the needed service, the coach remains responsible for helping the client identify concrete options for achieving her objectives or pursuing critical agendas.

What Is Malpractice?

Malpractice is a legal term that involves negligence resulting in injury or loss to the client. Such negligence is thought to "result from unjustified departure from usual practice or from failing to exercise due care in fulfilling one's responsibilities" (Corey et al., 2003, p. 181). In cases of malpractice, the coach would have failed to render appropriate professional services or failed to have exercised the degree of skill or expertise that would ordinarily be expected of similar professionals in the same situation. As summarized by Corey et al. (2003), malpractice generally falls into six categories, which have been modified here for the role of lifestyle fitness coach:

1. The coach employed a procedure not considered within the realm of accepted coaching practice.
2. The coach used a technique or method for which she was not properly or adequately trained.
3. The coach failed to use a technique or procedure that would have been more beneficial to the client.
4. The coach failed to warn others about a violent client and thereby did not act to protect these people.
5. The coach failed to obtain or properly document the client's informed consent about coaching activities.
6. The coach failed to explain to the client the possible consequences of coaching interventions.

For a client to succeed in a malpractice case, the burden of proof rests with the client. Four elements must be demonstrated for malpractice to be proved.

First, the client must show that a bona fide professional relationship existed between the coach and the client. Second, the client must prove that the coach acted in a negligent or improper manner, or deviated significantly from the usual standards of care in the coaching profession. Third, the client must document that he suffered harm or injury. Finally, the client must legally demonstrate a causal linkage between the coach's negligence or breach of conduct and the actual injury or damage claimed by the client (Corey et al., 2003).

Discussions of malpractice may seem more pertinent to the realm of medicine or psychiatry, yet all professionals must become increasingly vigilant about these matters. In isolated cases, practitioners deliberately set out to harm their clients. Most other instances in which harm or injury occurs are indeed the result of some oversight, a moment of inattention, or unconscious neglect.

An Essential Framework for Coaching

Three interwoven themes reflect the focus of this chapter: goals, boundaries, and ethics. Within societal constraints, individuals may be free to choose their goals and to pursue them by legitimate means. When individuals elect to work with lifestyle fitness coaches, professional considerations and ethical codes define the range of goals, the types of processes, and the nature of the coaching relationship.

For some people, goal statements resemble whimsical wish lists, yet in working with coaches amorphous intentions need to be shaped into specific objectives and ultimately described in contractual ways. Only in moving from abstract to concrete or from general statements to specific objectives can coaches fully understand what is expected of them and whether such expectations are reasonable and within their scope of practice.

In upcoming chapters, we will move from broad perspectives of coaching to an emphasis on specific coaching skills and tools. In this regard, the theme of mastery will frequently appear. A core requirement of practice is knowing what to do and how to do it well. Coaches best achieve this through ongoing learning, practice, reflection, and supervision. Ethical discussions contained in this chapter are critical allies to your success. They address issues of high-quality coaching more than they do adherence to arcane rules and regulations. Coaches should engage in continuing education and training in their desire to pursue excellence in practice, not from a defensive stance of guarding against malpractice. With this vision firmly in mind, let's now move forward to understanding your skill base and how best to develop competencies.

Coaching Stages and Processes

A coaching relationship generally proceeds from initial contact through the various phases of working together toward the achievement of the client's goals and then ends. Endings may be final or simply a demarcation between the completion of one process of working and the beginning of another. The processes of coaching relationships and those of change itself bear similarity. Some theorists have attempted to depict coaching processes according to logical sequences of steps moving from start to end, and others have explored stages of an individual's progression through the experience of change.

This chapter will review process issues related to three themes and then focus on the important matter of endings. We can generally describe the three process themes as follows:

1. *Stages of the coaching relationship:* In this section we will review some typical perspectives about the progression of stages a coach and client are likely to encounter in their contracted relationship when the relationship continues until the client achieves some goal or criterion.

2. *Stages of change, or the transtheoretical model:* This section focuses on a well-researched model that is both diagnostic of clients in their engagements with change agendas and prescriptive of the likely progression through the challenges of change and long-term commitment to change.

"It's not that some people have willpower and some don't. It's that some people are ready to change and others are not."

James Gordon, MD

3. *Learning processes in change:* This section examines an intriguing model that considers change as a learning process. It offers an inside view of a client's reality and accompanying needs as she deliberately or incidentally embarks on a significant process of personal change.

Endings in coaching relationships may be straightforward or complicated, depending on the agendas engaged, the dynamics of the coaching relationship, and the outcomes achieved. Clients and coaches may end their relationships feeling empowered and encouraged to work in this way again or demoralized and discouraged because of their experiences. Becoming a lifestyle fitness coach calls for a deep appreciation of the wide range of possible endings to coaching relationships and the implications for both parties involved.

Before delving into this material, you may want to know why it is so important. Coaching relationships are not linear in their development or processes. Things you should do at the outset may be inappropriate later on and vice versa. Moreover, clients in a process of change have different needs during the evolving phases of their work. If you are not keenly aware of these dynamics, you may respond inappropriately or be surprised by the kinds of behavior you experience with your clients. You will have an opportunity later to connect this material with your own processes of change and with those that you have witnessed among clients, friends, and family members.

Stages of the Coaching Process

We will begin our discussion with an overview of models that provide generic descriptions of the stages of change typically encountered by clients in helping relationships. From there we will consider a more recent framework, based in narrative theories (Ivey & Ivey, 2003; Monk, Wislade, Crocket, & Epston, 1997), for understanding the stages of change.

General Models

Although counseling processes may differ along such dimensions as the depth of the intervention or the scope of treatment, counseling nonetheless strongly resembles coaching in the stages one encounters in work with clients. Egan (1998) suggested one of the simplest descriptions of stages by dividing helping relationships into three stages: "relationship building, challenging the client to find ways to change, and facilitating positive client action."

Hackney and Cormier (2001) suggest five stages of professional counseling that have been reorganized here to reflect the language of coaching. A sixth stage, borrowed from Shebib's (2003) model, was added to reflect work that must occur before the coach makes contact with the client.

- **Stage 1—Preliminary:** Before they meet with clients, coaches need to prepare materials and space. They must arrange where they will meet the client and prepare questionnaires, assessment materials, or interview processes if they plan to use such tools in the first meeting (Shebib, 2003).

- **Stage 2—Rapport and relationship building:** The term *relationship* has specific meanings in the coaching context. Hackney and Cormier (2001) think of this as a time when the helper builds trust and psychological comfort with the client. Relationships are alive. Over time they change and evolve. Coaches are not likely to focus on building rapport only in one stage and ignore it in others. Early behaviors are powerful determinants of whether and how the relationship proceeds. Whatever conditions the coach creates in this stage must be maintained and even developed throughout the remaining stages of the relationship.

Shebib (2003) cautions that early stages of relationship are ones of great vulnerability. If a client talks too deeply about issues or if the coach probes beyond the client's comfort level, the client may never return for a second session. In this regard, coaches need to be sensitive to client cues signaling discomfort in this phase. A question that the coach might pose toward the end of an initial meeting would focus on the client's reactions to the process thus far. For example, the coach might say something like the following:

Coach: "We've talked about a lot of things in this meeting. I appreciate your openness and willingness to discuss these matters with me, and I fully believe we can work successfully together toward the goals you have outlined. But before we end, I want to check with you about any feelings or reactions you might have about our meeting today. Can you tell me how this meeting has been for you and any questions or concerns you might have at this point?"

- **Stage 3—Assessment:** Coincidental with the building of a relationship is a process of understanding or assessment. Assessment according to Hackney and Cormier (2001) depends on three interrelated considerations. First, assessment depends on the coach's unique background and frameworks for conceptualizing human behavior. Coaches have philosophies, deep-seated beliefs and values, and histories of working with clients. Objectivity takes on a different meaning in a coaching relationship than it does when a health fitness professional is conducting standardized biomechanical testing or measuring body composition. Second, assessment depends on what the client brings to the relationship in terms of agendas, background, values, and needs, and how well the coach is able to understand those matters. Clients may reveal critical data to the coach, but the coach may not have the experience or understanding to appreciate and use that information in planning. Third, the cultural **worldview** that the client represents conditions the assessment. Each client has a unique frame of reference based on cultural factors, and these will influence what is said, how it is said, what is requested, and how work is done in the relationship.

- **Stage 4—Goal setting:** As Hackney and Cormier (2001, p. 29) state, "The act of setting a goal involves making a commitment to a set of conditions, a course of action, or an outcome." Coach and client mutually determine the process of goal setting, recognizing that initial statements of goals may change as new information and insights become available. Like issues of rapport and relationship building, goal setting is an ongoing focus of coaching. This does not mean, however, that coach and client do not set clear goals or that they should modify those goals whenever the client has difficulty directing effort toward them. As we will see in the skill development chapters (chapters 6 through 8), what clients initially state as objectives may take on deeper meaning as the relationship develops. Clients may be reluctant to provide all their reasoning behind needs they express until psychological comfort, trust, and safety have developed adequately. In this light, initial statements of goals are good starting points that coaches and clients should continually revisit in the first few meetings until coaches feel that they have a solid appreciation of what clients want, why clients have chosen those goals over others, and how changes that clients want to pursue will create fulfillment and balance in their lives.

Stages 2 through 4 of this model are what Shebib (2003) identifies simply as the beginning of the helping relationship. In the beginning, the objective is primarily "to negotiate a working relationship that is goal directed and based on trust and mutual understanding of expectations. This relationship is time limited and based on a contract that outlines the objectives and terms of the relationship" (p. 26). Another task of this stage is "to acquire and deepen understanding of the client's situation" (p. 26).

Chapter 6 will review the specific communication skills appropriate to the beginning stages of coaching. You have already seen, however, how much detail may be required to draw up a reasonable contract between client and coach (chapter 4). How you achieve contracting and how well you establish the core conditions for coaching will largely determine whether coaching progresses or ends at this point. Although much of the work in the beginning stages may seem to be in service of agendas that the client wishes to address, bear in mind that this period of the working alliance essentially is a time when clients tell their stories to an empathic coach under safe and supportive conditions. The worth of these actions alone can hold significant value for the client.

Although a coaching relationship is more likely than a counseling relationship to move quickly into goal setting, some coaching clients will require a more prolonged period of trust building and relationship development before they are ready to consider action.

- **Stage 5—Initiating interventions:** Having established goals and objectives for the relationship in a coaching process in stage 4, coach and client in this stage implement the strategies agreed on. The coach provides support for the client and keeps the client focused on the agenda. Aspects of education and information exchange may occur during this period, because the relationship should have been established sufficiently for the coach to apply influencing strategies (see chapter 8). Some justification may be present during this stage for continued fine-tuning or even renegotiating the contract based on new information and a deepening relationship. In this respect, a back-and-forth relation may occur between the early stages and the stage of intervention (Hackney & Cormier, 2001; Shebib, 2003). Another framework that might make more sense in coaching would envision a cyclical relation between goal setting and intervention, whereby the client works on different agendas in a sequential fashion until she has accomplished all that she intended.

Although clients may rely on coaches for intelligent guidance and support as they engage the challenge of change, the coach bears no responsibility for making change happen. When clients show continued resistance to change, when they set up conditions for failure, or when they choose to direct insufficient time and energy to their commitments, the relationship will begin to resemble a process of counseling more it does than a process of coaching. Coaches must reassess in these cases their own competencies and skills, their contractual agreements with clients, and the boundaries of their professional training to determine whether to continue, whether to refer, or whether to work in conjunction with another professional qualified to address clients' core behavioral patterns.

- **Stage 6—Termination and follow-up:** Again, the significance of endings may differ between counseling and coaching clients. Coaching agendas tend to reflect the achievement of personal growth goals or self-improvement agendas rather than the resolution of difficult emotional concerns or troubling behaviors. Counseling clients may end their relationships at a point of normalcy where life is nonchaotic and manageable, whereas coaching clients will more likely have moved from normalcy to higher levels of functioning. In this respect, terminating the relationship with one's coach may not be as difficult as ending with one's counselor or therapist. Even so, there are important rituals and processes to observe in ending. Coach and client may choose to celebrate the client's achievements, as well as discuss the working alliance frankly so that both parties can profit from lessons that may be available through a reflective review.

Follow-up is generally a good idea. In fact, coaches might consider a formal structure for follow-up over a period of months. Depending on such factors as the length of the coaching relationship, the agendas determined, and the success of the process, coaches may vary their strategies for follow-up. When clients have been working with coaches for a year or more, a natural process of decreasing levels of contact may occur. Intervals between coaching sessions may lengthen from a week to a month to finally 6 months. In coaching relations of shorter duration, the work may be highly focused or time limited. Some coaches may prefer to work with contracts of 10 to 12 weeks and then schedule a 3-month follow-up.

Actual contact between coach and client will terminate long before trace elements of the relationship have run their course. Effective coaches will

have transmitted important messages of guidance and support that clients will call to mind to motivate themselves or to counter threats of **relapse.** In this sense, the coach's voice lives inside the client and continues to foster client growth long after coach and client have ceased to meet. Yet the scheduling of periodic checkups or at least one follow-up session months after termination can serve to increase the volume of the coach's guidance within the client's mental framework for continuing development.

Kottler (2000) offers a variation of the model just described. He identifies five stages of the helping relationship: pretreatment, exploration, insight, action, and evaluation. Kottler highlights the stage of insight, during which the helper may probe beneath the surface of the client's story. Because Kottler's exploration stage is about hearing and understanding the client's world from the client's perspective, the stage of insight refers to the helper's efforts to understand a client's unconscious desires; irrational beliefs or assumptions; discrepancies in thought, feeling, or action; underlying feelings; and possible secondary gains that the client experiences through the process of seeking help.

It may be all too easy to assume that the client's self-presentation of issues and history is a sufficient picture from which to formulate plans and goals. This is not to say that the coach should position himself in a questioning or doubting manner in relation to the client's story, but rather that the coach should remain curious (Whitworth et al., 1998). When information does not easily come together or when the coach has a hunch that he could follow, he should see it as part of his legitimate role to ask questions, provide feedback, confront inconsistencies, and use all appropriate communication skills to obtain a full and practical understanding of the client.

A curious coach might notice that a client uses words like "must," "should," and "have to" while describing her intention to become physically fit. The coach could reflect these expressions in a sentence like the following: "I think it's wonderful that you are so keen to begin your program, but I need your help in understanding what you are trying to communicate when you use expressions like 'I must,' 'I have to,' and 'I should.'" Inquiry along these lines might enable you and the client to gain further insight into her motivations.

Telling a New Story

Based in the framework of narrative theory (Monk, Wislade, Crocket, & Epston, 1997), Ivey and Ivey

(2003) offer a simple yet useful model for understanding the stages of coaching. The key elements in their model are story, positive asset search, restory, and action.

- **Stage 1—Story:** In coaching, one needs to hear about the client's world, her wants, needs, dreams, concerns, and relevant history. We will see in upcoming chapters exactly what skills are most appropriate in helping clients tell their stories and precisely how coaches need to reflect this information back to clients to deepen understanding to levels congruent with the clients' objectives

- **Stage 2—Positive asset search:** As Ivey and Ivey (2003, p. 27) note, "It is not enough to listen; it is vital that positive strengths and assets be discovered as part of clients' stories." Although clients may come to you in hopes of finding better ways of living and high-level functioning, the stories they tell may be replete with details of failure or unsuccessful change attempts. The coach needs to sort through these details to discover with the client what assets he has to pursue his dreams and realize his vision.

- **Stage 3—Restory:** Creating a vision or building a dream requires restorying one's life, that is, imagining living according to different patterns, or acting, feeling, and thinking in new ways. If a client is living with self-perceptions that exclude awareness of strengths and assets, then the possible stories that the client will tell about future scenarios will be necessarily and inappropriately limited. Creating a vision based on full awareness of the client's potential, of what the client already has, and what the client is capable of doing allows for dramatic, positive shifts in awareness. Planning and goal setting can now encompass the full spectrum of possible realities that the client may wish to create.

- **Stage 4—Action:** In this model, action follows a process whereby coach and client work together to identify all relevant elements of the client's character and capability that the client can apply to the creation of a new way of being in the world. Action planning and implementation logically derive from such steps.

As noted in reference to Kottler's (2000) model, some inclusion of a closure phase in the Ivey and Ivey (2003) narrative model seems appropriate. Of course, clients may well cycle through a number of repetitions of story–positive asset search–restory–action before deciding to end their coaching relationships.

Prochaska's Transtheoretical Model (TTM)

How ready for change are the clients with whom you will be working? The fact that someone has hired you as her coach provides concrete data that the individual has moved beyond the starting gate of change. Even so, you may encounter someone who is committed to exercising but smokes a pack of cigarettes each day or overeats at every meal. A person may be ready to change one behavior yet completely unwilling to change others.

The transtheoretical model developed by Prochaska and associates (Prochaska & DiClemente, 1984; Prochaska, Norcross, & DiClemente, 1995) offers practical guidelines for understanding a person's readiness for change and what you can do to assist the person wherever she is in the process. The model describes six stages of change into which you can classify people (see figure 5.1). Imagine a behavior such as exercising regularly or quitting smoking. If you were to interview people about these behaviors, their readiness for change would enable you to classify them into one of six stages:

- **Stage 1—Precontemplation:** Precontemplators have no current intention to change. They may have tried to change a particular behavior in the past and failed, or they may altogether deny that they have a problem. Perhaps they are demoralized, having given up on the possibility of ever changing.

- **Stage 2—Contemplation:** Contemplators acknowledge they have a problem and are willing to think about their need to change. Although they are open to information and feedback, they can remain in this stage for years, realizing that they have a problem but unable to generate sufficient energy to change.

- **Stage 3—Preparation:** People in this stage are on the verge of action. They are developing plans and may even have made small changes. They focus more on the possibilities for action than on the causes of their behavior. This stage may characterize a large number of coaching clients.

- **Stage 4—Action:** People in this stage are following the action plan that they developed. The better developed this plan is and the more attention they have devoted to the work of the contemplation and preparation stages, the more successful they are likely to be.

- **Stage 5—Maintenance:** Maintainers have been continuously engaged in their change

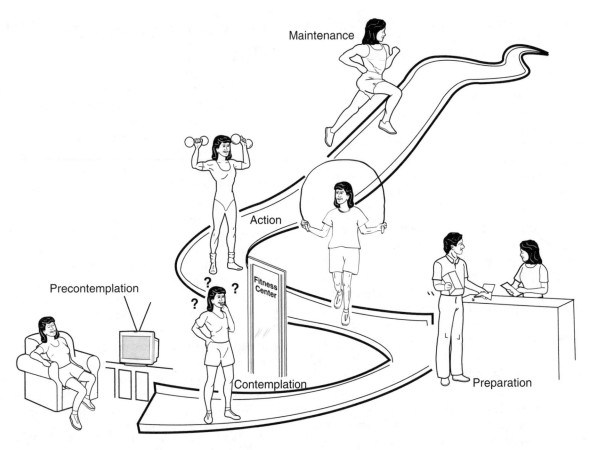

Figure 5.1 A representation of the transtheoretical model related to exercise.

Adapted, by permission, from J. Buckworth and R. Dishman, 2002, *Exercise psychology* (Champaign, IL: Human Kinetics), 220.

processes for at least 6 months. Although continuing in their programs or new behaviors feels natural in this stage, overconfidence and life stresses can lead to relapse (Marlatt & Gordon, 1985).

• **Stage 6—Termination:** In this stage the new behavior has become such an integral part of daily life that the likelihood of relapse is essentially nonexistent. Some professionals question whether people ever reach this stage, although Prochaska and colleagues (Prochaska, Norcross, & DiClemente, 1995) say that it is possible for a small percentage of people.

Intervention Strategies for the Six Stages of Change

How do you know which interventions are best suited to your clients? For each stage of change, several intervention strategies are recommended (Prochaska, Norcross, & DiClemente, 1995). The following is a description of nine interventions that you might apply at different stages of change:

1. *Consciousness raising.* This strategy involves intentional or unintentional exposure to information about oneself or the nature of problematic behaviors through such means as lectures, discussion groups, readings, advertisements, films, or even unexpected life events (e.g., health crisis).

2. *Social or environmental control.* External social or environmental forces may exert control over a person's behavior with or without consent. Examples include no-smoking areas, alcohol-free parties, broken elevators that force people to take the stairs, and sanctions including social ostracism for behaving in certain ways (e.g., neglecting personal fitness).

3. *Emotional arousal.* Often accompanying consciousness raising, emotional arousal targets the feeling level. Films, dramatic media presentations, and fear-arousing experiences including, for example, graphic depictions of diseased lungs or lives ruined through substance abuse, can generate emotional arousal.

4. *Personal revisioning.* Looking toward the future by imagining life after changing certain problematic behaviors captures the meaning of this strategy. Revisioning enables people to appreciate how their behaviors may conflict with core personal values and thereby generate motivation to change.

5. *Commitment.* Choosing to change, accepting responsibility for change, and then publicly announcing one's commitment to change are core features of this strategy. This approach typically includes clear delineation of the intended change through contracting or other means of making the commitment explicit.

6. *Rewarding.* This strategy relies on praise and other forms of reward to reinforce the positive change in behavior

7. *Countering.* In this strategy, one substitutes healthy behaviors for unhealthy ones, for example, doing tai chi for 5 minutes instead of having a late-night snack. This approach relies on identifying and controlling internal reactions, such as being aware when an urge arises and then substituting a preplanned healthy behavior.

8. *Environmental management.* Like countering, environmental management involves controlling one's world, but here the focus is more on the external environment. Environmental management involves deliberately manipulating one's environment to support change, for example, by placing exercise equipment and reminders strategically throughout one's home environment.

9. *Interpersonal support.* Involving friends, families, colleagues, and professionals can help people advance through the stages of change. Coaching relationships offer understanding, acceptance, and guidance through the challenges of change.

Applying Intervention Strategies From the Transtheoretical Model

Different interventions work more effectively at different stages of change. For example, consciousness raising is an especially helpful intervention for people in stages of precontemplation and contemplation. Consciousness raising might take the form of giving a sedentary person a pamphlet on the health risks of inactivity or suggesting that the person have an in-depth discussion about inactiv-

ity with her doctor. Sometimes unexpected events in a person's life, like learning that a friend who smokes was diagnosed with lung cancer, can serve as a wake-up call.

Another intervention helpful in the early stages of change (precontemplation and contemplation) involves social or environmental control. Here, surrounding conditions in the person's social or physical world influence the person's behavior. Nonsmoking laws are a good example of how this strategy works. At a social level, group pressure or support can also serve to influence behavior.

Although coaches may not be able to control social or environmental factors, they can use two other interventions that become available in the second stage—emotional arousal and self-revisioning. Here's how they might work.

Your expression of concern may increase clients' emotional arousal. Coaches serve as firsthand observers of the difficulties that clients experience because of poor diet, smoking, and other harmful behaviors. Your empathic feedback in these moments can help heighten clients' emotional concern for their personal well-being.

Emotional arousal may occur when a client views a film or reads a book related to the changes that he is contemplating. As a coach working with a client who is searching for motivation to change a life-threatening behavior, you might respond to that cry for help by recommending books, films, or discussion groups that can arouse emotions to direct the client's energy toward commitment.

The second strategy, personal revisioning, builds on the effects of emotional arousal. Here, you may focus the client toward a positive future image of life after a change has occurred. You can encourage the client to imagine himself after the change process has been successfully completed.

You should avoid some interventions in the early stages of change because they are likely to backfire. For example, encouraging someone to commit to action during precontemplation or contemplation stages would most likely fail. The client has not sufficiently worked through his internal connections to the problem or developed an adequate strategy to deal with all the side effects of self-change.

Interpersonal support is a strategy that applies to all stages of change, and simple actions represent it exquisitely. Listening to clients with compassion and warmth enables them to open themselves to their inner wisdom and self-caring. Listening to them without judgment or advice, but with concern and empathy, permits them to be their own judges and to find new strength to change.

Because many of your clients will already be on the path of change, they may have reached the stage of preparation or even action in relation to some aspects of their goals. In these latter stages of change, the most helpful strategies include rewarding clients for their accomplishments, helping them consciously manage their environments so that they can live up to their agreements, and enhancing their commitment through contracting.

People need feedback to grow, and positive feedback (reward) has the most beneficial effect on behavior (D. Johnson, 2003). Although some clients may be so dedicated to their programs that you take their commitment for granted, you should still regularly praise and reward their efforts. According to principles from the transtheoretical model, you may want to offer regular compliments and praise in client sessions for specific aspects of their efforts.

Another way to help clients in the more advanced stages of action and maintenance is to review and update their programs periodically, especially parts that deal with their training schedules and goals. In reviewing goals, you reinforce awareness of their commitments to action and to themselves. Because making public commitments increases adherence, you should encourage clients to tell others about their training plans and goals.

A third strategy for the advanced stages is countering, which involves substituting healthy behaviors for unhealthy ones. Especially when clients are working on changing other health-related behaviors (e.g., eating habits), you might encourage them to use exercise as their substitute behavior. For example, you could suggest to your clients that instead of giving in to an urge for a late-night snack, they could perform a short, relaxing sequence of stretches.

Although some clients may be entirely reliable to their commitments when they are on their normal schedules, holidays, vacations, and travel can create trouble spots for adherence. Working with clients to manage their environments in support of their change agendas will help them stay on the path. You should encourage them to plan for situations that previously led to relapse. For example, you might advise them to book reservations in hotels with fitness centers when they are traveling or help them design spaces in their homes where they can exercise when time is limited or when other factors keep them away from the gym.

Taylor's Learning Process Model

Committing to regular exercise or changing lifestyle patterns may involve deep-level restructuring of thoughts, feelings, and behaviors (Taylor, 1986, 1987, 1990). Observers may witness the results of long-term deliberations about change in a single moment when a person takes his last puff or chews his last bite of red meat. By contrast, we observe anew a commitment to positive actions like exercise each time a person shows up to train. In both instances, when a person commits to enacting new behaviors such as exercise or when he ceases old behaviors, the change process is in fact one that unfolds over time. We can rightly describe the change process according to different phases or seasons of change.

Taylor (1986, 1987) has developed a learning process model that is divided into four phases with critical transitions that usher the person onward from one phase to the next. Her model (figure 5.2) relies on the fact that mostly we live in a state of equilibrium in which elements of our personal worlds feel more or less in balance. The motivation for change may arise from an accumulation of experiences or from a single event. When this motivation reaches a critical mass, we move out of our comfortable world to encounter a cycle of

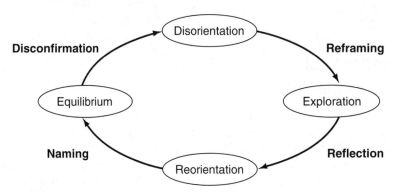

Figure 5.2 The Taylor learning process model.

Reprinted from M.M. Taylor, 1986, "Learning for self-direction in the classroom: The pattern of a transition process," *Studies in Higher Education* 11(1). By permission of Marilyn M. Taylor, PhD.

events (or phases) that eventually returns us to a new equilibrium, which, we hope, is an improvement over our old way of being.

The Taylor model has significant implications for the types of changes that clients in lifestyle fitness coaching may be contemplating. This model has been tested on people in university-based learning transitions (Taylor, 1987), elite athletes recuperating from serious injuries (Gavin & Taylor, 1990), individuals confronting unexpected unemployment (Taylor & Gavin, 1983), and postcardiac rehabilitation patients (Taylor, 1990), among others.

• **Transition 1—Disconfirmation:** Clients who voluntarily commit themselves to a coaching process do so with reason. Sometimes a big push comes from something like a medical report. At other times a gradual accumulation of dissatisfactions tips the scale and topples the person out of the phase of equilibrium. This first transition is called disconfirmation because

some aspect of the person's old world no longer works or makes sense. For example, a client may deny the effects of inactivity for years until a physical examination reveals warning signs of coronary heart disease. Less dramatically, a man may continue to believe that he is in shape until his 10-year-old daughter easily beats him in a mad dash to catch a bus.

• **Phase 1—Disorientation:** When excuses no longer work, when counterarguments trump rationalizations, or when the old reality no longer fits, people in a process of change may feel defenseless. They can no longer justify their behaviors. They cannot maintain their previous way of living. This first phase can be an emotional time. People may spin in confusion, anger, blame, sadness, frustration, or guilt (see figure 5.3). Taking a hard, cold look at themselves in the mirror, they may be saddened or repulsed to see what they have created over years of inactivity or personal neglect. They may

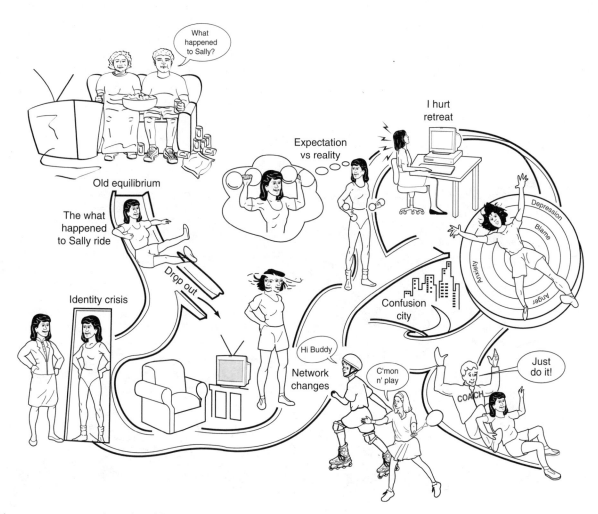

Figure 5.3 Moving from the old equilibrium into the disorientation phase.
Adapted from Gavin 1992.

seek someone to blame, or self-pity may overcome them. When clients drop the mask behind which they have hidden certain dysfunctional habits, they may feel extremely vulnerable. Although they may try to make light of their new awareness, the coach's best response is to show deep empathy for what these clients now realize. The first phase, disorientation, may last for days, weeks, or even months, depending on the nature and extent of the disconfirmation that they have experienced. (The disorientation phase generally corresponds to the stage of contemplation in the TTM model.)

• **Transition 2—Reframing:** Imagine someone who finally confronts the fact that she is out of shape and 50 pounds (23 kilograms) overweight. Perhaps she went to her 20th high school reunion and felt shamed by some of her athletic and slim former classmates. This disconfirmation (transition 1) may have pulled her out of equilibrium and thrust her into the phase of disorientation. This phase normally lasts until the person is able to reframe what is upsetting her without self-blame and without blaming others. As long as she spins in self-rejection or fails to get to the root of what bothers her, she will continue to ride the emotional roller coaster of the disorientation phase. With empathic listening and compassionate feedback, coaches can help clients

reframe what their challenges might be in a manner that implies neither self-blame nor blame of others.

• **Phase 2—Exploration:** Imagine that you have recently broken up with your spouse or lover. With the help of some good friends, you have moved beyond blame and out of an emotional spin. Is this the time to get into a new relationship? You will probably think that it's not, and recommendations based on Taylor's model support your belief. You should take time to explore what you need, what did not work in your old way of being in a relationship, and what changes you need to incorporate in future relationships. In the world of health and fitness, after a person has identified issues without blame and enters the phase of exploration, she can then consider options concerning how and when to exercise or, if she seeks another change, she can investigate what kinds of interventions or programs would be most beneficial (see figure 5.4). In this phase other people are important, especially those who are at a similar phase of change or perhaps a step ahead. People also usually welcome knowledge and information from books or other sources at this time. Clients will signal that they have entered this phase by their keen interest in facts and information, by their need to talk to you about what they are doing, and by their efforts to socialize with

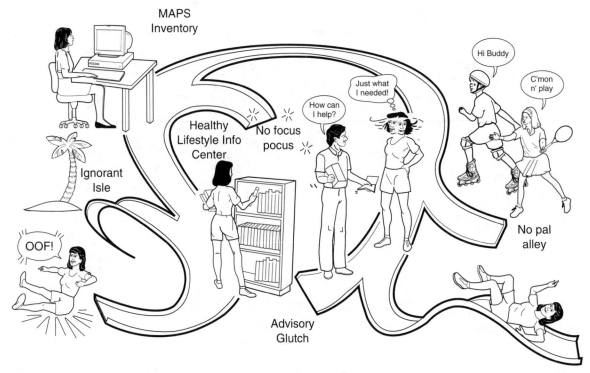

Figure 5.4 Moving from the disorientation phase to the exploration phase.

Adapted from Gavin 1992.

others who are walking a similar path. By having resources readily at hand and perhaps by scheduling extra time to talk with them, you will enable clients to efficiently move through this phase. (The exploration phase generally coincides with the stage of preparation in the TTM model.)

• **Transition 3—Reflection:** The exploration phase is typically an intensely social time. Clients who are trying to figure out new health habits and ways of functioning in a changed personal reality need other people with whom to examine their ideas, plans, and proposals. Reflection often marks the transition to the next phase in the cycle. The client may begin to withdraw into himself to consolidate thoughts and feelings and to begin piecing together a coherent strategy for action. From the outside, you will notice that the client may become more introspective. He may reduce his requests for feedback and no longer ask for readings or other sources of information. You should be sensitive to this shift by allowing the person to withdraw, rather than continuing to flood the person with ideas and suggestions or to encourage deep examination of issues.

• **Phase 3—Reorientation:** Clients enter reorientation with a plan. The plan may be rudimentary, but the client will be committed to testing it out and determining how well it works (see figure 5.5). Maybe the plan is a particular schedule of training, coupled with a variable routine for other activities. Perhaps it is a healthy eating program that the person has derived from explorations of how to lose weight sensibly and promote well-being. Your role in the reorientation phase often takes on dimensions of providing expert feedback and advice so that clients can fine-tune their programs. Your interventions may represent a more technical level of input during this phase. You are no longer helping clients decide whether to take up running or do weight training as you might have during the exploration phase. You are now engaged in providing precise data about programs to which clients have strongly committed themselves. A kind of shakedown occurs in this phase in which the client is making final adjustments to plans before solidifying them into ongoing routines. (The reorientation phase parallels the occurrence of the stage of action in the TTM model.)

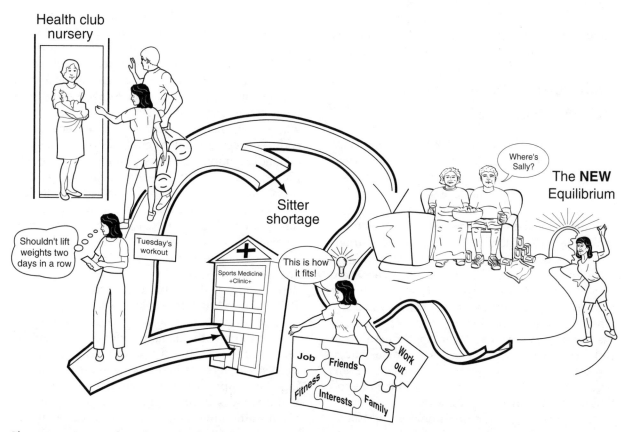

Figure 5.5 Moving from the exploration phase to the reorientation phase.
Adapted from Gavin 1992.

• **Transition 4—Naming:** You have undoubtedly met people who in the recent past succeeded in a smoking-cessation program or who have become regular exercisers. Usually, these people enjoy broadcasting their successes wherever they can. They want to help others who have struggled with what they have overcome. Clients who have made it through to this point are excited about their accomplishments and want others to feel as good as they do. Coaches can help by validating their successes, by acknowledging their achievements, and by making space for them to talk openly about their journeys. Creating opportunities for them to name publicly what they have learned and accomplished makes it more real for them and provides them reason to celebrate.

• **Phase 4—Equilibrium:** The learning process model is a cycle that begins and ends in equilibrium, although the new equilibrium normally is a healthier and happier way of being. The new equilibrium is the application of hard-earned learning that has been field-tested and refined. It demonstrates clients' capacity to grow and develop when they confront challenges informing them that their old ways of being are no longer viable. At this point in the change process, the coach's role may be close to ending, at least until the next challenge knocks at the client's door. (The equilibrium phase corresponds to the stage of maintenance in the TTM model.)

Applying Principles of the Taylor Learning Process Model

Taylor's (1986, 1987, 1990) work has encompassed a wide range of healthy adults confronting normal changes and life adjustments. Although we may see its phases as paralleling those of the transtheoretical model, the Taylor model reveals the layers beneath the surface of change. Clients who are catapulted into change may articulate goal statements without identifying underlying dynamics that have initiated the change process. Understanding why clients are deciding to address a particular change agenda at this precise point in time helps coaches identify where their clients are in the process of change. If the decision is recent and perhaps in reaction to certain life events (e.g., marriage or divorce, change in job, loss of a family member), a coach's interventions will need to reflect sensitivity to the turmoil that the client may be experiencing.

As clients progress through phases and transitions, Taylor (1999) indicates that certain patterns and needs prevail. To some degree, this may be reflected in the client's greater or lesser reliance on your coaching assistance. Rather than viewing these as indicators of commitment, coaches may come to understand that the varying needs clients have for coaching are related to their phases of learning and development. For example, following the exploration phase clients need to reflect more privately to create internal order of their thoughts, feelings, and actions. A client who has formerly been open and talkative may become more solitary and less needy. These kinds of shifts are natural and reflective of where the client is in a cycle of change.

You may find it useful to examine some of your own life transitions in relation to the processes described in the Taylor model. Learning activity 5.1 provides you with an opportunity to consider your own experiences. Through reflection, you may be able to identify signs that suggest phases and transitions. To expand your knowledge, you might further reflect on the work that you may have experienced with clients who have successfully cycled through a process of change.

Endings and New Beginnings

In some perspectives of life coaching (Whitworth et al., 1998; Williams & Davis, 2002), the relationship is defined as long term. Perhaps for this reason, discussions of endings are often overlooked or avoided, as if the relationship just continues. The fact is that all relationships have different forms of endings, even when some aspects of connection continue. People who live together over decades of time experience the endings of certain dimensions of their relationships and the beginnings of others. Through disease or the process of aging itself, sexual relations between two people may gradually diminish and end while new forms of intimacy are born. Parents may end their direct care taking of children and develop companionate forms of connection with their offspring.

In professional helping relations, endings are generally expected and, in fact, may be predetermined in the initial contracting. From the 1970s onward, the counseling field manifested a gradual transition from open-ended, long-term relationships with clients to brief or time-limited relationships. As the coaching field emerged in the1990s, diverse opinions were evident concerning the temporal nature of these relationships. Some writers defined ending according to the client's attainment of goals, whereas others imagined ongoing process-oriented relationships. But with the agenda of "action, action, action" (Martin,

Learning Activity 5.1 — Exploring the Phases of Change Through Personal Experience

This activity comprises two parts. The first is to examine a personal experience, and the second is to recall the path of change for one of your clients or for a close friend or family member.

Part 1: Your Personal Change

You may once have been inactive, a smoker, in an unsatisfying relationship, in a university degree program that didn't fit you, or in some other unworkable situation. Pick an experience that stands out clearly in your mind when you responded successfully to the call for change. Recall the sequence of events from beginning to end, that is, recollect when you first began thinking about changing and when you realized that you had successfully completed the process of change. Bring to mind as much of the history of this change experience as possible. Remember whether the change seemed sudden or whether a gradual awakening occurred. Recall what you felt like in the beginning of this change, toward the middle, and near the end. Then reconsider the phases and transitions described in the Taylor model. How much of it fits for you? Perhaps you might see close parallels in some places but not in others. Where your experience and the model do not correspond, you might examine other change processes you have experienced that more clearly illustrate a particular piece of the model. Remember that your experience and the model do not have to fit exactly. The principle task is to consider the seasons of change as you have known them.

Part 2: Someone Else's Change Process

If you have been working with clients for a while, you may be able to identify one you have known well who successfully changed a particular behavior, such as moving from a sedentary lifestyle to an active one. On the other hand, you may not currently be working with clients, in which case you might think about someone you know well who experienced a change process. This person might be a family member who stopped smoking or a friend who went through a significant life change. Your task is to explore your knowledge of this person's experience and, from the outside, try to determine any identifying behaviors that would reflect the phases and transitions suggested by Taylor. If this person is still available to you, you may wish to ask him or her for recollections of the process. Of course, you will need to be sensitive to whether the person is open to such reconsiderations. Remember that you are looking for examples of successful change efforts, so in this case the person is likely to have mostly good feelings about what she or he experienced.

You may wish to apply this process to several people you know or to a current situation in which someone is going through a change process. The goal is to be keenly observant of what they are experiencing, without being intrusive.

2001), a time would inevitably arrive even in coaching when clients simply wanted the space to "be" rather than to continue doing.

If we examine the likely agendas of clients in lifestyle fitness coaching, one can certainly imagine relationships lasting over a period of years. Similarly, it makes sense that some relationships would be shorter, measured in months rather than years. A person who struggles with regularity in exercise and with weight management and who wishes to pursue specific personal growth benefits obtained through sport and physical training could reasonably maintain connections with a lifestyle fitness coach for at least a year, based on knowledge concerning the time that people need to solidify new exercise habits (Buckworth & Dishman, 2002; Prochaska et al., 1995) and minimize risks of relapse (Marlatt & Gordon, 1985). In short- or long-term relationships, client and coach may not always meet weekly, but they are likely to have established some rhythm and regularity of contact such that the ending may be eventful.

Endings are also referred to as **closure,** a kind of relationship agenda rather than a static event. Closure is a process whereby the work comes to some mutually understood ending and whereby client and practitioner acknowledge and review feelings and perceptions and extract potential meanings for future relationships of the same nature. Walsh (2003) considers different types of endings in helping relationships, organized into three categories: endings initiated by the client, unplanned endings initiated by the practitioner, and planned endings. From these different types, we will consider only endings that are more probable in coaching relationships.

Tasks and Meanings of Endings

The end of the coaching relationship offers opportunity for the completion of certain tasks and for various assessments. As Walsh (2003) explains, the closing of the relationship may allow helper and client to achieve the following:

- Understand without ambiguity that the relationship is ending
- Reflect on their work from all angles
- Identify what was learned
- Acknowledge feelings about the relationship
- Consider the meaning of this relationship for potential future ones

Beyond these general agendas, Walsh (2003) highlights specific tasks, reframed here according to how they might pertain to coaching roles:

1. Recognizing that ending is a process, coaches must strategically estimate when and how to commence discussions of ending.
2. Acknowledging that clients will experience endings differently, coaches need to be open to a wide range of emotional reactions.
3. Reviews constitute important dimensions of ending and should focus not only on outcomes but also on processes, including relationship dynamics.
4. Helping clients transfer their learning to new situations or to other agendas can be extremely helpful in fostering client autonomy. Discussing with the client how to link what occurred in this process to what the client might be able to do independently in the future can be invaluable.
5. Unless the coaching relationship has persisted long enough to ensure that relapse or erosion of gains will not occur, the ending process should focus on concrete actions that clients will take to ensure the maintenance and enhancement of achievements.

6. In the coaching process, issues not covered in the original contract may emerge. The ending process could encourage exploration of these additional agendas and planning for future action.
7. The coaching process is a significant aid to personal growth and development, yet clients might use other means to foster personal fulfillment. The coach might help the client identify these additional resources in concrete ways.
8. Endings allow new beginnings. What are the ways in which coach and client might connect in the future? Closure should allow for a discussion of clear boundaries and guidelines concerning future contact, as well as for reinitiating the coaching relation.
9. Saying good-bye is the final step, with all other discussions and dialogues having been completed to the degree possible. Coaches are likely to experience their own emotions in ending yet will need to guard against projecting their own unfinished business about endings on their clients' processes of completion.

Whenever coaching ends, there is a need to reflect on both outcomes and processes. Ideally, coach and client should reflect on their experiences together, although this may not always be possible. Certain questions can help inform future actions of both the coach and the client (Walsh, 2003):

- How has the client changed? What is different? What goals has the client reached? Which ones has the client not achieved? What might have changed unexpectedly, for better or worse?
- How does the client feel about the work? Did the client see the investment as worthwhile? Was the general experience one of satisfaction and accomplishment? Does the client feel good about the coach?
- What's next? What will the client do now? What plans or new goals would the client like to consider? What would be the logical next step in the process of personal development? How should the client engage in this work?

Types of Endings to the Coaching Relationship

Knowing when to end a coaching relationship requires constant monitoring of the relationship.

Here are some guidelines to follow so that you are aware of the emerging need to end the relationship (Walsh, 2003; also, Gabbard, 1995; Hepworth et al., 2002; Herlihy & Corey, 1997):

- Having set clear objectives through explicit contracting, progress toward these goals will inform decisions about endings or the discussion of endings.

- Remaining aware of your own needs as a coach will help you understand whether you are prolonging or hastening the ending for personal reasons.

- Keep in mind that a metagoal of coaching is to enhance the autonomous functioning of clients. In this perspective, wherever you end in the process of moving toward goals, clients will at least have profited from your efforts to help them take personal responsibility, function autonomously, plan intelligently, and safeguard change processes to ensure success.

- Inform yourself of clients' specific histories regarding endings of relationships and their culturally linked expectations of ending processes.

Of course, the ending of the coaching relationship does not mean the end to learning. Learning is a lifelong process. Coaches may facilitate the ending of coaching sessions while engendering skills and processes for clients to continue their growth and development.

Unplanned Endings Initiated By the Client

In unplanned endings, the client terminates the relationship unexpectedly (Walsh, 2003). Such endings include some sense of surprise, and unfortunately the client may never share with the coach the reasons for ending. Clearly, the ambiguity surrounding these endings leaves matters open to interpretation. The following are possible scenarios occasioning abrupt endings:

1. **The client perceives that he has made enough progress but is unable or unwilling to talk with the coach about ending.** Studies assessing the rates of premature endings in various types of helping interventions show percentages varying from 20 to 50% (Sweet & Noones, 1989). An interesting dynamic explaining these results emerged from one study in which helpers expected that their clients would remain in the helping process two to three times longer than the clients themselves expected to stay (Pekarik & Finney-Owen, 1987). Results of studies do not fully support the belief that a process has been unsuccessful just because a client ends the relationship without warning and without communicating with the helper (Kazdin & Wassell, 1998). When helpers were asked what they believed to be the most significant moments in the relationship, they often identified experiences quite different from those that clients believed were most important (Stalikas & Fitzpatrick, 1995, 1996). One might say that the client is always right about his own experiences, but the reality is probably not that simple. Helpers may see things with greater objectivity, yet the client will ultimately decide. More to the point, helpers may be insightful, but they are unlikely to be mind readers. A client may experience certain effects from a session that only become evident in the hours and days after the meeting. Helpers cannot know this, even though they may hope for such epiphanies. When clients receive what they came for, they may just presume the coach will understand, without words, why they are ending. Perhaps clients attribute too much insight to coaches and helpers.

2. **The client ends the relationship because of dissatisfactions with progress.** If clients do not have early indications of progress, they may quit and go shopping for another coach. How long it takes clients to reach the point of quitting because of disappointment with outcomes varies. In some cases, clients stay too long; in others, not long enough. Strean (1986) offers several reasons why clients may end their relationships out of feelings of dissatisfaction:

- A feeling that the helper is not listening well

- Experiencing the helper as being too directive

- A sense that the helper does not like the client or is acting out her emotions on the client

- Complications from sexual feelings from either the helper or the client

- Experiencing the helper as identifying too closely with the client's issues

- Beliefs that the helper is uncomfortable with negative emotions like anger or expressions of dissatisfaction from the client

To prevent this kind of ending, coaches must not assume that clients have the same feelings that they do about the sessions. Coaches must ask for feedback from clients regularly, even as often as at the end of each meeting.

3. **The client experiences discomfort with some personal characteristic of the coach.** We might easily relate this to differences in cultural backgrounds, age, gender, or other obvious characteristics of the coach, but discomfort can result from something entirely peculiar to the client's personal history and experiences (Reis & Brown, 1999; Walsh, 2003). Coaches may sense how well clients connect with them based on nonverbal signals, or they may not. Clients can be highly skilled in "face management" (Gavin & Gavin, 2004), conveying to coaches positive impressions of their experiences while inwardly holding negative perceptions. Because the coaching relationship is not about healing the client's history but about working together in a productive alliance to assist the client toward identified goal attainment, clients who experience strong negative reactions to coaches based on their own idiosyncrasies should probably end the relationship rather than carry this extra issue into each of the working sessions. Although coaches may ideally want to know which of their personal characteristics triggered the client's reactions, ultimately its significance is minor so long as coaches do their utmost to convey the core conditions of helping relationships (chapter 3) to their clients, strive to be aware of their own behaviors, and seek regular feedback through discussions with colleagues and supervisors.

4. **The client ends the relationship during a hiatus in the coaching relationship.** Vacations, conferences, or unexpected life events may create a break in the rhythm of a coaching relationship. During periods like these, clients may consolidate lessons they have gained from the work, or they may come to realize that they are not as motivated to continue as they had felt originally. At a deeper level, it is also possible that if a coach breaks the regularity of meetings, irrespective of the reason, the client may feel abandoned or frightened by the sense of dependency that she feels in the relationship. In most helping relations, vacation periods or lengthy breaks in contact with clients bring with them increased probability of ending. Unless clients are open to a full discussion of their reasons, coaches may be left to wonder about the successes of their efforts.

5. **The client experiences discomfort about the coach's approach.** No matter what your title, clients will have their unique interpretations of what it is you do and how you should approach

the issues. Many clients in counseling expect the counselor to tell them what to do (Shebib, 2003) or believe that they can resolve issues in one or two meetings. Coaches may need to go to great lengths in describing their style and the processes of coaching. The more the client knows about the possible evolution of the working relationship, the more positive the outcomes are likely to be (Frank & Frank, 1993). Many clients may perceive lifestyle fitness coaching in ways similar to personal training. Although a fair degree of overlap may indeed be present in some cases, the agenda of coaching is likely to be broader. Moreover, the legitimacy of engaging clients in dialogue about issues, processes, and progress is a cornerstone of the coaching role that some clients may not immediately appreciate. They may believe that they should compensate a coach only when they are receiving training on machines or in physical activity. Otherwise, they feel, it is just two people talking.

Unplanned Endings Initiated By the Coach

Coaches may decide for a variety of reasons to end their relationships with clients. These reasons may arise because of issues in the relationship or because of specific concerns or experiences of the coach. Walsh (2003) describes several possibilities, discussed here as they pertain to coaching relationships.

1. **The client is not fulfilling her part of the agreement.** Clients commence relationships with coaches for many reasons. A client may simply come to that time of year when she renews intentions to change old habits, in the way that many people make New Year's resolutions. The client may be motivated by a sense of "should," that is, she thinks she should work on self-improvement, become active, lose weight, become more assertive, make changes, or whatever else inspires her in the moment to connect with a coach. Then reality sets in. Changing is not easy. It does not occur simply by hiring a coach. She has to do something, and that something requires effort and commitment that she is unwilling to give. Yes, coaches fire clients! An ethical issue can even arise here. Some clients may be willing to continue and to pay as long as they do not have to change and as long as the coach is willing to go along with the charade.

2. **The client oversteps the coach's professional boundaries.** As discussed in chapter 4, boundaries have to do with limits established to protect the welfare of the client and enable coaches to provide appropriate guidance and support for clients. Bruhn,

Levine, and Levine (1993) outlined five aspects of boundaries that are relevant to coaching: (1) contact time, referring to the amount of time coaches and clients agree to spend working together, including time spent in phone contacts and e-mail correspondence; (2) types of information shared, including the range of topics and discussions agreed to by coach and client; (3) physical closeness, concerning issues of touch and physical closeness permitted in the relationship; (4) territory, referring to the range of physical settings in which client and coach will work together; and (5) emotional space, dealing with the level and range of emotional feelings appropriate to the goals and purposes of the relationship. Some boundary violations may have to occur only once to justify a coach's decision to end the relationship. For example, a client may make an aggressive sexual advance, and the coach may decide that the relationship is not viable. Other violations such as repeated telephone calls late at night to a coach's home may be cause for termination.

3. **The client may engage in behaviors considered unacceptable to the coach.** Clients may behave in ways that are unacceptable to a coach. For instance, a client may use language that is racist, sexist, or foul. He may show up for appointments after having bouts of drinking, or he may show indications of other substance abuse. Clients may repeatedly come unprepared for sessions or may try to multitask during sessions (e.g., answering cell phone calls, eating during sessions). A coach may decide that the client's behavior is unacceptable based on a personal value code or professional judgment about client comportment.

4. **The coach has significant negative feelings toward the client.** As Walsh (2003) suggests, helpers do not like to admit that they may have strong negative feelings toward certain clients. Just as a client may discontinue the relationship based on the coach's personal characteristics, so too a coach may not want to work with certain clients. When the coach identifies this attitude at the beginning of the relationship, he might easily resolve the situation by suggesting that the client work with another coach. More problematic is the case in which the dislike develops over the course of the relationship. The coach is then in a difficult predicament of not wanting to work with the client either because of personality characteristics, the nature of the issues on which the client wants to work, or the way in which the client behaves in sessions. This kind of situation would probably require that the coach review matters with peers or a supervisor.

5. **The client makes poor progress and shows little capacity to improve.** Despite a client's best intentions and a coach's best efforts, the story may unfold that the client simply cannot successfully engage the process of coaching or implement the agreed-on steps to reach her goals. In these instances, the coach may reasonably wonder about her own capabilities, and that may be part of the problem. In other cases, the client may simply have other hurdles to contend with before being able to take on the challenges that she has set for herself in the coaching relationship. Although referring the client to another professional may be in order, the coaching relationship does not necessarily have to end. A coach can suggest a hiatus in coaching while the client works on an identified impediment to progress with another professional. An obvious example might be a situation in which a woman wants help in preparing for trekking adventures in Europe but has correctable foot problems that require surgery.

6. **The coach becomes overwhelmed.** Life happens, and coaches are as vulnerable as all humans are to disease, disability, stress, and strain. Although coaches might be expected to manage their personal and work lives well enough that conditions like burnout do not occur, coaches sometimes take on more than they can handle. Sometimes the unexpected happens. In general, it makes sense for coaches to plan for contingencies and perhaps work in alliance with other coaches who have compatible styles so that appropriate referrals can be made when necessary.

Planned Endings

As we have seen earlier in this chapter, a logical or desirable progression in coaching moves from beginning to end more or less according to plan. This does not always mean that the client has reached his goals; some other mutually determined criterion may become relevant to the decision (Walsh, 2003).

1. **The client has achieved the goals desired.** Clients may progress toward the attainment of objectives mutually determined in the coaching relationship until they feel they have achieved their purposes entirely or substantially. As suggested in the discussion of stages of the coaching relationship, some clients may recycle through goal setting and action stages so that they accomplish a number of objectives. In these instances, the end may come following a number of successes, and the client then makes a decision to integrate without further

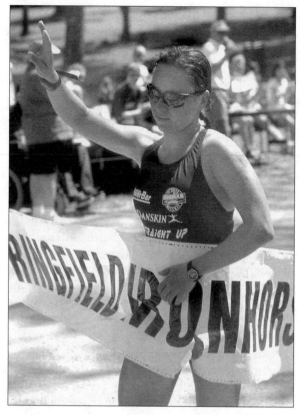

The coaching relationship may end when the client has reached her goal.

strategic action the lessons and benefits of progress to date.

2. **The client and coach reach an agreed-on time limit for the relationship.** Sometimes coaching is delineated according to a calendar of meetings. Clients agree to meet for a certain number of sessions to advance a particular agenda. They may not have concrete outcome goals as much as they have process goals of working in different ways or experiencing things differently with the assistance of a coach. For practical reasons, some clients may have budgeted a particular amount of money for coaching and thereby scheduled a specific number of sessions to work on an agenda.

3. **Issues have arisen in the coaching relation that suggest other avenues.** Although they do not initially intend to seek such information, a coach and client may discover through their working relationship a host of other concerns that the client should address. For instance, clients may have serious health issues arising from overeating, smoking, or substance abuse that jeopardize the client's abilities to pursue and attain activity goals. Through dialogue, coach and client may create a plan of action

for the client to address these matters with other processes or with other people. The coach might help the client develop a plan of action that includes other forms of treatment, which the client would pursue with other professionals before engaging in physical activity programming. Contact with the coach could continue during this period, with the coach reinforcing action planning and behavior commitments.

Some Potential Reactions to Endings

Feelings may vary when clients end coaching relationships. Ideally, clients would feel a strong sense of achievement from the goals they have pursued and attained. In so doing, clients would also have gained an enhanced sense of autonomy and personal efficacy. That is, they not only would have achieved specific goals but also would have learned how to learn, how to plan, and how to strategize for success. They would experience themselves more fully and be more satisfied with themselves in real-world interactions through having achieved important gains and by having successfully committed themselves to their important goals.

At a process level, clients would have reason to rejoice in their ability to work collaboratively with another person and to be open with that person, without negative consequence. Transferring this learning to other relationships would provide clients with yet another source of satisfaction.

Although clients may experience such emotions as sadness and regret in the ending of a significant coaching relationship, they may understand these experiences as normal and appropriate. If the client allows these emotions to be legitimate and without judgment, this too can create a meaningful benefit from the coaching process.

More problematically, clients may react with an extreme sense of loss when the coaching relationship ends. This circumstance is more likely to occur when coaching has continued over a long period and when the client has been unsuccessful in achieving process goals of increased autonomy and self-efficacy. Another problematic reaction that may be less obvious in its implications occurs when clients deny that the ending has any meaning whatsoever or when clients avoid discussion of the matter. In these cases, clients may be experiencing far deeper reactions that they are either unaware of or unwilling to address.

Of course, some clients may react with anger at the ending of a coaching relationship. Perhaps they accuse the coach of not helping or not being sensitive to their needs. Clients who have, for whatever reasons, not achieved their goals may react by expressing strong negative feelings toward the coach.

In ending, coaches need to be aware of what might seem a reasonable request by a client for continued contact with the coach through a new relationship, such as friendship or social connection. When clients are either unwilling or unready to end, yet cannot rationalize continuation of coaching, they may wish to transform the coaching relationship into a form that they can more easily justify.

Clients are not the only ones affected by endings. Coaches may experience enhanced feelings of self-efficacy through the work that they have done with clients, and they may take justifiable satisfaction in their clients' accomplishments. Just as clients who end long-term coaching relationships may understandably feel sadness, coaches may experience similar emotions in endings. Through those feelings, they may deepen their capacity for human compassion.

What happens when clients do not achieve their goals, when they blame coaches for their failures, or when they terminate after a long period of unsuccessful effort? In these instances, coaches might experience a lessening of professional competency, guilt, or a tendency to blame the client for perceived failures. In a problematic sense, the coach may go so far as to make an inappropriate offer of additional help to clients who are ending but are quite dissatisfied with their achievements through coaching.

Reflections on Stages, Phases, and Endings

Some theorists use deceptively simple terms to describe change processes. Bridges (2001), for instance, simply talks about the beginning, middle, and end. Although these terms are commonly understood, they mask a myriad of dynamics when applied to matters of personal change. In this chapter we have reflected on three distinct frameworks for understanding change in the coaching relation-

ship. The first pertained to stages of the coaching relationship, in which we looked at the kinds of agendas engaged by coach and client at different points in their relationship. The second concerned stages of readiness for change that might characterize clients at different points in their relationships with coaches. Indeed, clients may be in the stage of preparation regarding the contracted agenda, and through work with the coach, may advance the stages of a related agenda that was not part of the original agreement. Recommended strategies that coaches might consider depending on clients' identified stages of change accompanied this second framework. Third, we examined the personal dynamics of change as experienced by the learner, as Taylor (1986) would identify clients in a change process. The intriguing part of this model was the view that it offered of the evolving needs of clients as they progress through phases and transitions toward their goals.

The final agenda of this chapter was the matter of endings. Clearly, the initial stages of coaching are tenuous times, and coaches must proceed with extreme delicacy and sensitivity. The same is true of endings, although they are rarely presented in such a manner. As the client becomes a familiar face with predictable patterns and as interactions seem increasingly comfortable, coaches might think of endings as informal, almost matter-of-fact "see you later" kinds of experience. They are anything but that. Coaches may never truly know their effect on clients and might rarely grasp the full value, positive or negative, that they may have had. Coaches need to mange endings as carefully as they do beginnings.

None of the processes reviewed in this chapter are absolutes. Presented here are thoughts and reflections derived from extensive experience in the helping professions. Because all relationships are unique, coaches must engage them not in the manner of formulated procedures but as something new, unknown, and essentially unpredictable. Stage theories are not prescriptive; they merely provide models against which coaches can compare and contrast their reality-based encounters with clients.

Building Rapport and Gathering Information

You are about to begin a process of skill review and development for coaching. The dissection of skills in chapters 6 through 8 may create an artificial or at least incomplete sense of the normal flowing dialogue experienced in work with clients. Chapter 9 provides more of the continuing development of conversation between coach and client, but here and in the next two chapters you will be exploring segments of interaction.

You may not immediately grasp why certain skills presented in these chapters are relevant or how the information that you are reading applies in practice. So before you begin I invite you to complete learning activity 6.1, which will suggest that you tape-record either a real or a simulated interview with a client and listen to it a few times throughout the next three chapters as a way of grounding your understanding.

"To be in a life of our own definition, we must be able to discover which stories we are following and determine which ones will help us grow the most interesting possibilities."

Dawna Markova

93

Learning Activity 6.1   Creating a Dialogue for Understanding

A good way to apply information that you will be reviewing in chapters 6 through 8 is by examining elements of an interview that you create with a real or simulated client. Here's what you will need to do:

1. If you are currently working with clients, you may ask one of them for permission to tape-record, for your ears only, an interview in which you discuss with this client some of his goals, attitudes, thoughts, feelings, and behaviors related to exercise and physical activity. Ideally, the person you choose should be someone who is a relatively new client with whom you have had minimal prior contact. If you are not working with clients or if asking one of your current clients does not seem appealing, ask a friend or colleague to simulate an interview about exercise-related thoughts, feelings, and behaviors.

2. Agree to meet for about 30 to 40 minutes in a quiet place where you will not be interrupted and where external noises can be minimized. Tape recorders readily pick up background noise that can have an annoying quality, especially if you listen to the tape several times.

3. Think of a number of questions that you would like to ask your client and write these down in a sequence that makes sense to you. You will use these questions as a guide, but not as a rigid format for the interview. Essentially, you want to treat the interview as a kind of conversation in which you are gathering information from your client and creating as many opportunities as possible for him to speak. Your intention should be to direct the interview and keep the focus on the client. At times, you may need to answer questions that your client asks or provide information or personal data. For the most part, however, your job will be to keep your client talking.

4. Before you begin, ask again for permission to tape-record the interview, reassure your client that only you will listen to it, and promise that you will erase it after you have listened to it a few times.

5. Begin the interview and in your own style proceed to ask questions and discuss issues that come up in the conversation. When you feel that you are at a good stopping place, end the interview and thank your client.

6. Before continuing your reading of chapter 6, listen to the tape at least once.

7. From your own perspective, jot down any impressions you have about your style. Did you ask lots of questions? Did you share personal experiences? Did you provide the client with technical information? Did you make suggestions? Did you ever confront your client with things that you felt were inconsistent?

Now return to chapter 6 with these impressions freshly in mind. You may wish to listen to this tape again just before reading chapters 7 and 8, because the skills described in these chapters may apply better to some of the interactions that you had with your client.

Communication in coaching has a rhythm that must be respected. Clients begin from different places of trust and openness, and they unfold into the relationship at different rates and with varying regressions. Most theories of coaching and counseling assert that certain coaching processes or skills will predominate in particular stages of contact between helper and client, yet this framework implies not only a mechanical methodology but also a linear movement from beginning to end. To

say that a coaching relationship will assume any particular form is to assume that which you cannot know. You will not know who the client is, what he needs, how he will engage the process, and how you will work with him.

Effective coaches need to be ready to move at whatever pace best suits the client. The relationship exists only to serve the client's agenda, and the client and you may pass through the early stages of the working alliance in periods ranging from minutes to hours. What happens during the coaching relationship may involve delays, regressions, or circling back to address issues of information gathering or goal setting more adequately.

Three relatively distinct sets of processes capture the domain of coaching skills. Some of these processes tend to apply more at the beginning of the relationship, whereas others will have more frequent usage when the relationship has been established. One frame for understanding the flow of skill application suggests that coaches must first *attend* to their clients, gaining rapport and understanding, before they attempt to *influence* them in change processes (Ivey & Ivey, 2003). Perhaps more accurately, the skills that coaches might apply distribute themselves along a continuum ranging from rapport building and information gathering at one end to influencing change at the opposite end. In the framework used in this book, we will look at skills along this continuum in three clusters:

1. Rapport building and information gathering skills
2. Skills for developing insight and understanding
3. Skills for organizing, influencing, and guiding change

We will begin in this chapter by exploring the first cluster, rapport building and information gathering skills, along with presenting materials to develop competency in skill usage.

In everyday life, we meet people and sometimes begin a dance of relationship. We show interest, we ask questions, and we make sounds of understanding and empathy. At other times, we are not open or interested in a relationship, so contact is either functional or quickly terminated. Upon reflection, most people might be aware of the specific skills or techniques that they use in moving toward or moving away from others, although they would not likely call them skills but would instead say, "This is what I do."

Throughout the 20th century, dozens of theories of human behavior, communication, helping, counseling, and therapy were articulated and distinguished from one another based on philosophy, clientele, or technique. Yet from the vantage point of the early 21st century, we can now classify all these theories based on their relative emphasis on different types of communications or methods. Indeed, this kind of comparative analysis helps us immensely in simplifying what might otherwise be a bewildering array of seemingly different approaches (Cormier & Nurius, 2003; Ivey & Ivey, 2003; Prochaska & Norcross, 2003).

When life coaching entered the professional arena in the 1990s, it did what so many fields before it attempted. To distinguish itself from other endeavors, it created a new language to describe processes that had become increasingly refined throughout the 20th century in the work of counselors, social workers, communications experts, psychiatrists, and psychologists. Reading some of the emerging literature in coaching has the feel of tasting old wine in new bottles. A more likely characterization of the skill set of this emerging field of coaching is that it places different degrees of emphasis on core skills and methods that other disciplines have amply described. To borrow a phrase, there is little new under the sun.

Returning our attention to everyday life, we know that we do not ask certain questions or say certain things in a first meeting. These norms for behavior have a not-so-surprising overlap with recommendations for communications in the early stages of a coaching relationship.

In the upcoming sections, we must see the skills described as deriving from the broad domain of social and behavioral sciences rather than being unique to coaching. What ultimately makes coaching different is how we apply these skills, so our discussions will attempt to distinguish degrees of emphasis, especially between coaching and the more in-depth endeavors of counseling and psychotherapy.

The Unspoken World of Communication

Nonverbal communication holds a preeminent place in the field of coaching. Early research in this area estimated that nonverbal behavior conveyed 65% of the meaning of a message (Birdwhistle, 1970). Before client and coach exchange their first words, nonverbal communications feed impressions. In fact, in some cultures nonverbal messages receive primary attention with verbal content accorded far less importance (Sue & Sue, 1999).

Nonverbal behavior has been defined as "all human communication events that transcend spoken or written words" (Knapp & Hall, 1997, p. 32). Five dimensions of nonverbal behavior affecting the interpretation and meaning of communication are kinesics, paralinguistics, proxemics, environmental factors, and time.

Kinesics

According to Knapp and Hall (1997), **kinesics** refers to body motions and includes facial expressions, eye movements, gestures, posture, touch, and body movements. Birdwhistle (1970) also incorporates such unchanging aspects of the body as height, weight, and physical appearance in his representation of kinesics. Research on kinesics provides general ideas for extracting meaning from body movements, yet there is a risk of overinterpreting such behaviors. Common sense tells us that arms folded across the chest could mean that a person is cold, whereas the study of kinesics may suggest an attitude of defensiveness.

Eyes

Much of what we sense about another person comes from the eyes. Does the client look at the coach when speaking? What is the client saying with raised eyebrows or furrowed brow? Does the client blink often, or is his gaze more like a stare? How dilated are his pupils? When a great deal of mutual gazing occurs during conversations, one can interpret this as an expression of interest and interpersonal comfort. Obviously, the way the eyes appear as client and coach look at each other will influence interpretations. Eyes that are set and unblinking can convey challenge or upset, whereas eyes that appear soft and blinking at a normal rate (approximately 6 to 10 times per minute) may suggest warmth and interest (Cormier & Nurius, 2003).

When a client is not looking at the coach but rather shifting his eyes from side to side or look-ing down and to the side, the behavior does not necessarily imply avoidance or disinterest. Communication experts in the area of **neurolinguistic programming** (Grinder & Bandler, 1976) argue that eye movements correspond to neural thought processing, and that by observing whether eyes move up or down or side to side, we can obtain clues about how the individual is processing information and the types of thoughts that he is having.

For instance, when the eyes move on a horizontal level from side to side, this theory suggests that people are accessing verbal information, such as remembering the words of past conversations or constructing new sentences in their heads. Eye movements up and to the client's right or left side are thought to represent accessing of visual images, either ones from the past or ones that the individual is creating in the moment. Eye movements down and to the client's right or left may reflect either an internal dialogue (left side) in which the person is talking to himself or the experiencing of a significant emotion such as joy or sadness (right side). One of the more significant implications of this theory is simply that clients may move their eyes to access internal information that a coach may be requesting. For instance, if a coach asks the client to imagine himself doing a particular sport, the client may create a visual image (up and to the right) or remember a time when he had participated in this activity (up and to the left). In either case, neurolinguistic programming would argue that the client's eye movements parallel the information that he is trying to obtain (see figure 6.1).

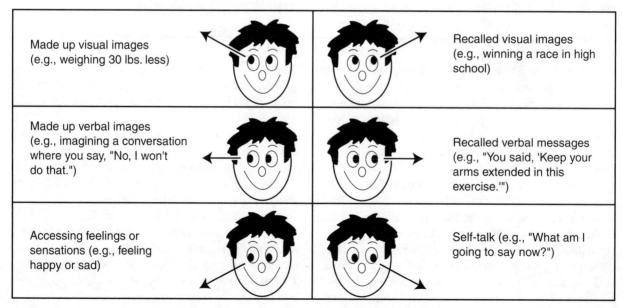

Figure 6.1 The neurolinguistic programming model of the relation of eye movements to internal experience.

Another perspective on eye contact comes from studies of cultural differences (Knapp & Hall, 1997; Sue & Sue, 1999). Many white North Americans equate eye contact with listening, whereas those in other cultures may see eye contact as bold and confronting. Lowered eyes while speaking may be a way that some cultural groups show respect and deference in conversations.

Mouth

When a client is not speaking, the expressions of lips and mouth may communicate a great deal. Common interpretations of being tight lipped suggest experiences of control, anger, frustration, or repression. When a person turns down the edges of the mouth, we may read sadness or disappointment. If the client's mouth drops wide open, we may interpret surprise or shock. Biting of the lips may express tension, and a relaxed easy smile may communicate satisfaction or pleasure.

Facial Expressions

Ekman's (1982, 1993) scientific studies of facial expressions and emotion have confirmed much of what we may intuitively sense when looking at another person. Although the face is one of the body areas that we learn to control most, in unguarded moments we often reveal more than we want. Ekman's work indicates that different facial areas tend to convey different emotions. We can usually see anger in the brows and lower face. Fear appears in the eyes. The mouth and jaw tend to display surprise and disgust, as well as the emotion of happiness. Although opinions vary, cultural differences usually do not influence basic emotional responses shown in the face.

Head

What does it mean when someone tilts her head to the side or plays with her hair? Some believe (Fast, 1989) that angling one's head to the side may represent a questioning or doubting attitude about the matter in discussion, but it could also mean that a person has a hearing impairment in one ear. Playing with one's hair has been linked to a kind of coquettishness or nervousness. A rigidly held head can reflect anger or tension, and hanging one's head down toward the chest may mean disappointment or sadness. Nodding the head up and down displays the more obvious message of agreement or compliance. Similarly, shaking the head from side to side may mean disagreement.

Shoulders

From a seated position, leaning into the conversation may express interest and attention, yet leaning too far forward could convey aggression. Shoulders that are sloped downward may indicate disappointment or depression, whereas shoulders turned inward toward the chest may represent nonreceptivity. Shoulders elevated toward the ears may indicate that a person is experiencing fear or anxiety (Dychtwald, 1977). A shrug of the shoulders could convey doubt, uncertainty, or indecision.

Torso

How a person stands may reflect attitudes of assurance, rigidity, dependency, or self-esteem (Dychtwald, 1977; Kurz & Prestera, 1976). A slouched posture with abdomen protruding may indicate dependency or lack of assertiveness, whereas a rigidly erect posture could convey defensiveness and a controlling attitude. A rounding of the spine may indicate lack of confidence and low self-esteem.

Arms and Hands

We can readily see tension or anger in hands clenched into fists, and fidgeting motions with the hands communicate messages of anxiety. Arms folded across the chest generally represent a defensive or closed attitude. Relaxed and easy movements of hands and arms suggest openness and involvement, whereas rigidly held arms and hands can indicate anxiety or self-restraint (Dychtwald, 1977; Kurz & Prestera, 1976).

Legs and Feet

Shifting one's weight from foot to foot in a standing position may indicate impatience, and standing on one leg with the other foot wrapped in front can suggest insecurity (Dychtwald, 1977; Fast, 1989). In a standing position, locked knees can indicate rigidity, as might be seen in a military brace. From a seated posture, crossing the legs toward or away from the other person may reflect intimacy (toward) or distance (away). Generally, people interpret foot tapping or a wagging foot as a sign of anxiety or impatience.

Total Bodily Movement

Ekman (1982, 1993) discusses the function of body movement as adaptive to the person's internal experience. Body touching, scratching, rubbing, or other repetitive body movements may reflect the person's psychological discomfort. When the body moves easily, in a rhythmic pattern in relation to the other person's movements, we can read harmony and synchronicity into the relationship. Conversely, when two people in communication display very different amounts of total body activity, the behavior suggests not only disharmony or conflict but also a kind of power dynamic in which the more mobile body conveys greater discomfort than the body that is steadier in movement.

Touch

A final dimension of kinesics to consider is the extent and manner of touching in a **dyadic relationship.** In more depth-oriented helping relationships such as counseling and psychotherapy, all forms of touching may be seen as problematic, but health fitness professionals may engage in various kinds of touching, sometimes for corrective purposes (e.g., postural alignment) and other times in more spontaneous expressions (e.g., celebrations of achievements). Handshakes in most professions are considered acceptable, and certainly the quality of handshakes may reveal much about the relationship. Two-handed clasps versus limp-handed shakes suggest something not only about the relationship but also about the personality dimensions of each party. The bone crusher is communicating something about an attitude of strength and perhaps dominance, as compared with the person whose handshake is lifeless.

Paralinguistics

We listen not only to the words but also to the "music" of speech. At what volume does someone speak? Where are the intonations, that is, what words or expressions does the person emphasize? When and how often does someone pause? Is the quality of speech fluid or staccato? Is a quivering present in the person's speech, or is it steady and strong? Although these **paralinguistics** may characterize a person's general speech pattern, they may also vary depending on the subject or shifts in the relationship. As Sue and Sue (1999) point out, we should also consider cultural background when interpreting paralinguistic features. North Americans are characteristically described as having louder voice levels than those of some other cultures.

Silence or pauses in speech can convey much meaning. The refusal to answer, a hesitation before responding, or the respectful silence following another person's self-revelation may communicate much more than the words themselves do.

A person hesitating before answering a sensitive question may reveal the truth before he speaks the words. Silence can be a means of control or a method of creating space for the other to reflect.

Effective coaches need to become comfortable with silence and learn to use conversational pauses to help clients shift perspectives or levels of communication. Different cultures have different norms about silence (Sue & Sue, 1999). North Americans often interpret a pause in the conversation as disruptive or indicative of discomfort, and therefore something to avoid. We strive to avoid the void, to fill the gap, and to disallow the pregnant pause. Coaches must learn to use silence in service of clients' agendas, and to quell their own anxiety in the absence of verbal communication.

The effective use of silence is a major component of skill development for coaches. Recognizing that many clients will experience some discomfort with silence, coaches need to manage this process. In the early phases of the relationship, an overuse of silence by coaches can unduly augment client anxiety. Later on, when coaches have established rapport and trust, clients may welcome silence as opportunities to reflect.

Proxemics

Most of us know at what physical distance from another we feel most comfortable. When someone moves beyond the outer boundaries of our personal space (Hall, 1966, 1976), we may experience anxiety, irritation, fear, or an agreement to become more intimate. In helping relationships in a North American context, physical distance of 3 to 4 feet between helper and client tends to be experienced as comfortable (Lecomte, Bernstein, & Dumont, 1981).

Proxemics involves both the consideration of personal space and the arrangement of environmental space. The positioning of seating in a room has great implications for communication and the interpretation of meaning. Furniture placed between client and helper serves as a buffer and may help increase comfort in some cases, whereas in other cases such a configuration can create a sense of distance or power dynamics, especially if the object is a desk. Coaches need to be sensitive to seating arrangements or office configurations in terms of how they may affect clients, especially those with a different cultural heritage.

Environment

Where clients meet with coaches has meaning and conveys intended or unintended messages. Health fitness professionals have traditionally operated from the bases of fitness centers, health facilities, or sport complexes. Lifestyle fitness coaches are likely to continue to rely on these locations for contacts with clients. Given the potentially sensitive nature of some discussions, however, coaches may need to meet with clients behind closed doors or in private areas of fitness complexes. Some of these spaces may have multiple uses so that extra care may be required to prepare the environment before a coaching session. As in the profession of personal training, coaches may also want to consider meeting at clients' homes and what conditions they might negotiate with clients for this venue to be viable. For instance, a client's private home fitness area may be appropriate. But if the client allows interruption by other members of the household or by telephone calls, contracting may need to include discussion of those elements.

Of course, two other environments are possible for coaching—the telephone and the Internet. Some coaching sessions may take place on the phone, and coaches may want to discuss boundaries with clients about times of telephone contact and the inviolability of the session. If a client is multitasking (e.g., working on a computer, driving a car, sorting through papers) while talking with the coach, the effectiveness of the session may be negatively affected. The Internet may serve as a means of transmitting guidelines, information, or other messages. Some coaches may even use processes like instant messaging or special chat rooms for real-time discussions with clients.

Time

Time can serve both as a framework for sessions and as a focus in discussions. Coaches and clients may have different perceptions of and preferences for meeting times. With the flexibility of telephone interviews, clients may have greater latitude in when they can converse with coaches. The dilemma in many helping professions is that clients generally prefer certain hours. Clients want to meet before or after normal 9-to-5 work hours. The options of telephone-based coaching and Internet exchanges may partially mitigate this difficulty.

Time also can be seen in regard to the duration of sessions and respect for agreed-on periods. Clients or coaches who are habitually late or who cancel at the last minute convey messages that may imply lack of commitment, interest, or regard for the other party. Cultural factors may affect how people view time (Cormier & Nurius, 2003).

Sessions that habitually run over may convey unintended messages and establish patterns. Clients may begin to interpret the 30-minute session as a 35- to 40-minute session and will come to expect it. Sessions sometimes run long because of the sensitivity of discussions, and clients may see coaches as more or less generous or considerate based on how they deal with time limits. In the older professions of counseling and psychotherapy, sessions tend to begin and end on time irrespective of topics discussed or the emotionality of clients at the end of the hour. Although rigidly enforced time

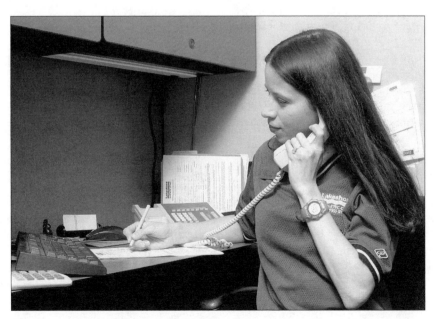

Coaches and clients may use the telephone and the Internet for occasional coaching sessions.

boundaries may adversely affect client perceptions of the coach's caring and support, lax boundaries are problematic in other ways. One specific issue is that open-ended meetings communicate to clients that the relationship is more like friendship than professional guidance.

A final consideration of time centers on where coaches and clients locate their discussions—in the present, past, or future. A hallmark of coaching is its emphasis on present and future rather than past. Knowing what a person has experienced, what has happened to him before the coaching relationship, or what has worked well for him in the past can be critically important. Coaches, however, tend to move quickly from this type of historical analysis into future-oriented planning. Some clients may come to sessions prepared to describe their successes and failures over the intervening period between sessions. Although this past focus may be necessary, the coach will typically move the discussion quickly into thoughts about how to improve the situation in the upcoming week, rather than dwell on potential causes or reasons through analysis of the past.

Clients express different amounts of energy for moving forward and varying degrees of resistance to leaving the past behind. Counseling and psychotherapy have been characterized as emphasizing the past to understand client behaviors, but even this stereotype is breaking down. With the advent of time-limited or solution-focused treatments (de Shazer, 1985; O'Hanlon & Weiner-Davis, 1989), the percentage of time directed toward unearthing potential causes of behavior is diminishing to permit greater investment in exploring action strategies for future behavior.

Coaches will nonetheless need to be sensitive to their clients' preferred pacing and their need to tell their stories. For some cultural groups, historical considerations carry greater weight, and coaches must allow for examination of the past in the coaching relationship (Cormier & Nurius, 2003).

Practical Implications

Lifestyle fitness coaches will benefit from increased awareness of and sensitivity to nonverbal communications, from both the client and themselves. Just as words can have different meanings, so too can nonverbal gestures vary in meaning according to context. As the coaching relationship develops, coaches will be able to discuss some of the hypotheses that they develop from clients' nonverbal behaviors. In the early stages of coaching,

coaches may need only to note these nonverbal cues without attributing absolute interpretations to them.

The most important message about the nonverbal domain is that it tends to function at a more unconscious level than verbal behaviors do. In this regard, coaches will need to be deliberate in their efforts to attend to and integrate these messages into their work with clients. Moreover, as a coach you must also study what you communicate nonverbally. In your training as a coach, you should arrange to be videotaped in simulated sessions with clients. The power of this experience is inestimable. You may discover habitual nonverbal patterns that heretofore you had never recognized. You may see how your nonverbal cues direct clients to speak either more or less about certain subjects and how you unintentionally communicate attitudes.

Some common guidelines are relevant to coaches in face-to-face sessions, yet the coach must always consider the unique characteristics and needs of the individual client. How far coach and client sit from one another, the degree of direct eye contact, the volume of speech, and the speed of speech may depend as much on who the client is as on cultural norms for such behaviors. The best feedback comes through self-observation and requests for information. As noted, videotaping sessions can provide a world of insight. In addition, asking clients about the meaning of certain nonverbal behaviors or requesting feedback from them about their observations may broaden understanding and increase coaching effectiveness.

Active Listening to Enhance Understanding

Different theorists discussing helper behaviors that promote understanding of clients have essentially identified the same set of core skills. The term *listening* is an encompassing concept that most of these theorists have identified (Cormier & Nurius, 2003). Each of us has our own definition of listening and the behavioral cues that imply whether someone is listening or not. Some writers prefer the term *active listening* (Ivey & Ivey, 2003) because it describes a process whereby listeners make deliberate responses to the speaker to communicate clearly that they are attending to what the speaker is saying. For instance, someone may be listening with rapt attention, but the speaker can nonetheless misinterpret the listener's body language as showing disinterest. To avoid this possibility, active listening involves such behaviors as verbal reflections, or directly mirroring back to the person the essence of their communications and feelings. We will review four skills under the heading of active listening and offer practice scenarios for the development of coaching competencies. These skills are minimal encouragers, reflection of content, reflection of feeling, and summarization.

Minimal Encouragers

Young (2001, p. 85) defines **minimal encouragers** as "brief supportive statements that convey attention and understanding." Often without awareness, we use minimal encouragers when we listen intently to another's story. Almost subvocally we say, "Mmm-hmmm." With more awareness, we attend to someone's story with words like "Yes, I hear you," "Right," or "OK." Another type of minimal encourager occurs in the repetition of key words in a client's message (Ivey & Ivey, 2003). A body posture reflecting attention (forward lean, good eye contact) and a nodding head typically accompany such expressions. Minimal encouragers have the advantage of supporting the client without interrupting the story.

Some important caveats attend the use of minimal encouragers. Coaches know when they themselves are listening to clients; clients, on the other hand, may not know they are being heard. Perhaps more importantly, clients may not know *how* they are being heard, that is, whether the coach is listening critically, judgmentally, or empathically. In an attempt to be objective and nonjudgmental, your face may be masklike and paradoxically create the exact opposite impression. Although you may believe that your nonverbal attentiveness adequately demonstrates your interest, clients who feel stressed by the encounter or by the disclosure of intimate details usually appreciate overt messages of support and encouragement. Although it may not be your habit to encourage with minimal verbal remarks, the practice has much to recommend it.

In a coach's interactions with a client, the timing of minimal encouragers may coincide with a certain content area of the story or a certain dimension of the client's self-presentation. For instance, whenever a client talks about a success or achievement, the coach may respond with an enthusiastic "Mmm-hmmm." Otherwise, there may be silence. Or perhaps, whenever the client expresses emotions or feelings, the coach may react with minimal verbal encouragers. Another way in which coaches may intentionally or unintentionally direct clients with minimal encouragers is by reflecting certain types of key words that the client uses (such as any word conveying success). If we take behavioral conditioning principles to heart, this response may unintentionally reinforce presentations of particular themes or types of content. Clients may begin to dredge up any remotely connected story of achievement in their histories to get the reward of the minimal encourager. Or, if the coach is responding to emotional content, clients may begin to dwell on their feelings. Coaches who are unaware of their influence on clients' communications may formulate impressions of their clients that are, in fact, distorted by their own unintentional behavior-shaping reinforcements. The point to bear in mind is that minimal encouragers serve to keep clients talking, yet because they act as behavioral reinforcements, they influence the direction of a conversation or the depth of the discussion. Selective use of minimal encouragers increases the client's presentation of whatever material the coach reinforces. Incidentally, a nonverbal behavior such as nodding or smiling will have similar effects of encouraging the client to say more about whatever is being discussed at the moment.

Coaches need to use minimal encouragers with awareness and in synchrony with the client's storytelling. Paralinguistic features of speed or volume may create entirely different client experiences of a coach's words. Saying, "I hear you" in a loud, fast-paced voice will have an entirely different effect on a client than saying the same words softly and evenly. In addition, a coach may easily convey impatience or even boredom through the overuse or untimely application of minimal encouragers. Coaches who repeatedly say, "Mmm-hmm . . . mmm-hmm . . . mmm-hmm" may seem to be saying to the client, "OK, I've heard enough about this. Let's move on to something else."

Another caveat is that coaches may tend to use minimal encouragers as a prelude to speaking. A coach may say, "Right" or "I hear you" just before interrupting the client's flow to provide feedback, instruction, or another kind of commentary. Clients who are sensitive to the timing of these interventions will soon learn to stop talking as soon as the coach utters the cue that she intends to say something.

Reflection of Content

Some writers refer to reflection of content as paraphrasing (Ivey & Ivey, 2003), and others call it mirroring (Hendrix, 2001). Paraphrasing is a skill whereby the coach "feeds back to the client the essence of what has just been said" (Ivey & Ivey, 2003, p. 125). The coach takes the principle words and content of the client's message and feeds it back to the client in a manner that in no way resembles parroting or mimicking. The term **reflection of content** is perhaps more precise than the term *paraphrasing* because it limits the feedback to the content of the message. Another skill to be discussed later, reflection of feeling, feeds back the emotional or feeling dimension of the client's message. Putting these two together often creates a more complete mirroring of the client's message, although a coach may have a strategic reason for reflecting content and not feeling, or reflecting feeling and not content.

Reflection of content is not, in Young's (2001, p. 98) definition, a "word-for-word reiteration." Rather, it is a distillation of the client's primary message. Reflection of content has greater effect than a minimal encourager in demonstrating to the client that the coach is listening attentively, without pressuring the client to respond in a specific way as might occur through asking questions. Reflection of content is probably one of the most misunderstood and underestimated skills in the helping professions. When it is well done, the client is mostly unaware that it is happening yet somehow feels buoyed by the conversation and encouraged to go deeper into the story toward self-discovery and clarity of vision. When it is done poorly, the client can experience paraphrasing as irritating, demeaning, or even mocking.

Ironically, the longer one works as a helping professional, the more likely it is that he will assume that the client knows he is listening, and jump to the stage of intervention because it is so obvious (to the helper) where the client is going in the story. In Rogers' (1951, 1961) model of the helping relationship, reflections or paraphrases are the central skills for helpers to master. Elegant paraphrasing nourishes the conditions that clients need to experience in order to unfold naturally and discover their own meanings and solutions.

Purposes of Reflection of Content

Reflections of content serve many functions in working with clients. For one, reflections enable clients to experience a sense of being heard and, thereby, to feel that the coach supports them. Second, as noted previously, by hearing their own words reflected back, they have opportunities to reflect on their thoughts and issues and to modify, evaluate, or acknowledge them for what they are.

Third, reflections that capture the essence of clients' communications focus them on the issues of greatest importance. Sometimes a client can be so caught up in thoughts and feelings that only through the coach's timely reflections can the client move out of a spin into a focused dialogue.

From the coach's perspective, a reflection of content can be invaluable in a number of situations. Sometimes coaches will have so much information before them that they do not know which path to choose. A competent paraphrase allows the coach to identify all the leads that a client has put out and thereby place responsibility for direction appropriately on the client's shoulders. In a related sense, a coach who is highly oriented to action may feel the compulsion to do something or to make something happen, even while realizing that the timing is wrong. To slow the process, coaches can rely on reflections to help clients complete their stories or fill in pieces that coaches sense are missing. Of course, coaches can overuse reflections, although the likelihood is greater that coaches will underuse them by favoring influencing skills (see chapter 8).

This skill has one additional value worth noting. When coaches experience conflicts with clients, verbal exchanges often accelerate at the expense of listening. Almost in an effort to prove who is right, each party details their evidence and impatiently awaits the termination of the other's litany to provide the conclusive argument. Even when the coach is factually correct, he must relegate the dynamic of proving the case to secondary status and focus on hearing the client's perspective. When clients become upset with coaches or seem to have a need to make the coach wrong, the use of reflection of content becomes a critical coaching aid. Allowing the client to experience herself as being heard takes some of the steam out of the argument, while also creating space for the client to reflect on her own words. From the stance of nondefensive listening, the coach empathically hears the client and accurately summarizes the client's thoughts and perceptions.

Steps in Reflection of Content

Training guidelines for novice helpers offer useful structures for developing competency in the use of reflection of content. Ivey and Ivey (2003, pp. 133-134), for example, indicate that an effective paraphrase comprises four elements:

1. **Sentence stem.** Saying things like, "What you seem to be saying is . . . ," "Sounds like . . . ," "What I'm hearing from you is . . . ," or "You're tell-

ing me that . . ." initiates the reflection of content. Sometimes the coach might add the client's name at the outset of the reflection; at other times the reflection moves right into the content without much of a sentence stem.

2. **Key words.** The coach identifies key words or expressions that the client has mentioned over the past few minutes and captures them in phrases and sentences. When the client's words may be ambiguous or are likely to have unique meaning, the coach will want to repeat them exactly rather than use synonyms or seemingly similar expressions.

3. **Expressing content.** In a timely fashion, the coach intervenes by summarizing the content of the client's most recent expressions. A reflection of content occurs in proximal relation to the time when the client presented the material. But the coach offers it at a point when the client may have paused or when the client appears to be seeking feedback or response from the coach. If the client seems highly charged in telling his story, a reflection could interrupt the flow. In this instance, minimal encouragers would likely work better. Essentially, the client's behavior will determine the timing, not the coach's need to paraphrase.

4. **Verification.** Reflecting content can be risky. The client may not realize what he has said, and upon hearing his own words fed back to him, he may reject the presentation as an inaccurate portrayal of the issues. Moreover, the coach may have used synonymous expressions that failed to capture the true meaning intended by the client. For reasons such as these, the fourth element recommended by Ivey and Ivey (2003) is an accuracy check. The reflection might end with such questions as "Is this what you were saying?" "Am I hearing you accurately?" or "Is this what you mean?" Sometimes a client's nonverbal communications make such accuracy checks unnecessary, while at other times they indicate that you are off track even before you have finished your summary. Coaches must not be invested in being right. Even when you have perfectly mirrored a client's words, he may reject the paraphrase because hearing it aloud is either too threatening or simply is not what he intended to communicate. Clients have the right to change their minds and to say things differently, and that option is one of the many benefits of reflections. Until someone verbalizes his internal world, he may not fully know it. Only in its expression may it acquire reality and value. In a process of self-discovery, many clients will find themselves contradicting things that they said earlier in a session as they come to fuller realizations of their deep-felt meanings.

Uses and Abuses of Reflection of Content

Too much of a good thing can turn things sour. Clients hire coaches to clarify and implement change processes directed toward goal attainment and life fulfillment. Reflection of content is a rapport-building skill that serves some other critical functions in the coaching process. Ideally, clients become more self-directing and self-motivating through the coaching process, but at the outset they may require direction, support, and external motivation. Becoming autonomous may be a lifelong process. Coaching provides clients with structures for identifying goals, clarifying needs, action planning, implementation, and self-evaluation. In so doing, coaches need to rely on more than a reflective skill set.

We have considered the intended purposes and uses of reflection of content, yet this skill has some problematic sides, such as the following:

- **Slow rate of progress.** If clients have to discover all their issues, needs, goals, and action plans through an introspective process encouraged by reflective techniques, they will need a great deal of time—often far more than most are willing to commit. Progress may seem slow, and consequently clients may become demoralized if this skill becomes the basis for coaching.

- **Intervening too deeply.** Reflection supports clients in looking inward and understanding their issues thoroughly. When coaches combine reflection of content with reflection of feeling (see next section), clients may become too introspective and coaching may begin to resemble psychotherapy. Coaches only need to know enough about clients' histories and internal worlds to support the structuring and implementation of robust and viable action planning. The reflective process can encourage clients to talk about issues far beyond the relevant working agenda for lifestyle fitness coaching.

- **Reflection as a defense.** You have surely been in a conversation in which you asked a question of another person and the person responded with a question back to you. You probably experienced this as a defensive strategy by the other person. A client might ask you a question, give you feedback, criticize you, or express a myriad of emotions, and you can choose to respond with a reflection. Sometimes this is appropriate, whereas at other times a reflection can be defensive and unwarranted. Rather than answering a client's questions or responding to his feedback, you may reflect his input, perhaps in the mistaken belief that it would be better for him to answer his own questions or to understand more about his concerns. Although this misuse occurs, it probably occurs far less often than the opposite case does, in which coaches respond to questions when they should be reflecting them back to the client.

• **Mechanical reflections.** Some discussions of paraphrasing or reflection place its usage in a sequence of communication (Young, 2001). Knowing how to integrate this skill with others to form effective communications is useful, yet if the coach applies reflection in a mechanical manner because that is what the textbook recommends, it will likely backfire. Reflection needs to be appropriate to the moment, not a formula application.

Reflection of Feeling

Paraphrasing or reflection of content generally pertains to the cognitive part of a client's message (Cormier & Nurius, 2003), while **reflection of feeling** is an accurate restatement of the emotional or affective part of the client's message. The coach must distinguish here between emotions that a client talks about having experienced as part of a story and those that the client is experiencing in the moment. To complicate this slightly more, another variation of feeling expression in a session occurs when a client says that she is experiencing a particular emotion while her nonverbal communications strongly indicate that she is experiencing some other emotion.

We may interpret reflection of feeling as representing all three of these types of emotional expressions, that is, historical experiences of emotional states, present emotional states, and conflicting messages (verbal versus nonverbal) reflective of emotional states. A historical account of feelings may be accompanied by descriptive details that minimize their importance (e.g., "Oh, it was silly to feel that way") or that in other ways distance the person from the emotion (e.g., "Well that was a long time ago—it doesn't bother me at all now"). In these cases, the reflection of feeling may be more like a reflection of content, or paraphrase. Here is an example:

Client: "I used to feel self-conscious and embarrassed about my weight, but I don't feel as sensitive about it anymore . . . Even so, I would like to lose about 30 pounds just for health reasons."

Coach: "So, you no longer feel sensitive about your weight, but for health reasons you still think it would be wise to lose about 30 pounds. Is that accurate?"

Another possibility is that the person describes an uncomfortable feeling in the past and expresses a similar emotion in the context of coaching. Here, the reflection would likely include a paraphrase of the experience and a clear reflection of feeling of the present emotion. This might happen as follows:

Client: "I have always felt self-conscious and embarrassed about my weight—ever since I can remember [blushes, shows obvious discomfort, eyes become moist] . . . but now as an adult my motivation to lose weight is primarily driven by health concerns."

Coach: "As you were describing your discomfort around weight issues, I was aware of how some feelings seem to be with you right now as we speak."

In this reflection, the emphasis is on the feeling more than on the content. The rationale for this might be that by addressing these emotions more fully, the client will be better able to make clear commitments and motivate himself to adhere to exercise agreements.

When clients experience emotions in a coaching session yet do not state exactly what the feeling is, the coach will first need to identify what the emotion is and second decide whether it is appropriate to reflect it. Coaches can show empathy for clients by expressing concern through nonverbal messages, but the use of reflection of feeling makes implicit issues explicit. Coaches need to have a clear rationale for directly focusing on emotional content in sessions. You will notice in the previous example that the coach deliberately focused on the client's emotions without labeling them. Although the coach might have thought that the nonverbal cues represented emotions of sadness, by avoiding direct labeling of the feelings the coach provides the client with wide latitude to address his feelings at whatever level or depth he feels comfortable.

Of the three types of emotional expressions noted in the preceding discussion, the case of conflicting emotional expressions will demand of coaches more than a simple application of reflection of feeling. When clients verbalize one emotion but manifest another nonverbally, coaches must choose how to deal with this information. Although coaches can reflect both the words and the nonverbal behaviors, the fact that they contain conflicting sets of information serves to caution coaches about the skills that they may need to use should they decide to address this matter in the moment. We will postpone this discussion until chapter 8, when we present the skill of confrontation and show how it applies to situations like this.

Purposes of Reflection of Feeling

Cormier and Nurius (2003) identify five purposes for using reflection of feeling in a helping relationship. First, a reflection of feeling helps the client identify what her emotional experience (positive or negative) might be in a certain situation, with a particular person, or about a specific topic. Emotions serve as key sources of energy for movement toward or away from people, situations, or activities. Knowing whether a client likes something is helpful, although it may not always be evident in the client's verbal descriptions. The coach may have to infer a client's positive or negative response more from nonverbal cues than from verbal cues.

A second purpose of reflection of feeling is to increase the client's capacity to cope with and manage emotions. Because some clients may believe that they should minimize emotional expression, especially when these emotions are labeled as negative, they may experience considerable tension in their lives from the ongoing repression of emotions. Containing emotions takes effort, and when clients fear others' reactions to their emotions, they may be doubly guarded against allowing their emotions to become visible. In this case, clients may develop unrealistic beliefs about the consequences of emotional expression without having opportunity to experiment safely with emotional expression. Although lifestyle fitness coaching is not counseling or therapy, it shares elements of empowering clients through validating their experiences. If a client feels disappointed about progress or perhaps anger toward himself for not following a plan, coaches can facilitate the client's expression of those feelings rather than ignoring them or allowing the client to deny their significance. As clients express emotions in a coaching process, they learn how to release these feelings safely so that ultimately they feel less controlled by them. Feelings are just that, but when people continually repress, deny, rationalize, or otherwise contain them, they may take on proportions far larger than the realities they represent. Just as a healthy grieving process will typically include the expression of a range of emotions, so too growth and development are likely to incorporate a variety of appropriate emotional reactions that serve to inform and motivate intelligent action.

A third purpose of reflection of feeling relates to the coaching relationship itself. At different times, clients may have reactions to the experience or to the coach. A common occurrence might arise when the client is not making progress and needs to find someone to blame. Perhaps the coach has misjudged some critical elements, or it might be that the client has failed to comply with the agreed-on plan. Resistance is usually a subtle expression of the client's emotional reactions (Ivey & Ivey, 2003). Behaviors such as lateness for sessions, nonpayment of fees, unreturned telephone calls, or a kind of passive–aggressive reaction to the coach's suggestions are forms of resistance. By taking the risk of identifying evidence of resistance, coaches can enable clients to deal with obstacles to progress. When feelings about the coach or the coaching process remain unexpressed, clients' abilities to address issues impeding goal attainment will diminish. Eventually, clients may terminate in dissatisfaction. A critical competency of coaches is their ability to face clients' emotionality toward them. In all cases, coaches must regard these emotions with respect and never turn them back against the client, even when the client is projecting blame on the coach.

A fourth purpose of reflection of feeling identified by Cormier and Nurius (2003) is educational. Often if you ask someone how she feels, she will respond with a thought.

Coach: "How do you feel about not finishing the race today?"

Client: "I feel that I could have if only I had prepared better."

We can characterize feelings in different ways. Hutchins and Vaught (1997) suggest five categories of emotions: anger, conflict, fear, happiness, and sadness. Within each category are different levels, with words representing degrees of those emotional experiences. Some examples of types and levels of feeling expressions are offered in figure 6.2. For instance, a person might express a low level of sadness as feeling *disappointed* or *low*. She might show a moderate level of sadness in words like *dejected*, *sad*, or *blue*. Words like *hopeless*, *depressed*, or *crushed* might communicate a strong level of sadness.

Coaches can help clients distinguish among different emotions they are experiencing as well as identify the levels of feelings they are having. With clients who underestimate or overestimate emotional realities, coaches who can distinguish levels of feeling can more effectively assess progress or understand reactions to the coaching agenda. Some clients may not even have a vocabulary for emotion, and they simply spin in undifferentiated states of feeling without knowing what the

Level \ Type	Glad	Sad	Mad	Distressed
Strong	Ecstatic Overjoyed Delirious Blissful	Depressed Crushed Disconsolate Stricken Tearful Hopeless	Furious Outraged Enraged Livid Infuriated Boiling	Frightened Terrified Scared Dreading Panicky
Moderate	Cheerful Happy Delighted Joyful	Dejected Cheerless Sad Down Blue	Mad Stormy Angry Antagonized Incensed	Agitated Frustrated Upset Flustered Rattled
Low	Pleased Glad Content Cheery	Low Bored Disappointed Dour	Upset Ticked Displeased Ruffled Vexed Disgruntled	Anxious Apprehensive Confused Dismayed Uneasy Bothered

Figure 6.2 Examples of levels and types of feelings.

implications might be or how to shift out of those feelings. Although the coaching agenda is not directly about developing emotional competency, such growth may be either part of the means of goal attainment or one of the ends itself. For instance, a client may need to be able to identify concrete feeling states about his experiences in doing different sports and fitness activities (means), whereas another client may wish to become more assertive through physical training and as part of that work become able to differentiate between such emotions as anxiety, fear, and excitement (ends). Figure 6.3 provides some practical distinctions between pseudoexpressions of emotions and genuine feeling statements.

The fifth purpose of reflection of feeling is similar to one for reflection of content, namely, to convey empathy and understanding. Think of the norms for everyday greetings. We normally respond to the question "How are you today?" with the response "Oh, fine. How are you?" Talking about emotional experiences is generally an intimate act. Even when we take risks to expose our feelings ("Actually, I'm kind of blue today"), the response we get may be minimizing or rationalizing ("Yeah, must be the weather" or "Don't worry, it will pass"). To be

Pseudoexpressions of feelings	may indicate the following	real expressions of feelings.
I'm feeling that you aren't really listening.		I'm feeling lonely. I'm annoyed.
I'm really feeling that you don't care about me.		I'm feeling sad. I feel rejected.
I feel like you're not going to help me.		I'm disappointed. I'm frightened.
I'm feeling that I'm never going to reach my goals.		I'm worried. I'm feeling hopeless.
I feel that everyone here is in a great mood.		I'm happy. I'm enjoying being here.

Figure 6.3 Pseudo- and real expressions of feelings.

heard with empathy when we express emotions can be tremendously validating and often helpful in enabling us to move beyond our present feeling states.

Steps in Reflection of Feeling

Guidelines for reflection of feeling are similar to those for reflection of content (Brammer & MacDonald, 1999; Ivey & Ivey, 2003; Cormier & Nurius, 2003). The structure might consist of the following four elements:

1. **Sentence stem.** Choose a way of introducing the reflection that is nonrepetitive and appropriate to your own style of speaking. Examples might include such sentence stems as these: "Sounds like you are feeling . . . ," "What I'm hearing is that you are feeling . . . ," "I sense that you are feeling . . . ," or "You're saying that you are feeling . . ." Note that these sentence stems are phrased in the present tense. Depending on whether the client is discussing past or present feelings, the tense of the verb needs to reflect the timing of the experience. So if the client is recalling a past emotion, the sentence stem might be "What I'm hearing is that you were feeling . . ."

2. **Key emotions.** The coach identifies the key emotions in the client's story or current experience. When clients report or are experiencing strong emotions that they accurately articulate, coaches will need to exercise care in how they reflect those feelings. Using synonyms may inadvertently minimize or exaggerate clients' emotional experiences and thereby diminish rapport between coach and client. Sometimes using the client's exact words when reflecting feelings is safest. When clients use words that either minimize or exaggerate their actual emotional responses, coaches may confront this perceived discrepancy, but this approach involves communication skills far beyond reflection (see the section on confrontation in chapter 8). In instances when the client only hints at emotions or conveys feelings through nonverbal behaviors, coaches would be wise to be even more tentative than normal in their reflections. In these cases, the coach might use different sentence stems, including ones like the following: "I can't be certain about this, but I'm getting the impression that you are feeling . . ." or "I have a hunch that you might be feeling . . ." As a rule of thumb, when clients do not explicitly state their feelings and coaches decide to reflect clients' nonverbal cues, slight underestimation of the level of emotion would likely work better than overesti-

mation. In general, clients have resistance to owning emotions that are less than positive, so reflections that potentially feed back stronger emotional experiences than clients are willing to own could cause clients to retreat into defensive intellectualizations or even criticisms of the coach.

3. **Expressing emotion combined with content.** The timing of reflections of feelings is critical. They need to occur close to the moment of the actual expression of the emotion or the telling of the emotion-laden story. Depending on whether the coach has recently paraphrased the client's content, the coach may want to embed the reflection of feeling in a content reflection. A reflection of feeling without content, as long as the coach offers it in a timely fashion, can be extremely effective in shifting the client's focus to the emotional experiences relevant to the discussion. Such a reflection communicates to the client the coach's sensitivity to and caring about the client's emotional world. Unlike reflections of content, feeling reflections may be effective when the coach inserts them in momentary pauses rather than when the client has more obviously finished a thought or a story. These reflections can be quick and supportive, as exemplified by such reflections as "Ouch, sounds like that hurt!" or "Wow, I really sense how happy you are." If a client is still in the midst of an emotion or the telling of an emotional story, the coach can use nonverbal indicators of awareness of the client's feelings or minimal encouragers to support the client in continuing to tell the story and communicating the acceptability of the emotional content. The use of reflections of feeling always needs to be appropriate to the agenda that the client is projecting and the client's readiness to face emotions. The main exception to this guideline would be when the coach reflects positive feelings such as joy or happiness.

4. **Verification.** Reflecting emotion can be even riskier than reflecting content. As noted earlier, clients may not be aware of their emotions, or they may not be ready to own them. Even if the coach has accurately captured the client's emotional experiences in the reflection, completing the reflection with an accuracy check may nonetheless be beneficial. The reflection might end with such questions as "Is this what you're feeling?" or "Do I sense your feelings correctly?" or "Am I right about this?" The client's response may be to give nonverbal agreement or continue in the discussion at a deeper level. When the reflection is inaccurate or the client is unready to acknowledge his emotions, the client's feedback will provide clear guidance

to the coach about how next to proceed. The client may want to clarify, justify, minimize, intellectualize, deny, or avoid. Rather than pursuing the subject or attempting to prove to the client that her (the coach's) perceptions are accurate, the coach needs to follow the client's lead. This approach does not mean agreeing with denials or minimizations but rather slowing down the process so that the client can regain composure and control in the moment.

Uses and Abuses of Reflection of Feeling

Capturing positive emotional expressions in clients' stories or experiences can be extremely valuable in coaching. Positive emotions provide rich sources of energy and reinforcement for goal-directed behavior. Yet when clients bring up more difficult or unpleasant experiences, reflection of feeling encourages clients to talk more about potentially troubling emotions. Although this method can be quite useful, there are some potential downsides to the use of this skill in coaching. Here are some issues to keep in mind:

• **Deepening the emotional agenda.** Clients in lifestyle fitness coaching will typically be focused on health and lifestyle changes. They may also wish to use sport and exercise programs as adjuncts to self-development efforts. Although any significant behavioral change is likely to have an emotional component, feeling issues are unlikely to be the central theme of the change agenda. By emphasizing emotional content, coaches implicitly sanction this kind of focus in sessions. Clients may believe, as a result, that they should be talking about emotions or that they may experience some personal benefit from discussing their emotions. But this is not a therapy relationship. Clients will ultimately evaluate their work with you based on the original agendas that they negotiated. Although they may feel better by talking about their feelings, they will not necessarily achieve their primary goals through that means.

• **Fostering emotional dependency.** When a coach proves to be trustworthy and caring, clients may feel encouraged to self-disclose at levels far deeper than necessary for achieving their stated agendas. If a client has a number of emotional concerns and few outlets for discussing them, an empathic coach could be a welcome resource in that person's life. The effective use of reflection of feeling fosters an environment of safety and support. Many clients may lack this kind of support, and when they find it with someone they have hired to help them, they may want to continue the relationship

not so much for the stated agendas but for unstated, emotional reasons. These remarks are not meant to discourage coaches from reflecting feelings but to caution against overemphasizing this skill. Coaches can sense that clients are implicitly shifting the agenda to a covert emotional one when conversations linger around emotional themes or when the client continually attempts to redirect the focus of discussions to life matters that are clearly peripheral to the agreed-on focus of the working alliance.

• **Encountering resistance.** Clients may segment their experiences with professionals in ways that define anyone working in a sport or fitness context as a technical aid to performance enhancement or exercise adherence. Although coaches should understand client likes and dislikes as well as how they feel about various issues, some clients will consider these areas off limits. They might be willing to tell you what they want to achieve, how they want to achieve it, and what they are willing to do, but they might discourage any attempt to move close to their emotional world. When a client tells a story with obvious nonverbal indications of emotion, coaches who choose to reflect the unstated emotional themes need to be prepared for the possibility that the client will ignore, discard, or reject this kind of input. In a therapy relationship, this behavior would be identified as resistance to the appropriate agenda of therapy; in the case of lifestyle fitness coaching, the resistance that the coach encounters may be entirely appropriate. The client may be giving strong signals that he does not want to advance in this direction. Coaches have at least two choices at this point. The first and most probable one is to follow the client's lead. The role of the coach is to work with clients' agendas to enable them to achieve their objectives. But if the emotional content that the client is denying or avoiding has a strong link to the stated agenda or if it obstructs the client's progress, then the coach may need to rely on other skills to work through this impasse (see the section on immediacy in chapter 7). Briefly, the coach may need to discuss her perceptions of the situation and review alternative strategies for continuing the work. One of these strategies may be to refer the client to a counselor so that he may address emotional blockages to his progress on health fitness agendas.

• **Being wrong when you are right.** As noted earlier, coaches can be right about the emotions that they detect in their clients' stories but wrong about either reflecting them in the moment or continuing to assert the validity of their observations. Sometimes it is a simple matter of timing. In the beginning stages of coaching, clients may be focused on developing comfort with the coach and the notion of needing help to do something that "should be simple." If coaches emphasize emotions too early, clients may feel that their coaches are implicitly communicating that something is emotionally wrong with them. Because the definition of *early* will always be client specific, coaches will know mostly through testing the waters. To use formula-like applications (e.g., use reflection of feeling only after the second session) will likely be unproductive for many clients. The second sense of being wrong when you are right has more to do with coaches who attempt to prove their point. "Watery eyes equal tears equal sadness" might be the kind of proof that the coach offers, while the client continues to deny. Pushing emotional agendas on clients when they are ill prepared will usually backfire. Remember that any signs of resistance represent sources of data that you can keep in mind as statements about who your client is, what the person needs, and what is most comfortable for him at this time.

Summarizing

Clients may meander through wide-ranging issues in coaching sessions. Most likely, this tendency will characterize early meetings more than it does later ones, because the coaching process requires a broad scanning of life matters in the first few meetings. In initial sessions each statement new clients utter may be fraught with potential interpretations, so coaches may need to reflect all the themes a client presents before narrowing the focus. Relying on the skill of **summarizing,** coaches can bring together diverse topics of discussions at strategic moments in a session. In another application of summarizing, coaches highlight central themes that keep recurring in a number of sessions at an appropriate time.

The skill of summarizing may be seen as a type of paraphrase, except that it occurs over a longer period of conversation (Ivey & Ivey, 2003). Another way of thinking about summarizing is that it brings together themes or topics in client stories that the client has repeated or referred to with particular emphasis (Cormier & Nurius, 2003). The coach tries to identify ways in which the client organizes his story and then frames this organization in a summary (Ivey & Ivey, 2003).

Purposes of Summarizing

Writers have identified several purposes of summarizing (Brammer & MacDonald, 1999; Cormier & Nurius, 2003; Shebib, 2003). For one, summarizing can be a way that the coach confirms general understandings and validates assumptions. By presenting the client with a review of issues, goals, themes, or other ideas, the coach can determine whether she has grasped the messages communicated by the client and at the same time permit the client an opportunity to reflect on the wholeness of his (the client's) message to ascertain whether some elements might be missing. Given that a client may present a range of information in a session, the client can more easily perceive progress when the coach reviews the major themes. A client who floods the coach with a myriad of ideas may have little clarity about the relative importance of his own themes. Through a summary statement such as the following, the client may have opportunity to reflect and then continue the discussion with greater clarity.

Coach: "Let me take a minute here to see if I've gotten all you've said about your reasons for wanting to work with me. As best I can recall, you mentioned that you have three goals you want to achieve. First, you said you want to feel better about yourself because right now you feel you're in 'a bit of a rut.' The second thing you mentioned may have been related to the first. You said that being committed to an exercise program would give you a sense of purpose in your life, and you really wanted to have this kind of focus. And the third thing I heard was that eventually you wanted to train for a 10K race, although you noted that was likely 'way down the road.' Were these the main points you made? Did I miss anything?"

Note that the coach is tentative in her summary and tries to repeat key words or phrases that the client used.

A second purpose of summarizing is to identify a particular focus of the client's communications. When a certain statement or issue continues to emerge in the client's remarks, the coach may attribute additional weight to that theme. At an appropriate point, the coach may bring together the different references to this single theme and through summarizing enable the client to consider the significance of the theme and how it relates to plans and processes. For instance, a client who has repeatedly mentioned the influence of family members on her ability to structure time for regular exercise may need to explore this issue. Here is how a coach might summarize this theme:

Coach: "Carol, I've heard you mention a particular issue a few times this session and in our last meeting as well. If I can capture it, it

109

sounded to me like you were saying that you have trouble thinking of yourself as a regular exerciser because of some of the expectations your husband and your parents have of you. You said just a minute ago that your aging parents were very needy and dependent on you—for you to be unavailable to them in case of emergency was 'unthinkable.' Last session, I remember your saying that your husband might feel bad if you took up part of your free time to devote to a regular exercise program. Have I put this together accurately? Is this something you've been trying to tell me?"

This second type of summary may have a different effect on the client than the first. The first is a review of various themes, whereas this type is like shining a beacon on a particular area of the client's messages. In this second type, the coach must have established adequate rapport with the client and have a solid rationale for raising the issue at this time. This kind of summary may seem confrontational to the client and cause her to retreat.

A third purpose of summarizing may serve the coach's needs as much as or more than it serves the needs of the client. When meeting a client for the first time, the coach may be overwhelmed by the amount of detail presented. A coach may want to slow down the process both to allow himself to think more clearly about what has been said and to permit the client an opportunity to reflect and concentrate. Clients may be anxious and therefore speak rapidly and possibly without a great deal of coherence. Other clients may stylistically define their task as one of downloading as much information onto the coach as possible so that the coach can quickly put things together in an action plan. In the paralinguistic dimensions of the client's speech, the coach will find cues about exactly how to pace this summary. If the client speaks in a rapid, nonstop manner, the coach's summary will have to be similarly fast paced and probably point by point. An example of the pacing and content of this kind of summary for a client who has swiftly given a life review and five reasons for working with the coach might sound as follows:

Coach: "Let me pause for a few seconds to make sure I've got it all. I heard you say you're generally healthy, happy, and highly motivated. You want to work with me for a maximum of 6 months, and you want to achieve these goals—one, lose 10 pounds, two, find an exercise plan you can stick to on your own, three, learn proper technique

so that you don't injure yourself, four, have fun while you train, and five, learn how to relax. Is this an accurate summary?"

The coach speaks in a manner to enumerate issues and give the most concise summary possible. The client wants to move quickly into action, and although this pattern may change as the relationship develops, the initial data dump suggests a no-nonsense, let's-get-down-to-business attitude that the coach needs to reflect.

Another example of regulating the pacing of a session by summarizing might occur in instances when clients seem scattered or are experiencing a high level of stress from life situations. Summarizing in this case might serve to signal safety and ease pressure rather than attempt to capture in list form all the themes that the client is presenting. Here is an example of such an exchange:

Client: [Speaking in a rapid, pressured way while showing nonverbal signs of tension and stress] "I'm sorry . . . I'm so sorry . . . I just couldn't do what I promised to do this week. My life has been totally out of control. My car broke down, so I had to take the bus every day. Things at work have been unusually busy, and my youngest child has been home sick . . . I am simply overwhelmed . . . Please excuse me . . . What a waste . . . I really intended to train. I don't mean to dump this on you, but I could not do what we agreed I should do."

Coach: "I hear you. Let's just stop here for a minute . . . It sure sounds as if you have had one heck of a week, and you're really feeling overwhelmed."

The coach uses the skill of summarizing to slow down the process and give the client room to reflect without the pressure of moving forward. Rather than reiterate the elements of the client's problematic week, the coach provides an empathic and encompassing summary. In so doing, the coach conveys permission for the client to simply be with her experience for a few minutes before addressing the coaching agenda.

A fourth purpose of summarizing is to bring all the themes and issues of a session together toward the end. This review serves as a confirmation of what has been discussed, as a kind of progress note, and as an opportunity to launch the next step from this platform. Clients need to experience forward movement in coaching. A summary at the end of the session firmly implants themes in the client's mind so that he may continue to develop these ideas over the interval between sessions. The coach should structure the summary in a manner that ties together diverse themes so that the client leaves with a sense of coherence rather than with fragmented thoughts. Although the coach may take notes as the client talks and thereby have a reasonably complete list of issues and concerns, unless the coach summarizes this information publicly, the client may not be clear about what he said or whether he was heard. By summarizing the session, the coach helps the client leave with a comprehensive review and a supportive sense of having been fully heard. The following is an example of how a session summary might sound:

Coach: "We're coming to the end of our time today, so I thought I would take a minute to try to capture what I believe you have been telling me. You gave me a great description of your progress on the program we laid out last week. You trained 4 days, exactly as planned. And you said that, for the most part, you felt good both during and after. You raised a couple questions that I hope I answered. You wanted to know about how long you should hold your stretches and whether you should ease off if you come into training feeling tired. I think the area we spent the most time considering was how to deal with training when you are traveling. You identified four strategies, as I recall. First, to book hotels with fitness centers or ones with fitness clubs close by. Second, to arrange your flights so that you can have time to get in a decent workout on your first evening. Third, to take your minispeakers so that you can play your yoga tape in the hotel room. Finally, to ask some of your colleagues whether they would like to train with you. This last one you thought would be important to help you with your goal of developing greater social contact through your exercise plan. Does this summary reflect what you remember as the major parts of our discussion today?"

Providing details on all areas of the discussion might be difficult or too time consuming, so shorthand acknowledgement of the topics covered can suffice. Simply listing topics that have been covered permits the client to take in all that has transpired rather than remain focused on the last thing said before the session ended. The summary serves to keep perspective on the whole of the process rather than the most immediate piece.

Steps in Summarizing

Because summarizing can be a somewhat longer piece than either a reflection of content or a reflection of feeling, coaches should time it so that it fits into the structure of a session. Depending on its purpose, the summary may occur at the beginning, middle, or end of a session. For instance, in bringing focus to a particular area of the client's messages, the coach should time the summary so that he and the client have adequate time to develop the theme. On the other hand, a closing summary needs to come shortly before, but not exactly at, the end of a session. If the coach offers the closing summary at the very last minute, no opportunity will be available for client reactions or modifications. The following four steps provide a structure for the form of summary statements (Cormier & Nurius, 2003; Shebib, 2003):

1. **Introductory sentence.** Find a way to introduce the summary that is appropriate to the material that you are summarizing. If it is a closing summary, you might say, "Before we end, it might help if we could review what ground we've covered today." Or you could say, "I'd like to end our session with a brief synopsis of our work together. These are the main points that I can remember . . ." If you use the summary to focus the client on a particular theme during the session, you might begin by saying, "I'd like to try to bring together some of the things I've heard you say (today or over the past few sessions)." Or you might say, "I think I'm hearing a theme in some of the things you've been telling me. It sounds like . . ." As with other skills, you should offer summaries tentatively so that the client can easily disagree with or modify your remarks.

2. **Identifying key elements, patterns, or themes.** The coach may need to keep notes during a session to produce an accurate reflection of the main themes or patterns over time. When the coach focuses on a theme that has emerged across a number of sessions, mental recall of details may be less precise than hand-written notes taken during those sessions. When coaching has progressed to stages in which the client is actively engaged in implementing plans, records of progress can be helpful. These might be charts that are reviewed each session. The degree to which the summary details the material it is purported to represent will affect the coach's credibility one way or another. If the coach says that he is going to review the entire session, then he must account for the entire process, although he may represent large parts of the

discussion as items on a list (e.g., "We discussed in detail your progress, and in your estimation you're 80% on track"). If the coach is going to focus on a theme, he should generally have at least two concrete instances of when this theme was mentioned. Note that detailing every instance in which the theme was mentioned may overwhelm the client and provoke a defensive reaction.

3. **Summarizing content and feeling.** The messages that the coach chooses to summarize will appropriately represent both the content and emotion expressed. The agreed-on agenda, the client's receptivity to emotional data, the amount of time needed for processing the summary, and the purpose that the summary is intended to serve determine what is appropriate. Coaches should never consider summaries to be topical checklists devoid of emotional content. The coach weaves feeling dimensions related to content into the summary so that the result is a well-rounded representation of the client's expressions rather than a one-sided one. Part of a summary that demonstrates the weaving of emotion and content might sound as follows:

Coach: "You focused some of your discussion today on finding reliable exercise buddies, although you sounded pessimistic about being able to do this . . ."

An exception to this principle might occur when the coach is summarizing action steps that the client has agreed to. Here, the listing of steps would be adequate because its function is primarily to reinforce the agenda in the client's mind.

4. **Verification and encouragement.** Summarizing can cover a lot of ground. Depending on how much material the summary represents, coaches will need not only to provide clients with opportunities to reflect on, react to, or modify the summary but also to encourage them to take an active role in these summaries. Although the coach needs to ensure that the summary adequately represents the client's messages, the coach wants to communicate that the responsibility for tracking the process is shared. In this respect, the coach may wish to add a few words of encouragement to the client to think through what the coach has summarized so that that client is not a passive recipient of lists of details. Examples of these kinds of verification messages are as follows: "Well, that's how I would summarize the session, but I'm interested in knowing how you would summarize it" or "Is this an accurate reflection of what you've said? Is there anything I've said that doesn't fit or that you'd like to put another way?"

These steps offer guidance, but you should not treat them as formulas. On occasion you will have to modify, abbreviate, or simply skip some of these steps.

Uses and Abuses of Summarizing

The skill of summarizing may come more or less easily to coaches. Although it is described here as a skill for developing rapport, coaches can use summarizing as a way to influence behavior change (Ivey, Ivey, & Simek-Downing, 1987). Clients need to experience increasing levels of self-direction in their work with coaches so that by the time the relationship ends, they are able to carry on independently and successfully. Summarizing is not a rote process of detailing elements of a conversation. Effective use of this skill requires a high degree of creativity, insightfulness, and planning. Learning to summarize a session concisely or capture a theme across sessions in ways that coincide with the client's energy, pacing, style, and needs may take a fair amount of practice. Some of the more common pitfalls that coaches may fall into when using the skill of summarizing are the following:

• **Mechanical summaries.** When a coach uses the skill of summarizing in a session, it must serve a specific purpose. Summarizing should never sound like a checklist or recital of elements of the conversation. Sometimes clients will summarize on their own, and coaches should encourage this practice. Other times, coaches will have a practice of concluding sessions with summaries. When that happens, the summary needs to engage the client in an interactive process. The summary may be structured as a mutual process in which coach and client conclude their work by collaboratively reviewing the session. The summary would sound like a back-and-forth exchange in which each takes turns identifying key elements of the session. If the coach invariably assumes responsibility for detailing a session and uses this listing as its concluding moment, clients may become more dependent on the coach and the process of the session will have a certain lifeless conclusion.

• **Inconsistent use of summaries.** Patterns emerge rapidly in relationships. They are part of what creates comfort and safety. The relationship becomes more predictable by its structure. If a coach uses summaries either to begin a session (e.g., "I'd like to begin by reviewing briefly where we were at the end of last session . . .") or to end a session, clients may come to expect this behavior. When coaches are inconsistent in their use of summaries, the possibility arises for clients to attribute meaning to this behavior. For instance, a client might think that not much happened in the day's session because the coach did not summarize her progress. If a coach establishes a pattern of closing sessions with summaries (which, incidentally, is generally recommended), then this style needs to remain consistent unless there is good reason to omit this aspect of the meeting.

• **Incomplete summaries.** Without intentionally deleting themes, patterns, or elements of what is being summarized, if a coach represents only part of the messages as a complete portrayal, his credibility and trustworthiness may diminish. Especially when a coach continues to represent partial summaries as the whole, the client's faith in the coach as an accurate source of information or as a competent listener will decrease. When a coach is not sure that he has all the elements of a summary, he needs to signal this uncertainty to the client. The strategy of cocreating a summary can be valuable for closures, and coaches might use this approach to ensure that the summary is complete. Coaches could use the following kind of opening invitation to the client:

Coach: "I wonder if we could end our work today by mutually putting together a summary of what has occurred in this session. I have my own review, but I think it works best if we can do this together. So, if I can start, the first area we covered was a review of your workouts this past week, which you described as 'great.' What do you remember as coming after this discussion?"

A collaborative approach, however, will probably be less appropriate when the coach is trying to bring focus to a particular theme. In these instances, if the coach has insufficient detail or examples, the summary may be more confusing than helpful. For instance, a coach may try to summarize the client's thoughts about body issues but lack the detail necessary to create client awareness of the theme, as shown in the following ineffective summary:

Coach: "I think there is an important theme of body image in what you have been saying today. You mentioned earlier something about how you feel when you exercise, and then there was something else you said about a kind of unhappiness with how you look. Do you remember?"

As absurd as this may sound, coaches and counselors have done far worse. They have possibly

tracked a theme at a subconscious level and then want to raise it to consciousness but neglected to record (mentally or through notes) accurate reflections of the theme.

• **Biased summaries.** Unlike the previous example, a biased summary has a degree of intentionality. The coach begins to focus on a theme and consciously or not listens for evidence supporting her hypothesis or concern. Whenever the client mentions this theme or something related to it, the coach eagerly notes it. Intervening topics receive less rigorous attention. When the coach offers a summary, key elements that may contradict the conclusions or summary statements that the coach has presented may be missing. When clients are aware of these deletions or omissions, they may become rightfully concerned about the coach's objectivity. Whenever you find yourself specifically listening for evidence or examples representing specific issues or themes, you will need to have strong justification for so doing. Coaches need to develop and test various hypotheses about client behaviors or processes, yet this biasing emphasis must be highly explicit. That is, the coach needs to articulate to herself that she is doing this. Sometimes she may even make her search for evidence known to the client so that it does not become a game of catching the client in the act but rather a collaborative strategy of gathering information to feed understanding and planning. By knowing exactly what your emerging belief is, you can instruct yourself to search just as vigilantly for evidence to the contrary.

• **Argumentative summaries.** A final type of misuse of summaries can be likened to courtroom arguments in which evidence is marshaled to prove a point. Summaries are rarely to be offered in a conclusive manner. Their primary purpose is to promote rapport, understanding, insight, and action. Because coaching is by definition a collaborative venture, the use of argumentative summaries implies more of an adversarial relationship. The following is an example of the inappropriate use of summarizing by a coach to prove a point:

Coach: "So far in this session, I've noted six times that you said equipment problems at your gym interfered with your program implementation. Three times the equipment was in use, two times it was during hours when use was restricted to 20 minutes, and the sixth time, the machine was in repair. It seems that you are blaming the machines rather than taking personal responsibility for not living up to your agreement."

This example may seem exaggerated, yet when coaches experience high levels of frustration with clients or they develop a belief that clients are not committed, they may try to browbeat clients into compliance. The strategy is likely to fail.

Review of Active Listening

Active listening is a highly engaged process of attending to the client's words and behaviors with exquisite awareness and then expressing back to the client in a timely manner the messages that you are receiving. Its functions for the coach are to increase understanding of the client and to establish essential conditions of trust and rapport for the work that lies ahead. From the client's perspective, active listening facilitates open and appropriate communication about issues that the client wishes to address and enables the client to perceive the viability of the coaching relationship as a means to her ends. Although use of minimal encouragers, reflection of content, reflection of feeling, and summarizing may be highest in the early stages of the coaching relationship, they will remain essential ingredients of any coaching session. Rapport may fluctuate throughout the coaching process. As clients encounter more difficulty in implementing plans, they may show signs of resistance or become more emotional about their perceived failures. These reactions and feelings need to be acknowledged, and the skills reviewed in this section are appropriate to apply to these matters.

Questioning That Promotes Understanding and Builds Rapport

If you want to know something, ask a question. A common way in which people express interest in one another is by asking questions. Where do you live? What do you do? What's your favorite food? As Antoine St. Exupery tells us through his characters in *The Little Prince*, people often ask the wrong questions. So there may be right and wrong questions, and there is also the matter of timing. When does one ask certain questions? And how can one phrase a question so that it is unbiased and encourages openness rather than defensiveness?

The skill of questioning is a means of fostering rapport and understanding, yet it could be equally well placed in chapters on skills for developing insight and understanding (chapter 7) or skills for organizing, influencing, and guiding change (chap-

ter 8). Questions have many purposes and forms. Although they are essential to the coaching process, as Kottler (2000, p. 64) remarks, "Asking questions is a mixed blessing. It does get you the information you want in the most direct fashion, but often at a price." Kottler suggests that if you cannot get the information that you need another way, then ask a question, almost as your last resort.

If you have been in a job interview recently, you might recall how frequently interviewers used this skill. They ask many questions, yet at the end of the process you may not feel close to them or have any sense that they have been interested in building rapport. True, they may have gathered a great deal of information, but at what cost? In common parlance, we refer to trick questions, leading questions, biased questions, closed questions, or questions asked when someone already has the answer. When a person asks you a leading question (e.g., "You like ice cream, don't you?" or "What are you going to do about this situation?"), you are likely to assume that the questioner already has her mind made up, that she expects a certain right answer, or perhaps that the situation is a bit unfriendly.

All of us may remember being cross-examined, grilled, interrogated, or otherwise required to answer a seemingly endless list of highly pointed questions. As a result we may develop extreme sensitivity to being questioned. In this light, how does questioning serve as a supportive, trust-building, empathic skill?

Purposes of Questioning

Theorists have widely explored applications of questioning procedures in helping relationships (Brammer & MacDonald, 1999; Cormier & Nurius, 2003; Downs, Smeyak, & Martin, 1980; Ivey & Ivey, 2003; Ivey, Ivey, & Simek-Downing, 1987; Kottler, 2000; Shebib, 2003; Young, 2001). Let us consider the most common uses of questions as they apply to coaching relationships:

• **Initiating interviews.** Clients generally expect coaches to ask them questions about relevant background factors, needs, goals, and preferences. Implicitly, clients may have a framework for determining whether a question is within bounds or probing beyond the legitimate domain of the relationship. For instance, when a coach asks, "How much money do you make a year?" the client may respond with a defensive posture rather than a direct answer, because the client may consider such information peripheral at best to the working alliance.

• **Encouraging client communication.** In the early stages of coaching, clients may perceive themselves as needing direction. For this reason, they may arrive at the first meeting, smile, and await the coach's questions. To encourage expression, coaches often use questions to get the client to talk about relevant topics. In conjunction with minimal encouragers, reflection of content, reflection of feeling, and summarizing, the skill of questioning promotes client communication. As Young (2001) illustrates, a cycle of communication occurs in the early stages in which the coach intersperses questions with active listening skills rather than stacks questions one after another in a seeming interrogation.

• **Assessing client issues.** As Ivey and Ivey (2003) point out, questions are invaluable to assessment processes. Coaches ask questions to determine conditions for goal setting or limitations to training. Questions may focus on the who, what, where, when, why, and how of different issues. As you might imagine, a client may be more or less open to questions intended to assess factors, depending on the degree of rapport between coach and client. If questioning starts too abruptly in a session, rapport may be insufficient to foster frank and candid responses.

• **Delineating issues.** Communications theory uses the term *complex equivalent* (Grinder & Bandler, 1976) to refer to cases in which the same word or phrase has distinctly different meanings for people. When someone says, "I was upset," we often think that we know exactly what that person means because, indeed, we too have been upset at times. But this is an assumption. Effective coaches check out the meanings of words and phrases to ascertain whether the meanings they have for words and experiences coincide with those expressed by the client. Often this process relies on the elicitation of concrete examples. When you were feeling upset, what exactly did you do? What would I have seen had I been observing you in the moment? What were you feeling inside? How strong was this feeling? What would you compare it to? The coach would not necessarily ask all these questions but would certainly pursue some clearer definition of the client's experience, assuming that this purpose was timely and appropriate to the agenda.

• **Expressing interest.** Asking questions at appropriate times and in a manner that shows concern can make evident to the client the coach's keen interest in helping him. As noted in the structure of reflections or summarizing, the last part of

the coach's message will usually be a question to check accuracy or request elaboration. Questions can be invitations to explore matters mutually (e.g., "Would you be willing to explore some of these issues in greater detail?") or to work together in a process (e.g., "How might I best assist you in your efforts to achieve your goals?"). These types of questions are likely to feel supportive to clients and to facilitate forward movement toward goal attainment.

• **Discovering meaning.** Coaches can use questions to probe for deeper meanings in client messages, in a way similar to their use of questions to delineate issues. As we will discuss in the section on reflection of meaning in chapter 7, skillful questioning enables clients to go beneath surface values and goals to discover embracing concerns that may serve to direct programming and motivate behavior. A possible exchange between coach and client in such a discovery process might sound as follows:

Coach: "You've mentioned that you want to lose 20 pounds and reduce your body fat to 18% during the next 6 months. These seem like highly important and relevant goals for you. Can you tell me a bit more about what you think these changes will bring to your life?"

Client: "I'm not sure. I just thought I would look better and probably feel better . . . But now that you ask, I think part of what this is about for me is that I feel like I don't belong . . . Most of my friends are trim and athletic, and I'm a bit of an oddball in the group . . . You know, the one who finishes last or does the cooking for the group while they go out for a run."

Coach: "So, changing your body is also about fitting in? Being part of the group, rather than being an outsider? Is that what you're saying?"

Without implying that anything is wrong but rather seeking deeper understanding, the coach probes through questioning and discovers client needs and interests that can serve either to modify goals or to create energy for their achievement.

• **Creating focus.** Questions can be used to focus a client on specific issues or concerns. We will consider this use in detail in chapter 7. The coach can do this covertly or overtly. For instance, the coach can gradually shift the focus of the interview from broad topics to specific interests that the client might have in sport and fitness programs. A topical shift of that nature would be entirely legitimate in the work of lifestyle fitness coaches, whereas a shift to another kind of topic (e.g., inquiring about the client's financial investments) might be off limits. A more overt way of using questioning to shift the focus of a session involves an explicit announcement by the coach of a requested shift. This might sound as follows:

Coach: "So far, we have been talking about sport and fitness activities that you've done in the past. I'd like to shift our focus now to the future, if that's OK with you. [Pause for verbal or nonverbal response.] If you can imagine yourself 3 years from now, what sports and other activities might you hope to be doing then?"

- **Controlling the process.** Sometimes clients provide too much information or use the session as a sounding board for all kinds of issues. Although disregarding a client's comments and launching into a new direction of inquiry is rarely appropriate, coaches can guide clients back to the agenda by asking questions. Although this use of questioning has a manipulative dimension, we can justify it in the early stages of coaching because clients may simply not know what they are supposed to talk about and so they talk about everything. The following intervention is an example of bringing the discussion back into focus without disregarding the content of a seeming digression by the client:

Coach: "Would you help me understand how these things you have been mentioning in the past few minutes can be applied to the goals you want to achieve in your work with me?"

No doubt, there are other purposes of questioning, but these capture most of the uses in a coaching process.

Types of Questions

The most prevalent types of questions are **open questions** and **closed questions.** A third type appears in statements that function as questions.

Closed Questions

Closed questions lead the client to respond in a word or short phrase rather than an expansive answer. They are typically used to obtain facts, to verify information, to close off lengthy explana-

tions, or to control the flow of the interview (Ivey, Ivey, & Simek-Downing, 1987; Ivey, Ivey, & Simek-Morgan, 1997). They may begin with such words as *do, is, are,* or *have.* Their form is best recognized by the implicit demand of the question to answer directly and briefly. Here are some examples of closed questions:

- Are you ready to proceed?
- Is this the machine that you wanted to buy?
- Do you agree?
- Are you interested?
- How old are you?
- Where do you live?
- What is your job title?
- Do you want to do one more?

Open Questions

This form of questioning invites exploration and conversation. An open question may direct the client to a theme of discussion, but it permits the client ample latitude to explore thoughts and feelings. Some kind of reflection is more likely to follow an open question than a closed question. Because closed questions generally produce short answers, you have little need to paraphrase or summarize what the client has told you, whereas when you ask open questions, the response you receive may be lengthy. Open questions may begin with words like *how, what, would, could,* or *why.* Some examples of open questions include the following:

- How has your training been going lately?
- What kinds of sport and fitness activities interest you most?
- Why do you want to get involved in a coaching relationship?
- Could you tell me what you have learned thus far?
- Would you describe what an ideal training week would look like to you?

Indirect Questions

Sometimes the coach makes statements that include a request for a response. This kind of question, known as an **indirect question** (Shebib, 2003), is a less intrusive way of seeking information. Especially when the coach has been asking many questions, the use of indirect questions may break the pattern and serve to ease the pressure of questioning for the client. Here are some examples of indirect questions:

- I wonder what you hope to achieve through this work.
- I would like to know your opinion about this.
- I am curious to hear how you reacted to this.
- It would help me to understand more about your experience here.
- I don't know exactly what you mean by that last statement.

Each type of questioning has a function. Knowing when to use each type will help you work more efficiently with clients. Most writers in the field believe that a lengthy questioning process can diminish rapport between coach and client and may reinforce unproductive power and dependency dynamics in the relationship (Ivey & Ivey, 2003; Kottler, 2000; Shebib, 2003; Young, 2001).

Ill-Formed or Problematic Questions

The structure of a question affects both the answer that you receive and the quality of the relationship that you are attempting to nurture. The following review of some common errors in questioning will help you formulate questions that will better serve your purposes for obtaining information and fostering the relationship (Downs et al., 1980).

- **Leading questions.** When the way in which you phrase the question influences the likely response, the question is known as a leading question. Often these questions are phrased as negations, making it difficult for the client to disagree or deny the possibility. These questions take forms similar to the following:

  - Wouldn't you like to try this?
  - Isn't it a lovely day?
  - Why don't you come along with us?
  - Don't you think it would be a good idea to . . . ?

- **Loaded questions.** This type of ill-formed question almost demands a specific answer. A loaded question makes saying no or disagreeing seem wrong, illogical, nonsensical, or unwise. Examples of loaded questions include the following:

  - Everyone else in the club is going. You're coming too, aren't you?
  - Is this so difficult that you won't even try it?

- What is the matter with you?

- **Bipolar questions.** A question of this sort not only contains embedded assumptions but also limits responses to the options provided, even though these options do not include all the possibilities. In some forms, it is a forced choice in which both answers are potentially incorrect for the individual. Examples include the following:

  - Would you rather have a green shirt or a red shirt?
  - Are you going tonight or tomorrow night?
  - Do you have one or two bicycles at home?
  - Do you want to meet Tuesday or Wednesday?

- **Double-barreled or multiple questions.** This form of question is not so much leading or biased as it is confusing. The coach asks more than one question at the same time, and often the questions may be unrelated to one another. The client may not know which question to answer first, or may answer one and get so involved in answering that the second question gets lost. Some examples include the following:

  - Why do you think you need a coach, and who recommended me to you?
  - How long do you imagine we will work together, and what are your principle objectives?
  - Is this program working for you, and would you tell me again about the difficulty you're having with that exercise?
  - What I'd like to know from you is what motivates you most, what turns you off, what's the longest you've ever been regular in exercise, and what is your vision for the future?

- **Interrogating questions.** Guidelines for questioning often caution against the use of why questions (Shebib, 2003). For many North Americans, the why question comes in the context of a perceived interrogation. Parents ask their children, "Why did you do that?" Teachers frequently use the why question in trying to get to the bottom of things. By the time we become adults, we may be oversensitized to why questions and react defensively, even though the intent of the questioner may be to help. Coaches need to be aware of the possible effect of why questions, but they should not necessarily refrain from using them in all instances. Defensiveness in response to a why question may be as much a reflection of the level of rapport between coach and client as it is of the type of question. Nonetheless, a safer approach to the issue is to use an alternative phrasing for why questions. Here are some examples of why questions and possible alternatives for them:

- "Why do you want to lift weights?" Alternative: "What do you imagine you would get from lifting weights?"
- "Why do you want to work with her?" Alternative: "Help me understand what your thinking is behind your choice to work with her."
- "Why did you answer me that way?" Alternative: "I'd like to understand your thoughts behind the way you just responded to me."

Ironically, no matter how well-phrased questions are, clients will often answer the question that they want to address, although it may bear little relation to what coaches have asked. No doubt you have had exchanges similar to the following, in which the question requires a simple answer yet the respondent uses the question as an opportunity to tell you something completely different.

- Person A: "What did you do last night?
- Person B: "I've been having a rough time in general. Things simply haven't been going well for me. Last week, I tried to . . ."

Here's a simpler example:

- Person A: "What time is it?"
- Person B: "I think it's late. I better get moving. I have an appointment at 3."

Some communication theorists (Grinder & Bandler, 1976) make the point that the "meaning of the communication [or question] is in the response you receive." You may ask about a person's health, and he may tell you all about his family history. When clients are highly motivated to tell you certain things, what questions you ask them are almost irrelevant. They will somehow find a way to turn your question into a means of telling you what they want you to hear.

Careful structuring of questions is nonetheless an essential effort for effective coaching. At the very least, if a client responds with a tangential remark to a well-formed question, the coach will have gained significant though unexpected information about the client. If the coach asks a confusing question and the client makes a seemingly irrelevant response, the coach cannot be sure whether the response generates from the client or from the coach's poor question.

Steps in Questioning

Guidelines for asking questions may seem obvious. Nonetheless, let us review some steps that you might wish to consider (Cormier & Nurius, 2003):

1. **Understand the purpose of your question.** Sometimes we ask questions out of curiosity, and that motive can be valid for coaching as long as what we are curious about has a direct link to the client's agenda. Questions need to serve the client's needs and interests, not answer our own concerns or speculations. Another aspect of this step applies to instances when you might be tempted to ask a question although you already know the answer. Using a question to influence a client to make public significant commitments, feelings, or ideas can be important to the coaching process. For instance, a client who schedules an appointment and shows great interest in the process throughout the first session might nonetheless be asked the following closed question to confirm her commitment to the process:

Coach: "What I have gathered from your remarks today is that you're committed to working with me for the next 6 months on the issues that we broadly outlined. Am I correct?"

Client: "Absolutely. I really want to work on this, starting right now!"

2. **Determine the type of question that best serves your purpose.** Recognizing the different purposes of questioning, do you want to modulate the pace of the session, refocus the client, have the client explore an issue, or get a simple answer about something? Asking an open question will likely facilitate client expression, and if this is what you want to achieve, then you have chosen the right type of question. Asking a closed question will likely provide a specific detail or answer.

3. **When possible, embed the question in reflections.** Asking a series of questions without reflecting content or reflecting feeling can be intimidating or create distance between coach and client. Framing the question at the end of a paraphrase or reflection, rather than asking question after question, is often helpful. This strategy may not always be feasible,

but when it can promote ease and comfort in the session, try using it.

4. **Evaluate the effects of your question.** Nonverbal cues may provide some appreciation for how your client is receiving your questioning. Verbally, the response you receive will either meet your intentions or yield other information. When the client uses your question to present information about other issues, you will have a choice of assessing through additional questioning whether the client understood your question or pursuing the topics that your client seems energized to discuss. All answers are helpful, even when they do not correspond to the specific questions that you ask.

People respond differently to questioning. Coaches may need to be sensitive to how clients time their responses. Some clients may pause for a seeming eternity before answering. If the coach is not in touch with the client's need to reflect, he may ask the client another question or repeat the question, thereby confusing or pressuring the client. Generally, coaches should ask the question and pause patiently until the client responds. Note also that paralinguistic qualities of the client's response may tell you as much as verbal responses do. If a client normally answers quickly but responds after a long pause to a particular question, you may want to reflect on the potential interpretation of this pause.

Another point to bear in mind in the steps of questioning is that clients who are more introverted will likely have a slower response pattern than those who are extroverted (Quenck, 2000). Depending on your own style, that is, introverted or extroverted, you may have different reactions to these patterns. Introverts generally like to reflect and engage in internal self-talk before expressing their opinions. In this respect, their answers to probing questions may come after lengthy pauses. Extroverts, on the other hand, are likely to shoot from the lip or think aloud. Their responses will probably seem more spontaneous. If you are extroverted, you may occasionally need to caution yourself to slow down the questioning process. Your own tendency to think aloud, to speak without extensive reflection, could run counter to the needs of your client. If you tend to be introverted, you may want to reflect internally on what your client has said before you ask the next question. If you are working with extroverts, however, you may want to process your thoughts aloud by reflecting content or reflecting feeling so that your extroverted clients experience continuous engagement in the coaching process.

Uses and Abuses of Questioning

We have highlighted some of the issues associated with questions in coaching. As necessary as questions are, coaches should use them judiciously. A process of caring and supportive questioning can affect clients positively, but overuse or inappropriate use of questioning can adversely affect the coaching relationship (Brammer & MacDonald, 1999; Cormier & Nurius, 2003; Hackney & Cormier, 2001; Ivey & Ivey, 2003; Kottler, 2000; Shebib, 2003; Young, 2001). Let us review some of the more problematic aspects of the questioning skill:

- **Feeling interrogated.** Clients may be highly compliant in sessions with coaches and continue to answer questions even though they experience increasing levels of discomfort. Coaches need to attend to nonverbal cues from clients when they are using the skill of questioning, and they should vary their approach to information gathering. Indirect questions may be less intrusive, and by using reflection skills, coaches can often lead clients to explore issues without ever asking a question.

- **Reducing client autonomy.** When questioning is one-sided in social communications, people generally perceive that the person asking the questions is in a position of greater power. When clients are repeatedly on the receiving end of a questioning process, they may eventually abdicate responsibility in the relationship and allow the belief that the coach has all the solutions to grow to dysfunctional levels. In so doing, the client may become more dependent on the coach. A powerful question that returns control to the client might be the following:

Coach: "I've been asking a lot of questions, yet I'm not sure that what I'm asking is as useful as it could be. So, may I approach it this way? What questions would be most helpful for me to ask so that I can best help you achieve your goals?"

- **Fostering socially acceptable answers.** We discussed ill-formed or biased questions in a previous section. An adverse effect of these types of questions may be that the client comes to believe that she has to present a socially appropriate image to her coach. Asking, "You want to improve your appearance, don't you?" leads the answer, conveys the coach's bias about physical appearance, and perhaps expresses a judgment that she is making about her client. Clients who perceive their coaches as highly effective and having it all together may be reluctant to share their true feelings, especially when they might differ from what they imagine the coach believes. When coaches sense that clients are presenting overpositive, socially acceptable answers to questions, they might use a number of strategies. As we will discuss in chapter 8, the coach can use the skill of self-disclosure to demythologize herself. In addition, engaging the client in a here-and-now conversation using the skill of immediacy (chapter 7) can help ground the relationship in reality rather than in fantasy.

• **Increasing vulnerability.** When two parties share information in a disproportionate manner in a relationship, the person who has shared the most may feel more vulnerable than the other does. In normal contexts, the principles explored by Jourard (1964, 1968) suggest that one person's self-disclosure induces the other person to self-disclose, and that this process becomes cyclical in an ever-deepening way. Because of the nature of client–coach relationships, coaches usually reveal far less of their personal values, beliefs, needs, and history than clients do. Although this is as it should be, coaches need to be aware of the responsibility attached to obtaining extensive information about clients. Coaches need to guard client information with confidentiality and may need to reassure the client of their nonjudgmental acceptance of the client. On occasion, the coach may wish to level the field through relevant and timely self-disclosures.

Frameworks for Considering Client Information

This chapter has emphasized skills that help coaches build rapport and gather information about clients. Two useful frameworks can help you conceptualize the information that you gather from clients. The first is a schema for categorizing information, and the second is an analysis of the depth of data gathering.

The Johari Window

At the outset of a coaching relationship, you probably know little about the client who calls for an appointment or who contacts you at your place of work. Over time, you will learn much more. Clients may know a great deal about themselves, but they may nonetheless have significant blind spots. Even when they are highly self-aware, how much they are willing to share with others will depend on a number of factors including the nature of the relationship, the trust level that they experience, personal values regarding intimacy, and even their ability to describe their internal states and processes. In a simple yet enduring model of the relationships among self-disclosure, feedback, and self-awareness, Joe Luft and Harry Ingham (Luft, 1969) described a matrix of awareness or self-knowledge. This model, known as the Johari Window, can help coaches conceptualize their knowledge base about clients and thereby strategize to augment areas appropriate to their clients' agendas (see figure 6.4).

• **The public self.** What clients share with their coaches is part of the public self. They may not discuss this information with everyone, but by describing it to coaches, clients make certain aspects of themselves public. Coaches may use questions and other information gathering skills to broaden the dimensions of this quadrant of awareness.

• **The private self.** This area represents self-knowledge that clients are unwilling to discuss with coaches. Because clients need to share only what is necessary to assist the coach in their collaborative efforts, large areas of a client's life may be off-limits to the coaching relationship. On the other hand, if clients have secrets that interfere with successful collaboration, then the effectiveness of the coaching process may be limited from the outset. Coaches may ask clients if there are issues or historical matters that they need to know about so that they can offer the best assistance possible, but if clients hold

	Known to self	Unknown to self
Known to others	Public self (What I know about myself and make public to others)	Blind self (What I don't know about myself but others have observed)
Unknown to others	Private self (What I choose to keep private)	Unconscious self (What I don't know about myself and what is also unknown to others)

Figure 6.4 The Johari Window: An awareness model for coaches and clients.

back important information, chances of success will diminish proportionately according to the centrality of the information to clients' agendas. If, for instance, a client has an eating disorder or a serious substance addiction, the coach will need to be aware of this information in order to proceed in the most appropriate manner or, in some cases, to determine whether the relationship is viable.

- **The blind self.** We often see things in other people about which they seemingly have little awareness. These may represent our secrets about them, but in a coaching process the task is usually to help clients become aware of aspects of themselves that they manifest through actions or unconscious communications. Of course, coaches should not always disclose information about clients of which the clients themselves are unaware. Timing is always critical, as is a regard for the legitimate agenda of the relationship. If the information is relevant to the coaching process, then the coach will need to use various skills to enhance client self-knowledge at an appropriate point in the relationship. Such skills as immediacy, reflection of meaning, confrontation, and feedback, discussed in chapters 7 and 8, will be useful in bringing about this objective. When the information is irrelevant to the coaching agenda, the coach may well decide to contain that information instead of sharing it.

- **The unconscious self.** Much of the early work in psychoanalytic theory (Freud, 1964) was premised on the belief that each of us has significant areas of unconscious experience, or that dimensions of ourselves may remain virtually unknown to us or to anyone else until a pivotal event brings to the surface the previously unconscious elements. Freud thought dreams represented the "royal road to the unconscious" because a careful analysis of dream content held the possibility for bringing to conscious awareness aspects of our previously unknown selves (Freud, 1964). In our highly psychological world, most of us know that people repress memories of traumatic experiences. Some people have little recollection of significant periods of their lives, typically periods in childhood and adolescence. One of the functions of certain types of psychotherapy is to enable clients to bring forth these memories so that they can deal with and resolve to the degree possible the presumed effect of these repressed experiences.

When we consider the agenda of lifestyle fitness coaching, this unconscious domain is never the focus of direct intervention. That is, the coach will in no way deliberately attempt to unveil aspects of the client's unconscious. This does not mean, however, that the unconscious self is irrelevant to coaching. Any process of change that has substantive effect on an individual's functioning stands some chance of bringing to light certain memories, experiences, sensations, or awareness of which the client may have had no prior knowledge and that the coach had not expected to emerge. This simple yet poignant story illustrates the point:

A client who was working with a health fitness professional decided that, as part of her program, she wanted to commit to drinking more water, specifically, at least eight glasses of water a day. Working through all the processes of establishing a SMART goal, action planning, relapse prevention, and creating social support brought no great awareness to this client about any underlying issues related to this simple goal. She merely thought that drinking more water would be important to her health, and she was aware that when she was thirsty she sometimes forced herself to ignore this need.

During a stressful period at work, she noticed herself sitting at her computer with a bottle of water and a glass within arm's reach yet persistently refusing to pause long enough to quench her growing thirst. Awareness of such blatant self-denial stunned her. The experience so profoundly affected her that she began recalling other instances of self-denial in her life, and she eventually recalled critical messages from childhood. When this woman was a young girl, her mother, perhaps as a way of coping with her own life stresses, repeatedly labeled her daughter as selfish. Her mother's words came back to mind with resounding force: "Stop thinking about your own needs so much. . . . You're too selfish." These messages became so ingrained over time that they formed a way of life for the client.

All this from a simple intention to drink more water!

The story is true. The likelihood that coaches will encounter these kinds of revelations is hard to estimate. In the situation with this female client, the coach only needed to be supportive. The client had uncovered a major influence on her behavior of ignoring or denying her needs over a lifetime. She not only reached her goal of drinking a daily quota of water but also set other goals for health improvement that she engaged thoughtfully and successfully during the following year. Should she have wished to discuss this matter further, a lifestyle fitness coach might have considered referring her to a competent counselor.

The Johari Window (Luft, 1969) is a practical guide that coaches can use to review the knowledge they have about clients versus what they perceive they need in order to do their work effectively. When knowledge remains in the area of the client's blind self, effective coaching calls for an assessment of the appropriateness of bringing this information to the client as an integral part of the cocreated database about the client. When the client seems to be withholding information that the coach can only speculate about, then skills of immediacy, reflection of meaning, confrontation, and feedback discussed in chapters 7 and 8 may be required to ferret out the necessary details. When the public self of the client is too large for the agenda of the coaching relationship, the coach may need to work with the client on defining appropriate areas of self-disclosure and dialogue.

Levels of Intervention

Diagnostic or assessment information is gathered only at the level required for the contracted coaching work. Coaches should avoid probing for information in a discovery process that goes beyond the client's needs and intentions. Although it may seem that the more you know about a person, the more effective your work will be, the philosophy of coaching emphasizes action far more than it does diagnosis and reflection. Put another way, coaching focuses more on the present and future than it does on the past, and the future is something that the coach and client cocreate through the coaching relationship. The future is not something that the coach needs to spend time discovering through extensive questioning and probing. Reddy (1994) and Harrison (1970) offer sage advice for coaches who are considering levels of client behavior toward which they intend interventions. For lifestyle fitness coaches, the legitimate arena for intervention pertains to sport, physical activities, and active-living possibilities. Coaches gather necessary information to inform their actions with clients, and they guard

against pursuing a deeper understanding of clients for its own sake or for speculative possibilities.

Cornerstones of Effective Coaching Technique

In this chapter we focused on fundamental coaching skills that facilitate client openness and expression while providing necessary support and guidance. In professional communication, we too often assume that we understand accurately what a client is saying because we think we hear clearly what she is saying. Active listening is a process that not only allows the coach to verify information that he is receiving but also enables the client to feel validated and perhaps to modify or elaborate messages that she has put forth. We explored these primary areas of active listening and questioning in this chapter both for their benefits and for their potential for misuse. A key principle emphasized throughout is that these skills become detriments to the coaching process when coaches use them mechanically or without full awareness of their effect on the client. In this respect, these skills have their greatest effect when coaches weave them into the fabric of communication with the client. You might wish to listen to the tape recording that you created as part of learning activity 6.1 to determine how often and how effectively you used the various skills described in this chapter.

As we consider other skills in chapters 7 and 8, you will have the opportunity to consider how best to combine all these skills to serve client needs and develop the necessary support structure of the relationship. Although upcoming chapters present approaches to working with clients that are more advanced, do not underestimate the power of these fundamental skills. They can take you and your clients a long way toward the goals that your clients want to achieve.

Developing Insight and Deepening Understanding

seven

"You have to leave the city of your comfort and go into the wilderness of your intuition. What you'll discover will be wonderful. What you'll discover will be yourself."

Alan Alda

Relationships are rarely static. In coaching processes, clients want to move toward their goals. For the most part, they do not hire you to discuss the past. They want to actualize their dreams—with your help. In more traditional work between health fitness professionals and clients, trainers may accept clients' stated goals for exercising at face value, or, if discussion occurs, it may be around the practicality or viability of stated outcomes. A client who wants to train a couple times a week and lose 50 pounds (27 kilograms) in 6 months may receive guidance about modifying either the goal or the level of commitment.

Lifestyle fitness coaches may have the advantage over other types of life coaches by encountering potential clients in sport and fitness facilities where they normally work. Sometimes the client is a new member of the facility who is looking for guidance and support. Other times, the coach knows the client well. For clients already involved in sport and fitness, the urgency for new programming may not be as important as it is for newcomers who are eager to get started. In the latter case, the coach may need to mix initial discussions with interim action strategies so that the client can begin to engage the world of sport and fitness. With both novice and experienced exercisers, the process of discovery of needs, goals, and congruent approaches to action continues throughout the coaching relationship.

Coaches are less likely to employ the skills described in this chapter at the very beginning of the coaching relationship. Unlike traditional approaches to fitness advisement, this approach involves using initial goal statements of clients as intentions to explore, test, and possibly modify as the relationship develops. Coaches want to take the broadest possible view of client issues and goals before narrowing down information toward the formulation of action plans. The process is likely to be iterative. Initial understandings lead to preliminary planning. Further discussions develop deeper understandings that lead to more grounded decisions for action.

This chapter will cover three skills. Each builds on skills previously reviewed in chapter 6. Focusing, reflection of meaning, and immediacy move the client and the coaching relationship closer toward engagement with a more embracing agenda and goal-directed activities. All three skills rely on the

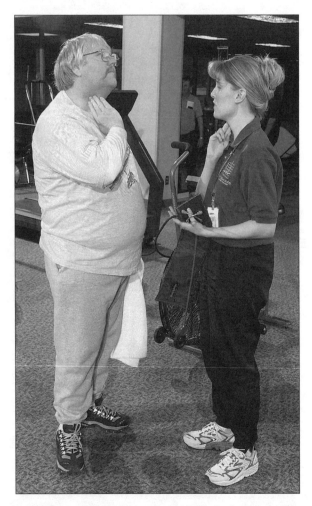

Establishing an atmosphere of trust will help develop insight and understanding between coach and client.

use of questions and on processes of reflection, but coach and client must establish sufficient connection and trust before the client can experience security and safety in discussions involving these skills.

Using these skills involves a higher degree of risk—for both the client and the coach. Moreover, coaches must formulate a solid appreciation for who their clients are before they can begin to put together pieces of the puzzle in these more engaging and probing approaches. The goal of all three skills is to deepen understanding and, in some cases, to facilitate insightful connections for the client.

Focusing

Different theorists define focusing in interrelated yet distinct fashions (e.g., Parrott, 2003; Young, 2001). A popular interpretation of focusing is based on the work by Eugene Gendlin (1981), who represents this skill as a type of awareness enhancement in which clients direct their attention toward a specific theme or, at times, on their felt experience, almost as a meditative act. Within the realm of sport and competition, attentional focus or concentration has also been widely explored as a strategy for performance enhancement (Abernathy, 2001).

The perspective on focusing represented here derives more from the works of Jean Baker Miller (Baker Miller, 1991; Baker Miller, Stiver, & Hooks, 1998) and interpretations of her meaning of focusing by Ivey and his colleagues (Ivey & Ivey, 2003; Ivey, Ivey, & Simek-Morgan, 1997).

A coach can take many angles when responding to a client's messages. Consider, for instance, a client who is expressing difficulty in adhering to an exercise plan to which he firmly committed in a previous coaching session:

Client: "I'm simply not doing what I agreed to, and it's not just because of me. . . I don't mean to make excuses, but work has been rough, way too much traveling . . . and my kids have needs, too. I can't always expect my wife to shuttle them around to all their sports and lessons, but I'm disappointed nonetheless . . . Maybe you should have come up with a more flexible plan for me."

A comprehensive paraphrase would reflect all elements of this client's message to the coach, yet if the coach has been working with this client for a while, he may have a hunch about the most productive lead to follow. A coach might have the following set of ideas about the client's issues from this one remark:

- The client is simply having a rough time meeting all his objectives. He feels disappointed, and perhaps demoralized. The coach can choose to focus on the client's felt experience, empathizing with the dilemma in which the client finds himself. A focusing response of this nature might sound as follows:

Coach: "Sounds like you've had a rough week. Work, family, and no exercise. I hear your disappointment and imagine it's hard to believe that things can get better—even though you really want to follow through on your commitment to yourself."

- The client is blaming others for not doing what he agreed to do. The coach could focus the client on his responsibility both for the contracted agreement to exercise and on his tendency to excuse his behavior. A response of this sort might sound as follows:

Coach: "I hear you. You're feeling disappointed, and there are a number of reasons you're suggesting for why you didn't follow the plan. Would you be willing to explore with me what you might have been able to do this past week to deal with the problems you've identified? What could you have done differently to live up to your commitment to yourself?"

- The client has a highly unpredictable job that requires him to adjust plans continually to accommodate emerging needs in his company. He may plan to train at his lunch hour but instead find himself on the way to the airport. Based on knowledge that the coach has about this client, he might have chosen to focus this way:

Coach: "I can truly empathize with your disappointment. You planned to exercise according to the schedule we laid out but instead you ended up traveling. With the kind of quick business trips you take, it doesn't leave much time for going to the gym. What do you imagine would be possible for you to do when you have uncontrollable events take over your schedule?"

Even if the client responds by saying that there is nothing he can do, the effect might be to enable him to reduce his sense of self-disappointment and, along with the coach, to brainstorm contingency plans for the future.

- The client has young children with busy schedules and is married to a woman who also holds down a demanding full-time job. Family responsibilities have to be considered in determining the likelihood of success for different training options. The coach could choose to focus on family demands, as represented in the following response:

Coach: "Sounds like you really have your hands full. Not only the demands of your job, but also what you believe is right to do in sharing responsibilities for your children. I admire your commitment. Yet, I wonder if we can think creatively about ways that you can meet your own goals and at the same time make sure your children get to their activities. What ideas come to mind?"

- The client shines the light of attention on the coach in his final sentence, when he says, "Maybe you should have come up with a more flexible plan for me." This statement provides the coach with an opportunity to explore feelings that the client might have about the coach or the efficacy of the coaching agreements. The coach should engage in a discussion of this nature based on a clear sense of rapport with the client and with consideration of the timeliness of this type of intervention. In focusing the client on the ongoing relationship and on his feelings toward the coach, the coach will employ the skill of immediacy. A later section of this chapter will describe this skill, but here is a sample of how it may sound:

Coach: "I hear you. You're feeling disappointed, and work and family responsibilities played into your problems with exercising as you had planned . . . I also hear that you believe I should have come up with a more workable plan for you. I'd like to hear more about this. Would you be willing to share any other thoughts or feelings you have about our work together?"

- The client may be feeling up against a wall with few options and not much hope. The coach could make a decision to inject new ideas or perspectives into the interaction by either sharing personal experiences, providing information, or offering advice. The next chapter will describe skills involved in this type of focus when we discuss self-disclosure, directives, advice or suggestions, and information. Here is how this focus might sound:

Coach: "Sorry to hear about your week and how disappointed you feel. Based on your experience this week, I have some ideas I would like to share with you . . . There are some things you may be able to do that will help you reach your goals even when you can't follow your plan to the letter. Here are a couple ideas . . ."

Another response of this sort, which involves the coach's self-disclosure, might sound like this:

Coach: "It sounds as if you're having real difficulty finding time to do your training. I certainly can relate. A few years ago, with a new baby at home and work commitments piling up, I just couldn't seem to be consistent about my training either. It took some effort—and lots of patience—to rearrange those aspects of my life that I had control over so that gradually I could move from no training at all to two reliable sessions a week. That wasn't ideal, but it was the best I could do—and, given the circumstances, it was plenty good enough!"

Ivey and colleagues (Ivey & Ivey, 2003; Ivey, Ivey, & Simek-Morgan, 1997) describe seven types of focus that a helper can consider in formulating a response to a client's message. Briefly, these are as follows:

1. Client focus means responding to the client's general experience.

2. Problem focus refers to emphasizing the problems or difficulties that the client is experiencing, as opposed to focusing on the client himself.

3. Other focus directs attention toward other individuals who might be involved in the client's issues, concerns, plans, or actions.

4. Family focus is similar to other focus except that the other individuals are members of the person's present family or family of origin.

5. Mutuality or "we" focus involves an emphasis on what is occurring in the relationship between coach and client (see discussion of immediacy later in this chapter).

6. Coach focus revolves around the coach's behavior of sharing personal information, providing information, offering suggestions, or giving advice (see chapter 8 for discussion of instructions, information, and advice or suggestions).

7. Cultural–environmental–contextual focus may include a number of different emphases, including situational considerations,

environmental matters, or such aspects of the client's makeup as sex, race, economic status, educational background, or religious orientation.

Framing these suggestions about focus within life fitness coaching relationships suggests potential avenues for the dialogue. To consider these in both theoretical and practical terms, we will use the following client profile as a reference for dialogue and proposals for potential focus.

Ted is a 45-year-old man of eastern European heritage who has been a heavy smoker since his teen years and has never been involved in any sort of regular exercise program. He is a self-made millionaire who generally works 60 or more hours per week. He has never married, although he occasionally goes out on casual dates. He is fiercely competitive and driven to succeed in whatever he does. A recent medical examination showed evidence of cardiovascular disease, and under doctor's orders he decided that it was time to start exercising.

In the initial interview, the following exchange takes place between client and coach.

Coach: "I'd like to know as much as I can about your reasons for wanting to work with me—particularly what you identify as your goals or objectives for coaching."

Client: "Well, it's simple. The doctor told me I should exercise and I've never done it in my life. I'm a very busy man so I need to find the most efficient way to exercise, and since I know nothing about proper exercise, I wanted the best help I could get, and I heard you're the best."

Coach: "Well, thank you. So, if I understand you, you want to do as much as you can in the least amount of time possible, strictly to address your doctor's advice."

Client: "That's it—but it's for me, not for my doctor. I get bored easily. I am very impatient. I want to see immediate results. And I have to keep my mind stimulated at all times. You already know that I smoke—two, maybe three packs a day. So, you're going to have your work cut out for you."

1. **Focus on the client's immediate experience.** Who is the client, and what is he experiencing right now? What messages are you receiving from the client in the present moment? You may be trying to absorb many details about the client's history, needs,

and goals, but how does all this information coalesce into a useful image of the person before you? From the client's profile and the segment of dialogue just described, you may surmise that this client is seeing you "under doctor's orders" and is initiating this process with a perceived life-or-death threat hanging over his head. Your focus could reflect what you are hearing from the client as follows:

Coach: "I'm beginning to get a picture. Tell me whether it's right or not. Your chief motivation is your health—your doctor told you that you needed to start exercising. You are willing to comply and will do whatever it takes, as long as it meets certain criteria. You probably feel like a fish out of water here because you say you know nothing about exercise, so you've hired the 'best' to get you on the right track. And you had better see results quickly, or else you'll find someone else to work with. Is this a reasonable synopsis?"

2. **Focus on the problem.** Turn attention not so much on the client as on an aspect of the client's experience. Separating the person from the problem is not always easy, yet by depersonalizing the client's messages and focusing on the problem to be resolved, you and the client may be able to dissect the matter with more objectivity, or at arm's length. Here is how a problem-focused response might sound.

Coach: "Let me take some of the information you've given me and feed back to you the situation as I hear it. Your doctor told you that you have early indications of cardiovascular disease and that a good exercise program would be your best treatment strategy. Yet I also hear that you are a heavy smoker, so we need to understand how that figures in. The third piece I hear is that you have little time, so your program needs to fit into your already packed schedule. The final element is about how you need to exercise: Your program has to engage your mind, not bore you, and produce immediately discernable results. Is this accurate?"

3. **Focus on significant others.** When other people may affect a client's commitment to the process of coaching and its prescriptive elements, the coach may wish to draw out the client's awareness of these influences. Sometimes, as suggested in this client's profile, significant others are almost

absent, so that this kind of focus might explore the client's present social connections or his desire for social contact related to his prospective program. To put this another way, the absence of significant others in a client's story does not necessarily mean that they do not exist or that social connections are unimportant. The lack of detail about relationships should provoke coaches to at least ask a question or invest time exploring this area before drawing conclusions. Focusing on significant others for the client Ted might sound as follows:

Coach: "Ted, you told me that you weren't married and have no children. I don't have a clear enough picture yet of how other people may play into your plans to exercise or the way that you'd like to exercise. For instance, we can codesign programs involving other people or not. And, if there are other people who may influence your plans to exercise, I would like to know about this so that whatever we come up with has the highest chances for success."

4. **Family focus.** What are the client's family relationships and responsibilities that might affect goal setting or program implementation? What is the client's family history that might have bearing on beliefs, attitudes, or behaviors? The attitudes of family members toward a client's commitments to exercise or pursue other self-improvement goals can either hinder or help. In Ted's case, exploration of family history or parental habits and injunctions might be helpful. Little of what Ted has said thus far suggests this focus, but if a coach were to explore the matter, it might sound as follows:

Coach: "Ted, you told me that you weren't married and had no children. Are there other family members who might somehow influence your involvement in exercise, either in terms of attitudes or needs they might have?"

Ted may possibly have a large extended family and bear responsibility for much of the care taking. Perhaps in his family of origin, exercise was eschewed except as a form of productive work. If Ted is to engage in exercise in a joyful rather than begrudging manner, examination of this avenue may be productive.

5. **Focus within the coaching dyad.** Sometimes it is valuable to bring the focus closer to home, that is, to the relationship between coach and client. This focus might mean emphasizing expectations,

attitudes, roles, or feelings. When coaches have indications from clients that they have strong but inappropriate expectations of the coach or when coaches sense that clients are experiencing certain feelings toward them that may have implications for the working alliance, coaches then must decide whether it is timely to bring these matters into focus. In Ted's case, his last sentence to the coach was "So, you're going to have your work cut out for you." Ted's remark implies that responsibility for success rests with the coach. Although coach and client share responsibility for the process, clients ultimately bear responsibility for implementation of the agreed upon program. Responding to Ted's challenge at the very beginning of the coaching process may be untimely, but at some point the coach will need to address role expectations. A possible response to Ted's comment might sound as follows:

Coach: "Well Ted, there's a lot in what you're saying. You realize that you need to exercise for your health, and you have some very clear parameters for exactly how you want to do it. Also, you have the additional issue of smoking. In your words, I'm going to have my 'work cut out for me.' It would help me to understand how you see this relationship working. What do you expect of me, and what do you expect of yourself in this coaching process?"

The coach does not comment immediately on the challenge but rather acknowledges first the framework for the client's comment. Then, instead of saying, "Ted, it's your responsibility to exercise, not mine to make you do so," the coach opens the way for clarification of the client's feelings. Perhaps Ted recognizes his responsibility while also acknowledging that the coach will have to work hard to help him. Or Ted may expect the coach to use some sort of magic to make things happen. Only by focusing on this comment can the coach be sure what expectations Ted holds about the working alliance.

6. **Focus on the coach's world.** In listening carefully to client stories, coaches may hear many distortions, fallacious beliefs, or seemingly irresolvable problems. Drawing on either professional knowledge or personal experience, coaches may have important points to add to clients' perspectives. The next chapter reviews this type of focus under skill discussions for self-disclosure, directives, information, and advice or suggestions. Here we explore a coach's deliberate choice to focus the client on

ideas or other forms of contribution from the coach that relate closely to the messages just presented by the client. In Ted's case, the coach might offer a number of possible responses, based on either professional knowledge or personal experience. Here are samples:

Coach: "Ted, I'd like to address a number of issues here, if that's OK with you. [Pauses for response.] First, there are some minimum time commitments that I would see as necessary for you to accomplish your goal. As for structuring exercise so as to keep your mind engaged, I think that will be something we can successfully discover together. I guess the third piece I want to comment on is your smoking. I estimate that it will be difficult for you to engage in certain exercise programs because of the amount you smoke. Also, I would suggest that after we talk you schedule another appointment with your doctor to get her opinion on the effect of smoking on your health—and on your exercise behaviors."

Another response involving the coach's self-disclosure might sound as follows:

Coach: "Ted, I think we will both have a challenge. I used to be a smoker myself. When I began to exercise, I realized how much my smoking affected my ability to exercise, particularly in aerobic activities. I have real concerns about your being able to reach your health goals without addressing your smoking. I sure had to."

7. **Focus on contextual or background factors.** When trying to locate the client in a matrix of sociocultural, gender, geographical, occupational, and other contextual variables, the coach may become aware of influences on the client's attitudes, beliefs, and behaviors that will continue to function unless the coach and client somehow account for them in strategies for working together and implementing action plans. A clinically obese woman with a negative body image may not do well in a mixed-gender fitness center. A client from a fundamentalist religious group may have certain concerns about dress codes not only for herself but also for others attending the same health club. Clients with strong gender stereotypes may restrict themselves to pursuing only certain kinds of sports or exercise programs. Those who live far from the nearest fitness center may need to incorporate plans for home-based training. Coaches need to under-

stand as much as possible about the ethnic and cultural backgrounds, sexual orientations, religious or spiritual associations, socioeconomic status, and other relevant contextual factors that might affect normative expectations that clients hold for coaching, programming considerations, and relationship dynamics. Ted's profile suggests at least two relevant contextual or background factors that the coach might choose to explore. One concerns his relationship to work, including his work ethic and probably the way in which he measures success in life. The second has to do with his eastern European heritage, which may have influenced his lifelong orientation to exercise and fitness. Focusing on these matters, the coach might say the following:

Coach: "Ted, I understand that throughout your life you have never exercised on a regular basis. It would help me to understand, based on your background and the place that work occupies in your life, what perceptions you hold about involvement in exercise and sport."

If Ted has been raised to believe that exercise is frivolous, or if his work ethic is so dominant that its demands subjugate all other values, then the coach should cocreate active-living options that Ted will perceive as productive (e.g., manual labor) or perhaps that allow him to do other things while exercising (e.g., a home treadmill that allows him to make telephone calls, watch news briefings, or possibly read documents while exercising).

Focusing may be considered more a matter of strategy than simply a coaching skill. For this reason, we have not dissected it as we did other coaching skills (namely, purpose, steps, and uses and abuses). As illustrated in the preceding examples, depending on the focus, the coach may have to use different processes of communication, including reflection of content, immediacy, self-disclosure, and giving advice and suggestions. In this regard, focusing speaks to the internal process of the coach in his decision about how to respond to a client's messages. Multiple options for responding will always exist. Some will prove more productive than others. Knowing which to pursue derives from accurate knowledge of who the client is and what he needs, coupled with the coach's self-awareness of agendas or biases that may drive his own behavior.

Our histories shape us as much as they shape our clients. In the fields of counseling and psychotherapy, many writers have noted that the theoretical orientations of counselors significantly influence the interpretations and interventions they make (Capuzzi & Gross, 2001; Gladding, 2000; Parrott, 2003; Prochaska & Norcross, 2003). A psychoanalytically oriented counselor will search for underlying drives and motivations based in early childhood experiences, whereas an existentialist counselor will focus on questions of meaning, value, and current experience.

Although the profession of coaching may be less theoretically driven (Williams & Davis, 2002), individual coaches typically formulate their own worldviews (Kelly, 1955; Frankl, 1969). Their own experiences will influence them, and they come to value certain things more than they do others. When working with clients, if coaches are unable to embrace diversity and consciously put aside, at least while they are listening, their worldviews in order to receive and comprehend those of their clients, they will likely fall into the trap of being lifestyle converters (Cormier & Nurius, 2003).

The choice of focus is strategic in the sense of deciding what path of discourse will best serve the client's needs, not in determining what should be done to meet the coach's objectives. The coach must always understand strategy from the perspective of how best to serve the client's agenda. Learning activity 7.1 provides you with an opportunity to explore your worldview and how it may influence the work you do in coaching

Immediacy

Immediacy is variously described as a skill (Egan, 1998; Ivey, Ivey, & Simek-Downing, 1987; Shebib, 2003) or as a component of empathy (Ivey & Ivey, 2003). Irrespective of whether it is seen as a condition for establishing trust and empathy in a coaching relationship or as a communication skill initiated by the coach, immediacy is a critical process in coaching. Immediacy involves the coach's sensitivity to the immediate situation within the relationship, a comprehension of what is happening in the moment, and the initiation by the coach of a dialogue to consider openly and directly the here and now (Capuzzi & Gross, 2001; Egan, 1998, 2002). Turock (1980) further notes that immediacy is likely to include expressions of the coach's desires, needs, or wants. Simply noticing what a client is doing or saying and bringing it into direct awareness can be seen in the following illustrations:

- "I see you smiling broadly and I imagine that you are feeling pretty good about yourself right now."

Learning Activity 7.1

Understanding the Influence of Your Worldview on Coaching

A worldview is a personal set of values, beliefs, attitudes, and opinions about people and the reasons things are the way they are in the world. In relation to lifestyle fitness coaching, you may wish to examine some of your assumptions about people who come to you for coaching and what you think is most important to know about them. Answer the following series of questions in a thoughtful, reflective manner. Write down whatever comes immediately to mind in response to these questions, and when you have finished answering them all, take time to study what you have written to derive greater appreciation for your personal worldview.

1. What do you believe to be the most important motivations for human behavior?

2. Aside from your personal beliefs, what do you think are the most predominant motivations in our society?

3. When people experience personal difficulties in their lives, what do you think the wisest paths of action should be? That is, how do you think they should ideally address their problems?

4. What do you assume to be some of the root causes for people to seek the assistance of a lifestyle fitness coach? This question isn't about whether they want to lose weight or be healthy; it concerns their reasons for choosing to hire a coach. What beliefs about themselves or about coaches do you think might be embedded in this decision?

5. Why do you believe that some people are successful in achieving goals they set for themselves in processes like coaching?

6. Why do you think that some people are unsuccessful in these endeavors?

7. To what degree do you believe that people can change any behavior if they set their minds to it?

8. How much of what happens to people in life do you believe to be a result of fate? If fate doesn't determine life experiences, then what does?

9. If you really wanted to get to know someone well, what five questions would you ask her?

10. If you were to identify some of the things that people need most to stick to an exercise program, especially if they have been sedentary for many years, what would they be?

- "I heard that deep sigh when you finished that story. I wonder what that means."

- "I sense your disappointment in me for not helping you more. I really want to hear more about this."

- "I know you are pressed for time right now, so I'll get right to the point."

- "I, too, am feeling excited about all the great results you've been getting from your efforts."

Immediacy, like the skill of focusing, builds on other skills. It is not a specific communication skill per se. Locating immediacy in the stages of coaching is difficult because it may be applied at

different points depending on what needs to occur to foster the client's identification and attainment of goals. In this book, it is located in the context of deepening understanding and developing insight because it will most likely serve those objectives directly, while indirectly assisting action planning and program implementation. As Shebib (2003, p. 77) comments, "Immediacy is a tool for exploring, evaluating, and deepening" the relationship. Its goal is essentially one of strengthening the relationship. The use of immediacy often combines the skills of confrontation and self-disclosure (see chapter 8) and may require that the coach discuss his own feelings and reactions (Capuzzi & Gross, 2001; Turock, 1980).

Purposes of Immediacy

Coaches may apply the skill of immediacy for a number of reasons, as suggested earlier. To highlight these, we might consider the following potential purposes for expressions of immediacy (Cormier & Nurius, 2003; Shebib, 2003):

• The coach deems it relevant to say something about himself, the client, or the relationship that may already be understood but perhaps would have a positive effect if the coach expressed it overtly. Coach and client may have various implicit understandings, or they may be developing norms for the relationship without having discussed them verbally and agreed on them. Coaches, believing in the importance of open acknowledgement of their own feelings, their observations of the client, or their sense of the relationship, may choose to direct attention to these issues by making the implicit explicit.

• The coach believes that she must directly address some pivotal experience in the relationship. If a client has a strong but unexpressed (verbally) reaction to a situation or to the coach's intervention, the coach may choose either to allow it to pass or to bring it to conscious awareness for both parties by describing her observations, thoughts, and feelings.

• The coach experiences a dynamic in the relationship that applies to how the client ineffectively manages other relationships and that relates to the client's agenda. The coaching relationship is potentially a microcosm of how the client engages with other people (Teyber, 2000). Although the specific relationship issues may not be disruptive to the working alliance in coaching, they may be interfering with how the client engages with others who are crucial to successful goal attainment. Coaches must always evaluate interventions in relation to the legitimate agendas of coaching. For instance, a client may have a somewhat dysfunctional interpersonal style that in no way affects the agreed-upon coaching agenda. Although it may be irritating to the coach and by extension to others who are involved with the client, this fact alone does not justify raising the agenda in the coaching relationship.

Types of Immediacy

Egan (1998, 2002) identifies two major types of immediacy: relationship immediacy and here-and-now immediacy. Cormier and Nurius (2003) suggest a slightly different typology: immediacy involving the helper's thoughts or feelings, immediacy involving feedback to the client based in the present, and immediacy focused on the relationship. If we explore these themes as they apply to coaching, the following types of immediacy seem relevant:

• **Immediacy related to the coach.** When the coach expresses thoughts or feelings reflecting his in-the-moment experiences, the skill of immediacy is involved. Expressions of this nature may range from simple statements of welcome or greeting to admissions of personal reactions or feelings. Some examples include the following:

Coach: "I feel flattered by your feedback."

Coach: "I feel excited by the work we're doing."

Coach: "Sorry, I have a headache and I can't seem to focus."

Coach: "I honestly don't know how I feel about that."

These examples of immediacy may be difficult to distinguish from self-disclosure as discussed in chapter 8. One way of distinguishing between immediacy and self-disclosure derives from the purpose of the intervention. When the coach intends to focus on the relationship per se, it is more likely that he will employ the skill of immediacy.

• **Immediacy related to the client.** This interpretation of immediacy is one facet of the skill of feedback, described in chapter 8. Although feedback encompasses more than this application, when coaches decide to tell clients about their perceptions or observations of client thoughts, feelings, or actions as they occur in the moment, they are using the skill of immediacy. Unlike immediacy related to the coach, this form of immediacy focuses entirely on the client, without additional input concerning the coach's reactions. Immediacy related to the client may serve multiple purposes, including increasing client self-awareness, acknowledging the client, or pursuing an issue through the coach's feedback about the client's nonverbal messages. Examples include the following:

Coach: "Seems like you're struggling to understand what I'm saying. Your brow looks furrowed, and you're looking very intently at me."

Coach: "I imagine that you're feeling very pleased with yourself for having discovered that fact. What a wonderful big smile you have."

Coach: "I wonder if you're upset with yourself. I see you wringing your hands and shaking your head from side to side."

- **Relationship immediacy.** What is the climate of the working alliance? How well are coach and client functioning together? Shebib (2003) thinks of relationship immediacy as focusing on the way the relationship is developing rather than on a specific incident or here-and-now occurrence. "The relationship is evaluated or reviewed, and relationship strengths and weaknesses are examined by explor-

ing the respective feelings, hopes, and frustrations of the parties involved" (Shebib, 1997, p. 114). Relationship immediacy might be called for when evident feelings or resistance to the work by either party are adversely affecting successful goal attainment. This application of immediacy should not be an end in itself but rather a means for enhancing the working relationship between coach and client (Cormier & Nurius, 2003). Coaching dialogue 7.1 provides some background for, as well as a simulated conversation representing, an expression of relationship immediacy.

Coaching Dialogue 7.1   Relationship Immediacy

Read the following dialogue to understand how a coach can use the skill of immediacy to address emergent concerns in the coaching relationship.

Background Information

The coach and client have been working together for 6 months, meeting at a regular time each week and having intermittent telephone contact. Although the client seemed to be highly motivated at first, increasingly over the past month the client has been showing up late for appointments and behaving like a truculent adolescent. Whenever the coach asks for information about the client's progress, the client seems reluctant to provide details. If some obstacle to progress is identified in the process of discussion, the client resists any ideas or suggestions that the coach puts forward.

Dialogue

Coach: "I have been noticing some things about how we are working together lately that might be worth discussing. Would you be willing to talk with me about how the coaching process seems to be going?"

Client: "As long as it doesn't take too much time. I want to make sure we deal with some problems I'm having in my training today."

Coach: "I can't be sure how much time it will take, but we can set an initial time limit of 10 minutes and then reassess at that point. After 10 minutes, we can talk about the specific agenda you're bringing today or continue. I'll leave that decision to you. Does this work for you?"

Client: "Yeah, 10 minutes would be OK, but not more."

Coach: "Agreed. Let me start since I brought it up. I've noticed a few changes over the past month in our coaching relationship. Before last month, you always came on time—"

Client: [Defensively interrupting the coach] "Yeah, well, I've been real busy this month so if that's it, then let's not bother discussing it because I can't control my boss, and that's why I've been late."

Coach: "So, you're telling me you've been late entirely because of work reasons so we needn't go any further in this discussion?"

Client: "Well, not entirely . . . But I'm sorry for interrupting. Let me hear the rest of what you wanted to say."

Coach:	"Sure, because the lateness piece is only part of what I want to discuss. The other parts are about how we seem to connect in these sessions."
Client:	[Again interjecting defensively] "Connect? What do you mean? I don't notice anything different. I come here, we talk, you tell me what to do, I try to do it, and then I give my report the following week."
Coach:	[Noticing that the conversation is being redirected, yet also aware that what the client is saying may be related to the perceived difficulties] "That's helpful to know. You're saying you haven't been aware of any changes in our relationship—"
Client:	"Well, maybe a little . . . But I'm sorry, I interrupted again. Finish what you were saying."
Coach:	"Hmmm. Maybe if you had a chance to tell me about the 'little' changes you notice, we could accomplish the same objective. Would you be willing to do that?"
Client:	[Looking energized and leaning toward the coach] "Yeah, sure. It's no big deal, but it feels to me like this is all about business these days. When I first started, you used to ask me all kinds of questions about my life, my work, my family, my friends, my interests—you name it, you asked me about it . . . And now it seems all you want to know about is whether I did what I said I would do. It's like somewhere I became a laboratory rat in an experiment."
Coach:	"I am so sorry that I'm coming across to you this way. I can see that the way you see us relating really upsets you."
Client:	[Minimizing the importance of what he has just said] "Well, I said it was no big deal."
Coach:	"I guess then it's just a big deal to me. I was wondering what had changed, and now you've given me a picture of how I'm coming across to you . . . Thanks, I believe we can deal with this. I am so appreciative of the fact that you told me how you were feeling. I had been concerned about this for weeks."

(The dialogue continues.)

Steps in Using Immediacy

The effective use of immediacy depends on the relational foundation of trust and rapport between coach and client (Gazda et al., 1999). Especially in a health fitness context, some clients may not be willing to address conflicts, differences, or feedback about behaviors that they define as irrelevant to their training. In this regard, initial discussions in coaching need to establish clear parameters for the working alliance. If a potential client indicates an unwillingness to consider any input other than performance and adherence reports, then the coaching process itself may not be a viable option for this client. If the client understands that feedback may be broader than what might occur in a personal training context, the question of timing remains. Timing concerns when it might be appropriate to use immediacy as a strategy, both within an individual session and within the larger context of the core conditions of the coaching relationship.

These cautionary words refer, of course, to applications of immediacy in which the coach raises significant and potentially sensitive issues. Saying to a client, "I am so happy to see you today," is a form of immediacy that is far simpler in its dynamics.

The following sections describe the steps that coaches may wish to follow in applying the skill of immediacy. The steps are based on the works of Egan (1998, 2002), Hepworth and associates (1997), and Cormier and Nurius (2003), and modified for applications in lifestyle fitness coaching.

Step 1—Awareness

The skill of immediacy begins with an awareness that something is happening in the relationship that pertains to its agenda, but it exists at a covert level or in a way that has been insufficiently articulated to capitalize fully on its saliency to coaching. More simply put, something significant is going on, and no one has dealt with it. Awareness means that the coach is not likely to be projecting, not experiencing countertransference, and not using the relationship to meet his own needs. Stated in positive terms, awareness implies ongoing monitoring of the relationship, of nonverbal messages as they relate to the client's verbal messages, of the coach's internal states and intuitions, and the analysis of all this information as it relates to the legitimate agenda of the relationship.

Step 2—Formulating a Response

How would the coach best express his awareness? What wording will produce the most positive response, or at least reduce defensiveness? How can the coach present a mental representation of issues in a factual, nonjudgmental, or nonevaluative fashion? A well-formulated response might have a structure that considers these elements (see "Judgmental Versus Nonjudgmental Examples of Immediacy" on page 135):

• **What have you observed factually?** The coach would frame for the client an objective or unbiased wording of what he is experiencing. Imagine, for instance, that the client rejects every suggestion that the coach puts forward and later decides to do something that the coach had suggested earlier, as if the coach had never mentioned it. How might the coach deal with this in a manner that isn't emotionally charged?

• **What are the potential effects or meanings of what you have observed?** In the situation just described, the effect and meaning could be that the coach is feeling frustrated and resentful, and that the client is living in a delusional world. If the client invariably chooses a solution originally suggested by the coach that proves to be effective, then does the coach need to address this issue? What is at stake? The coach's ego or the client's well-being? The case just described may seem extreme, but situations of this nature do occur. Whether the coach raises the issue and whether he includes his personal feelings or his imaginings of the meaning of the behavior for the client depends on the contract, the length of time the relationship is likely to continue, and the coach's personal needs and values. If the client acts in a denigrating, critical fashion with the coach, this circumstance alone may be important to discuss. Being a coach does not require that you allow clients to abuse you verbally even though they are

successfully addressing their agendas. In the preceding example, the coach might have included an additional statement reflecting effects, such as the following:

Coach: "And I also want to say that I felt upset when this just happened."

or

Coach: "This situation concerns me because I don't know whether what I observe here happens with you elsewhere . . . because when it happens to me, I feel really bad and upset, and other people in your life might have similar reactions."

• **What do you think will be achieved by addressing this matter?** In modern-day jargon, we get triggered when someone hits a sensitive area with a comment or behavior. Coaches must carefully manage reactivity in a coaching relationship. Clients are likely to push your buttons at various times, intentionally or not. Part of being a professional is referencing all your interventions to the goals of the relationship and the values that you wish to represent in your actions. If your immediacy will serve little other than your getting something off your chest, the intervention may not be justifiable. You need to have a well-articulated reason for your behavior, and this reason needs to serve the relationship and its objectives.

• **How will you know whether the response of immediacy had a desirable effect?** Clearing the air between coach and client can have its merits, yet the more relevant criterion might be whether the identified behavior changes. The feel-good response of having addressed a difficult issue may produce an immediate payoff and confirm that the process had value, but if the behavior recurs then what has been achieved? Coaches who use immediacy hope to realize improved functioning in the relationship and in client behavior directed toward goal attainment.

Step 3—Timing the Response

In more emotionally laden uses of immediacy, timing is of utmost importance. Raising issues of this nature toward the end of a session or when a client seems highly motivated to pursue something else may be unwise. The client's response to your guidance may be far less or far more than you anticipate; in either case, you need to make allowances. Additionally, if a client comes into a session with a passionate interest in discussing a particular topic or in accomplishing certain work, rarely would

Judgmental Versus Nonjudgmental Examples of Immediacy

The coach has noted the following pattern: His client seeks advice about how to handle various situations, yet when the coach provides suggestions, the client invariably rejects them by finding fault with some aspect of the suggestions. Later in the session, the client suddenly discovers a solution, always something that the coach had suggested earlier, and congratulates himself on answering his own dilemma. At the same time, the client wonders aloud why the coach couldn't be as creative.

Immediacy That Is Judgmental, Evaluative, or Critical

1. "I am feeling a bit frustrated here. I don't think I'm being given due credit. The solution you just came up with was something I told you 10 minutes ago, yet you're acting as if you never heard it before!"

2. "Can we talk about something? [Pauses for agreement.] I've been noticing a pattern that whenever I give you advice, you reject it, and then later come up with the same idea as if you've just discovered it."

3. "I need to say something here. I think you are feeling insecure in this relationship. Even though I give you good advice, you ignore it and then come up with my ideas as if they were your own. This suggests a kind of insecurity on your part. Am I right?"

Immediacy That Is Neutral, Factual, and Nonjudgmental

1. "I want to discuss something with you. Would you be willing to take a few minutes with me now? [Pauses for agreement.] I'm not sure what this is about, so I really need your help. When you just came up with an answer to the problem you raised earlier, I felt glad for you. I hope it will work for you. My puzzlement is that earlier in the session I said what I thought was the same thing, and in your words, you replied, 'That's stupid and crazy. That will never work.' Do you remember this happening? Do you have any thoughts about what's happening here?"

2. "Can we take a minute to look at something that may be happening between us? [Pauses for agreement.] I have been noticing what I think is a pattern, and because it just seemed to happen again, I thought I could get your thoughts about it. You just came up with what you described as a 'great' solution to your problem, and I agree with you that it seems to be a good one. Yet, I remember saying the same thing to you 10 minutes ago, and you told me the idea was stupid and crazy and wouldn't work. Do you remember this? Am I describing this accurately in your view? It seems like a pattern, and I sure would appreciate your help in figuring it out."

you sideline the client's agenda to address matters that the client may be unwilling, unmotivated, or resistant to consider.

Step 4—Being Open to a Variety of Responses

Because people may behave with a general lack of awareness of their influence on others, the use of immediacy could serve as a significant wake-up call for some clients. They may begin to make connections between what just transpired in coaching and similar issues in other relationships. Although coaches do not need to address these matters, they may need to make space for clients' insightful reflections. Should clients be highly motivated to pursue these new avenues of awareness, coaches may need to remind them of the boundaries of their relationship while also offering information about referrals to other allied health professionals. Of course, another response that coaches will want to prepare for is defensiveness or denial. Clients may deny awareness of the matter or attempt to discredit the coach. Rather than attempt to prove the correctness of their observations or perceptions, effective coaches will recognize this impasse and consider it in determining how best to proceed. When the coach's observations are unquestionably valid and relevant to the viability of the working alliance or to goal attainment, termination of the relationship may be one of the options to consider.

Step 5—Emphasizing the Relevance of Immediacy to the Goals of Coaching

If the meaning of the immediacy intervention is not entirely clear to the client, the coach may wish to review why he brought this kind of information into discussion and how it may relate to the goals of the working alliance. This particular step would occur after the coach has offered the observations or perceptions and has adequately discussed them with the client. In concluding this dialogue, the coach may then summarize by providing the client with perspectives about his use of immediacy.

Uses and Abuses of Immediacy

The power of immediacy for moving the relationship toward more productive dialogue cannot be underestimated. Conversations of this nature are very real. They capture the spirit of both coach and client, and these moments may produce a strongly felt connection and the discovery of deeper meanings. But such intensity may also be a liability. Let us review a number of problematic uses of immediacy, some of which we have touched on in earlier discussions:

• **Immediacy as an end in itself.** As Egan (1998) among others advises, immediacy is not a skill that coaches should employ for its own sake. In intimate relationships, people may talk about their feelings and their mutual effects quite regularly. The function is to deepen the relationship and reduce misunderstandings, misinterpretations, and the potential buildup of negative feelings. Expressions of caring, love, concern, or affection play an important role in increasing interpersonal attractiveness and connection. How much of this is critical to a coaching relationship is questionable. Certainly, when misunderstandings and misinterpretations affect the ability of coach and client to work effectively together, the coach could appropriately address these issues through the skill of immediacy. But the satisfaction that may result from increasing the intimacy level of a coaching relationship needs to be weighed against how central it is to the achievement of the client's goals—and what the long-range implications of this behavior might be. Even seemingly innocent expressions such as "I was really looking forward to

our session today" may represent minor boundary crossings (see chapter 4) that could eventually lead to ethical violations.

• **Immediacy as countertransference.** Just as clients may project thoughts, beliefs, or feelings onto their coaches, so too the reverse may occur. When coaches do not allow for periods of reflection about their coaching relationships, they may fail to observe how certain assumptions or even fantasies that derive from other pivotal relationships in their lives shape their experiences with certain clients. The tendency to see issues of countertransference as pertaining to the more in-depth domain of counseling and psychotherapy needs to be deconstructed. These types of reactions are common to virtually all intense, ongoing professional relationships. Here are two simple manifestations of countertransference that might easily occur in the client–coach relationship:

- **Situation A.** A male coach recently had an argument with his wife in which she accused him of not living up to his part of the bargain in the relationship. She criticized him for shirking his responsibilities at home. While still in turmoil about this argument, the coach meets his first client of the day, who subtly shames him for forgetting to call her during the week as they had agreed. He finds himself getting angry and feeling resentful toward his client.

- **Situation B.** A female coach has a young client who physically resembles her son. Her son happens to be a bit of a sneak. Although he hasn't gotten into serious trouble, the coach often finds out about her son's wayward behavior from neighbors or occasionally from authorities. The coach finds herself asking her client questions like "Are you telling me *all* I need to know in order to do the very best with you?" The client seems puzzled by the question, especially because she has asked it more than once.

• **Immediacy as a fallback for indirection.** When in doubt, we always have the present moment on which to focus. Current experience is fluid and ever-changing. In counseling and psychotherapy, the entire treatment can be framed as awareness training wherein the client is continually focused on the here and now (Yalom, 1980). When a coach does not have a clear plan of action or when she does not know what to do next, it may be all too easy to focus on the immediate experience. "I see you looking at me intently, like you want to ask a question. Can you tell me what's happening for you right now?" might be an appropriate intervention at certain moments in the coaching relationship, but as a means of deflecting attention from oneself to the client, it is probably inappropriate and ineffective. The coach must use immediacy strategically and in a way that relates to the client's agenda, not as a spontaneous reaction to her own uncertainty.

• **Effect of immediacy on client dependency.** When coaches provide immediacy interventions based on feel-good experiences with the client ("You are such a joy to work with") or when they deepen the relationship through intimacy-creating dialogues, clients may be enticed to continue in coaching more for the emotional boost they get than for the contracted growth agendas. If coaches forewarn that they may end the relationship because the client is now doing so well, clients who have become dependent on their coaches may begin to sabotage their own performance to show how much they still need to be involved in the coaching process.

Summary of Immediacy

Some applications of immediacy require great courage and equanimity. Even simple statements (e.g., "I like you") can be more problematic than imagined, and developing the capacity to be on top of relationship dynamics almost all the time can be demanding. In coaching relationships that endure over many months, occasions are likely to arise where the use of immediacy will be helpful. Either in terms of celebrating a client's achievements or in addressing an undercurrent in the relationship, coaches will need to be astute in how they frame their remarks.

The more comfortable that coaches feel with being in the moment with their clients, the more ease they will convey to clients about issues they choose to address. Coaches who approach any here-and-now interaction as potentially explosive will no doubt convey their fears through nonverbal messages to their clients, and the resulting communication will fulfill the negative prophecy, much as might the dreaded confrontation of a topic that has simmered for months. The key is to reduce the emotion related to the issue and to detach from particular outcomes. The client does not have to get it. Great insights do not have to result. There need be no epiphany or significant catharsis. The centrality of this skill to coaching suggests that coaches become as comfortable with it as possible in their daily lives so that when they use immediacy in coaching, it will come across as naturally as any of their other interventions do.

Reflection of Meaning

To what degree is the coaching process about meaning in a client's life? As a health fitness professional you may be familiar with the scenarios described in learning activity 7.2. Assuming that these clients are presenting their issues to you, would you begin to plan a strategy for helping them work toward their stated objectives, or would you want to know more about them and their goals?

Learning Activity 7.2   Exploring Meaning

The following scenarios indicate the stated agendas of four new coaching clients. What thoughts come to mind when reflecting on their agendas? What information might you want to obtain? What questions would you ask?

- Scenario A: A 42-year-old male client with a 26% body fat composition approaches you after his testing and asks whether you can design a program for him to reduce his percentage of body fat to 18%.

- Scenario B: A 26-year-old female who has been relatively inactive for most of her life wants you to help her train for an Olympic-distance triathlon.

- Scenario C: A 34-year-old client tells you that he wants to make friends through his fitness activities. He says that he spends too much time alone and wants to socialize more—and what better way than with people who like to be active as he does?

- Scenario D: A 50-year-old man in reasonably good shape wants to take up martial arts. He's not sure which one to pursue and wants your support in finding the right martial art and in helping him develop the strength and flexibility to perform well in this new activity.

If we review the literature on life coaching, we will find various propositions for why people pursue coaching rather than some other process such as counseling or psychotherapy. Customary thinking is that coaching is for people who are functioning well and want to do even better (Williams & Davis, 2002), whereas counseling and psychotherapy are for people who are experiencing adjustment difficulties or more serious psychological disturbances (Capuzzi & Gross, 2001; Parrott, 2003; Prochaska & Norcross, 2003).

In lifestyle fitness coaching, clients are likely to hire you in relation to some physical activity or active-living pursuit. Their goals may sound straightforward. The fact that they are interested in sport or exercise does not guarantee that they are functioning well at a psychological level. Although ample evidence indicates that people who exercise regularly show more positive indicators of mental health than those who are inactive (Buckworth & Dishman, 2002; Morgan, 1997), generalizing from population statistics to individual cases can be misleading.

We might at least assume two things when lifestyle fitness coaches meet clients within health clubs and fitness centers. First, these clients have an interest in doing something that will most likely have significant benefits for physical and psychological functioning. Second, if a client has psychological concerns that go beyond the boundaries of the coach's training and the contracted agenda of coaching, the coach can refer the client to appropriate mental health professionals while the client continues to work in association with the coach on the activity agenda.

Taken at face value, the interests of the four clients portrayed in learning activity 7.2 might be the norm for fitness advisors or personal trainers. Lifestyle fitness coaches may choose to go further beneath the surface. Whitworth and colleagues (1998) view clients' initial objectives as likely to be superficial, concrete, and object oriented. That is, the client may want to build muscle, lose weight, learn yoga, increase flexibility, make friends, test limits, experience adventure, or compete successfully. The magical thinking that is often incorporated in these objectives is that having or obtaining these ends will then make the client feel fulfilled. After the client has bigger muscles, less fat, more friends, or greater success at sports, life will be better and the client will feel fulfilled. Of course, in portraying the matter this way, you are likely to realize that achieving goals does not necessarily make people happy, that happiness or well-being is a state of being that a person

must realize in each moment, not just when he finds the pot of gold at the end of the rainbow.

Asking a man with 26% body fat why he wants to reduce to 18% may seem pointless. As a health fitness professional you might tend to jump right on the bandwagon in support of his goal. Obesity is rampant in North America. Why not reduce his body fat? Herein lies the dilemma. Although a goal may seem to have inherent value, as a coach you may still want to inquire about the values the person associates with his current state as compared with those related to his desired state. What will the change do for him? Why does he want to do this *now*? How does he feel about his 26% body fat self? In essence, what is the meaning of this issue for him?

Perhaps more out of curiosity than for any other reason, a fitness advisor may want to discover what has suddenly inspired a 26-year-old woman to train for a triathlon. For a lifestyle fitness coach, understanding the motivation would be essential to working with this client. Similarly, the 50-year-old man who wants to train in martial arts may see some important value in this arduous undertaking, or he may perceive it as a means to some end. Exploring this client's thinking might reveal important dimensions of his personality, needs, life experiences, hopes, and visions.

Finally, presented with the question of how to advise a client who wants to socialize while training, most fitness advisors can immediately produce a list of activities that are solitary and those that invite interaction. Yet, for the lifestyle fitness coach, the issues may run deeper. What is this client's current social style? What kinds of interactions is he seeking? How much of a stretch will it be for him to enter a highly interactive fitness environment? Do his interaction needs have other aspects? For instance, does he want to be playful with others, compete with them, engage in aggressive encounters, or go off on long adventures with a group?

The Meaning of *Meaning*

Human beings are meaning-creating creatures (Frankl, 1969). Others may not ask us the somewhat taboo why question, although we will often ask it of ourselves. Why did I do that? Why is this so important to me? Why do I want to do this? Why does this have to happen to me?

Existential psychologists indicate that crisis and tragedy prompt many people to search for meaning (Binswanger, 1963; Bugental, 1965; Frankl, 1969; May, 1977; Yalom, 1980), although any process of change suggests a meaning shift within the person.

An obese client who decides to lose weight may be responding to self-perceptions or the perceptions of others and seek to change those views. A recreational athlete who decides to go all out in a performance enhancement program so that she can compete as an elite athlete is likely to have had some internal change represented outwardly in her goals and the actions required to achieve them.

As Prochaska and Norcross (2003, p. 122) comment in their description of existential therapies, "One does not discover meaning in life; one creates meaning out of life. The question is not what is the answer to life; the answer is that life is an ongoing process to be experienced, not a problem to be solved. The meaning of our existence emerges out of what we choose to stand for."

The coaching process involves understanding what meaning clients are creating out of their experiences, what new meanings they want to create, and what they want their experiences to stand for. In the early stages of a coaching relationship, clients will be encouraged to tell their stories. The way they tell their stories may reveal meanings that they attach to their experiences or to their visions of future realities. As Ivey and Ivey (2003, p. 282) suggest, "If we can help clients find what they really want and mean, their decisions and actions will flow more easily."

The search for meaning may run quite deep, but coaches need only enough understanding to work with the client's more potent motivations and drives, and to ground the client's objectives in reality rather than fantasy. For instance, a client who wants to bulk up to overcome a sense of insecurity may need to find other supportive processes, such as reading, counseling, or human development workshops, to achieve his goal. Alternatively, he might discover through dialogue with a coach that his reasons for focusing on this particular means to his end merit reexamination. Through such dialogue he may discover less fear-driven reasons for engaging in physical activities.

Purposes of Reflecting Meaning

Reflection of meaning is a skill process that incorporates a number of other communication skills, including reflection of content, reflection of feeling, and questioning. This skill has appeared in the coaching literature under such headings as *powerful questions* and *curiosity* (Whitworth et al., 1998), although the focus is quite similar. Coaches use reflection of meaning to discover the personal significance of events, thoughts, needs, or objectives of clients (Young, 2001). Reflection of meaning serves purposes such as the following:

- **Developing a fuller understanding of the client.** Perhaps the most straightforward purpose for using reflection of meaning is simply to understand the client better. If someone says, "I want a new car, and I'd love to have a summer cottage," you might immediately identify with those interests because you, too, would like to have those things. The trap in thinking arises from the fact that the same objective phenomenon, whether it is a car, a house, a new job, or 12% body fat, can have substantially different meanings for different people. Assuming that these objective things represent the same internal motivations can be problematic. Using reflection of meaning allows the coach to discover what clients' experiences, desires, or goals mean to them. When a client tells a story about certain life experiences, we may say things like, "I can certainly relate to that." But can we really? Again, the same external events or incidents can have widely different personal interpretations. Someone says, "I just finished my first marathon." The listener responds, "Oh, you must be so proud of yourself." The speaker replies, "No, I feel sort of disappointed and depressed." In a less candid conversation, the speaker might give the socially acceptable response because she knows that she should be proud of herself. As some coaching books repeatedly emphasize (Martin, 2001; Whitworth et al., 1998), coaches need to be curious. They need not only to hear the story but also to probe for the story behind the story. Only by doing so can they develop processes and activities with their clients that have a kind of ecological validity, that is, that they make sense for the whole person, not just for one isolated dimension of the client's identity.

- **Clarifying the meaning of intended behavior changes.** When clients are identifying their intentions or goals for working with you, although they may be clear and even conform to the structure of SMART goals, understanding what the goals mean to the person will be helpful. What will these intended changes enable clients to do differently? How will the changes affect their lives? What personal values do these goals represent?

- **Addressing myths and fallacies.** In listening to clients' stories, we sometimes hear assumptions about the world, about themselves, about the effect of their behaviors, or about what will happen in the future if certain things do not change. Some examples of client mythologies include the following:

  - "If I am more fit, my wife will love me more."

- "If I exercise regularly, I will lose all my old friends who don't exercise."
- "If I have no energy to begin with, how can I possibly think of exercising? I will be exhausted afterward."
- "If I exercise regularly, I can eat all I want and still lose weight."
- "If I exercise regularly, it will make up for smoking a pack of cigarettes each day."

Reflection of meaning involves a different process than directly contradicting a person's erroneous beliefs. A coach could tell a client who believes that his wife will love him more if he is more trim and fit that this assumption is not necessarily the case, or the coach could reflect this belief back to the client in such a way that the client becomes more likely to dissect this assumption and, in the process, find more personal, self-serving motives for exercising. Imagine, for the moment, that the client based his program on this motivation. No matter how much progress he makes, unless his marital relationship changes, the client is unlikely to achieve his goal. Moreover, the coach would have no way of assessing the viability of this outcome or influencing it directly through the coaching process.

- **Identifying motivational sources for behavior change.** As reflected in the case of the man wanting to improve his marriage through exercise, establishing the motivational roots for initiating and maintaining regular exercise or for pursuing some other athletic goal is critical in the early stages of work with clients. Although coaching may be a long-term process, the eventual goal of coaching is to empower the client to be self-directing and autonomous in addressing life's challenges and opportunities. The questioning process that is part of reflection of meaning enables clients to discover what core values their actions serve and how they can continually find the energy and commitment for their actions by referencing plans to these deeper motives. Coaching dialogue 7.2 demonstrates how a coach would endeavor to discover clients' deeper meanings and core values that will support all their efforts to achieve their goals. As the dialogue indicates, through the coach's use of reflection of meaning, the client realizes the "reasons beneath her reasons" that will likely serve her better in attaining her objectives.

- **Exploring complementary paths to goal attainment.** When coach and client explore meaning in a coaching process, clients are able to appreciate better who they are, what they need, and the full-

ness of their agendas. Fitness involvement has been advanced as a modern-day panacea for all kinds of problems and life dilemmas. The fact is that exercise, helpful as it is, is only one avenue to health and personal fulfillment. Lifestyle fitness coaches work with clients not only to help them formulate action strategies involving sport and other active living options but also to assist them in discovering sustaining motivation and shaping their expectations for change more congruently with the actions that they undertake. Clients who expect that exercise will make their social lives prosper, improve their mental health, develop their physical health, and build their bodies into beacons of health and beauty could be right. On the other hand, they may need to consider a few other factors to achieve these objectives.

Coaches can support clients in creating goals that are profoundly encompassing. They can also help clients frame their expectations more realistically based on what they are willing to do or support them in finding other avenues along which to work in tandem with their sport and fitness agendas. As indicated in coaching dialogue 7.2, the 36-year-old client may choose to address her smoking and eating issues as part of her overall strategy for developing that strong, healthy glow. Alternatively, she may decide to proceed in a stepwise manner, dealing with her exercise involvement first and then, having gained confidence and motivation from addressing that agenda, take on the serious challenge of quitting smoking and eating better.

Steps in Reflecting Meaning

Ivey and Ivey (2003) think of reflection of meaning as comprising four interrelated components: thoughts, feelings, behaviors, and, of course, meaning. Meaning implies values, beliefs, deep-level motivations, and the significance that a person attributes to different facets of life and human action. Clearly, what someone does is likely to represent personalized meanings. Thoughts, feelings, and behaviors, however, do not provide perfect reflections of meaning. People must discover meaning through a process of inquiry, whether they do this privately or in a dialogue with another person.

Reflecting meaning relies on other skills, notably, reflection of content, reflection of feeling, summarizing, and questioning. Other skills, reviewed in chapter 8, may also be pertinent and could in fact be the signal to the coach that reflecting meaning may be required to advance the client's process. For instance, the skill of confrontation includes noticing discrepancies between different things that a

Coaching Dialogue 7.2   Discovering Core Motives
Through Reflection of Meaning

Read the following dialogue to understand how a coach can use the skill of reflection of meaning to help a client understand deeper dimensions of her goals.

Background Information

The client is a 36-year-old single woman in a highly demanding executive position. She has exercised irregularly over the past 15 years and now wants to "get really fit and healthy." She smokes a half pack of cigarettes a day and wants to quit. She eats reasonably well, although when she notices herself gaining a pound or two (a kilogram), she immediately goes on a starvation diet.

Dialogue

Client: "So, yes, I want to be really fit. I want to be able to run 10K races without even having to think about it. I want to wear sleeveless shirts and have great arm muscles showing . . . and I want people to cringe with envy when they see my abs."

Coach: "Well, this is getting a bit clearer for me. It sounds as if you want to be in peak form, so that running a 10K would be easy, and your body would be so fit that it would really make people notice. Are these your goals?"

Client: "You've got it. That's what I want."

Coach: "Tell me this. If you were able to run a 10K race with ease, and if your body looked like the models on the covers of fitness magazines, what would this give you? What would it mean to you?"

Client: "Well, it would mean that I look young and athletic . . . and people would look at me differently."

Coach: "OK, go on. You'd look young and athletic and people would see you differently . . . and what would that mean for you?"

Client: "Well, I'm 36, you know . . . and I'm beginning to notice some changes in my skin and in how firm my body is."

Coach: "Am I hearing your concern about aging and some worries about not looking young?"

Client: "Well, it's more than that. I used to take pride in my appearance. I counted on it, but I notice some mornings I have to use a bit more makeup than normal. I guess my smoking doesn't help that, nor does the way I eat sometimes."

Coach: "It sounds like your emphasis is on looking healthy, and that you believe exercise can help, yet you also seem to be aware that your eating and smoking behaviors may need to be modified as well."

Client: "Well, yes. I've been ducking this. I thought I'd get that great healthy glow from just exercising, but you're right, smoking doesn't do a lot for my complexion."

Coach: [Nodding agreement] "Uh huh."

Client: "But, you know, now that you've said it, I want more than just looking healthy. That's my real goal. I guess I can have a perfectly sculpted body and still be unhealthy unless I'm willing to deal with the whole package."

Coach: "So, you're saying that a deeper desire is to be healthy, and that having a fit-looking body is important, but looks could be deceiving unless you're dealing with other factors, like eating and smoking."

Client: "Yes, that's it for sure. I like the idea of looking young and fit and healthy and strong and sexy, but I want it to be for real, not just an external show . . . I want to be that way from the inside out."

person has said or done, or between what a person says and how she says it (nonverbal communications). By observing discrepancies, the coach may realize that the client's words do not reflect her true feelings or experiences—or that something deeper is occurring.

Whatever the stimulus for initiating a process of reflecting meaning, coaches need to be aware that the client must perceive such explorations as legitimate. A reflection of meaning reveals what lies beneath the surface, and although this method is generally accepted as appropriate terrain for the coaching relationship, clients who expect coaches to function more as personal trainers may not welcome questions like, "Why do you want to do this?" or "What does this mean to you?"

You might want to consider the following steps when using this skill.

Step 1—Determination of the Need and Timing for Discovering Meaning

Using a reflection of meaning will be eminently more successful when coaches have clarified their credentials, identified appropriate boundaries for their work, and discussed their methods of working with clients. With these tasks accomplished, clients should understand the ways in which coaches work, and they should feel safe within well-defined boundaries (including the promise of confidentiality). When some clients tell their stories, they may be aware of the meanings beneath their objective goal statements, in which case coaches will not need to probe and explore. More likely, many clients will offer only the surface objectives, which, depending on the client, may have little potential for generating and sustaining the necessary motivation to engage meaningful behavior change. After the need to probe for meaning is established, the second question is whether the timing is right. Reflection of meaning optimally occurs on the foundation of trust and rapport between coach and client. This connection may develop easily, or it may take time. Recognizing that clients may feel uncomfortable exposing what they consider sensitive personal information to someone who is a relative stranger, the coach may need to postpone for a session or two the deeper process of reflecting meaning until he feels that core relationship conditions (see chapter 3) have been sufficiently established.

Step 2—Formulating a Theme for Reflection

Coaches need to have a general direction for the use of reflection of meaning. Inquiring out of general curiosity what meaning a client attributes to life, relationships, or exercise is inappropriate. Clients may perceive such questioning as "What do you think is the meaning of life?" as entirely inappropriate, unnecessarily philosophical, or simply out of bounds, perhaps thinking or saying, "It's none of your business!" When clients offer straightforward goals, such as "I want to learn how to exercise regularly and efficiently so that I can maintain my weight at the level it is now," a coach could easily offer support for this objective, while at least wondering, "If the client achieved this, what would it mean to her?" Moreover, the client does not necessarily have clear definitions of words like *regularly* or *efficiently*. So, at a minimum, the coach could explore the client's meaning of those words.

Step 3—Introducing the Theme of the Reflection

In simple reflections of meaning, such as "What does the word *efficient* mean to you?" a straightforward question may suffice. But when coaches are aware of a theme that has weaved its way through a number of sentences or even sessions, it is likely, first, that the theme has more bearing on the client's agenda, and, second, that the client will need some opportunity to hear a summary of messages that the coach has been collecting and that warrants reflection. The coach may begin the process of reflecting meaning through the skill of summarizing. Coaching dialogue 7.3 illustrates this initiation of a reflection.

Step 4—Appropriately Blending Skills in the Search for Meaning

When an issue, concern, or objective is easily accessible to the client, a coach may only need to ask one or two questions to discover the client's meaning. In this case, the client knows the meaning, but the coach does not. Bringing this information into the public venue of their relationship will foster progress. More often, neither the coach nor the client fully understands the meaning of some issue, and therefore the process of discovery is likely to take some effort. If the coach barrages the client with probing questions, the client might experience the process as a kind of interrogation. Defensiveness and emotional distance might result. A more effective strategy might rely on the considered use of a variety of skills that pace the client in the process, that encourage openness, and that minimize defensive reactions (see coaching dialogue 7.3). The use of paraphrases may follow initial probes, and these paraphrases, in turn, may lead to additional questions. Some questions that have been suggested

dialogue

Coaching Dialogue 7.3 Integrating the Coach's Perceptions Through Reflecting Meaning

Read the following dialogue to understand how a coach integrates perceptions obtained over time and employs the skill of reflection of meaning to help a client gain fuller understanding of his aspirations.

Background Information

A 59-year-old man in relatively good health has recently retired from a well-paid position as a research scientist. He feels that he has denied himself the opportunity to follow many of his dreams throughout life, but he now has the time and the financial security to pursue them. Many of these dreams involve high-risk sports and, being wise and cautious, he wants to make sure that his body is in the best possible shape before he embarks on these adventures. After three introductory meetings and some preliminary action planning, the coach wishes to address a theme that he has heard several times in the client's messages.

Dialogue

Coach: "Phil, would you be willing to allow some time today for me to summarize a theme I think I'm hearing from you—and for us to discuss it together?"

Client: "Sure, sounds like fun!"

Coach: "The picture you have drawn of yourself, if I'm correct, is of a highly successful scientist who got where he did by being careful, conservative, and never taking chances. Is this part accurate?"

Client: "Yup, that was the old me."

Coach: "OK, and now what I've been hearing is that you want to train for some pretty rugged and even dangerous sports because they have been your dream and you never took the time for them."

Client: "Right again. Keep going . . . I'm getting intrigued."

Coach: "Great. So this seems to be a kind of shift in the way you have lived your life, and I'd like to understand more about what you are seeing in this new direction, especially when you contrast it with your previous patterns."

Client: "Great question . . . Frankly, I'm not 100% sure about this, but I think I lost an important part of me playing the scientist all these years, and I want to start having fun."

Coach: "Umm hmm. You're saying that you were playing at being a scientist, and that you didn't have very much fun?"

Client: "Well, I had fun discovering things but not like the fun I think I could have had climbing Mt. Kilimanjaro. I've been a stodgy scientist and I had to stuff a lot of my wilder side all these years."

Coach: "I hear you . . . And you imagine that climbing Mt. Kilimanjaro or something like that will allow you to get to know that wilder side better."

Client: "Sure will. And I'm not being crazy about this—that's why I hired you. I want to go about this carefully, but I need to break out of the box that I've allowed myself to live in all these years."

Coach: "Hmmm, so it feels as if you've been in a box for a long time?"

Client: "Maybe that's an exaggeration. I've had a good life . . . It's just time for a change. I'm still young enough and healthy enough to push the envelope a bit, and that's what I intend

(continued)

143

(continued)

Coach: "So, why not?"

Client: "Yeah, why not? I realize some of this sounds crazy and I hope you can help me keep things in balance, but this isn't just about doing wild things, it's about me and how I see myself. I want to get reacquainted with that young kid I once was who was a great student, but, man, he also knew how to have fun. I want to rediscover that kid and go play with him!" [eyes growing moist]

Coach: [Pauses for a few seconds to allow the client to compose himself and to be ready to listen.] "This seems real important to you, and I'm glad you helped me with this. I hear that all of this is about being your whole self, the way that you have always seen yourself but have not always allowed yourself to be . . . And it's not about being crazy, it's about bringing more excitement into your life in a careful way, even though it looks a lot riskier than what you've been like for the past 30 years . . . And I hear you want me to be your safety belt—to keep you from going over the edge by reflecting the capabilities I think you have and the risks of what you're considering."

Client: "Wow. What a great way of saying it! Thanks. I'm going to think about this some more because having talked about it, I now understand it better and I feel more in charge of it. At times, I just felt this urge to do it all, whatever it was . . . and now I have a better sense of where this is coming from. So, again, thanks."

---

for accessing clients' meanings (Ivey & Ivey, 2003) include the following:

- What values do you see in this for you?
- What will this mean to you if you are able to achieve it?
- What is it that makes this so important to you?
- Tell me how you see this making sense for you?
- If you were to put this all together, what would it all mean to you?
- Why do you want to do this?
- Why this (goal) and not that one?

Step 5—Relating the Derived Meaning to the Goals of Coaching

Because the purpose of reflecting meaning is far less philosophical than practical, the coach must ensure that the derived meanings from the reflective process can be connected to the coaching process and the client's goals. Clients may have moments of insight in this kind of dialogue and will readily link their discoveries with the goals that they have for the coaching process. In other cases, the connec-

tion may not be as evident, so the coach may need to continue working with the client to establish the connection.

Uses and Abuses of Reflecting Meaning

Helping clients find deeper meaning and values in their desires to change can not only assist coaches in costructuring interventions that are more likely to succeed but also provide clients with a source of ongoing motivation for action. If we think of the popular approach of having clients identify positive affirmations that through constant repetition serve to direct and energize behavior change (Goldman, 2001), then we can readily imagine how critical it will be to find the words or images that will reliably fuel healthy action. Using the skill of reflecting meaning enables clients to understand better why they are choosing certain goals, why they feel the need to change *now*, and what they fundamentally want to achieve through the coaching process. Yet, as with all other skills, certain uses of reflection of meaning can become problematic. Here are some issues to bear in mind:

- **Reflection of meaning as an end in itself.** Coaches contract with clients in relation to agendas that clients deem important to pursue. A process of reflecting meaning can be rewarding in itself. Some clients may revel in processes of self-discovery, yet because coaching is intentionally action oriented, such discovery processes must always serve the client's orientation toward action and goal attainment.

• **Taking over the agenda.** Imagine a client who states certain objectives with which the coach, for personal reasons, disagrees. For instance, a client may want to do whatever it takes to become an elite amateur bodybuilder, but her coach may subconsciously disapprove of this agenda. By using meaning reflections, the coach could lead the client to question her own values and goals. Implicitly, the coach may convey disapproval of the client's agenda by the way in which she asks, "Why exactly do you want to do this?" The discovery process may continue until the coach determines that the client now has the right agenda, and then the work of implementation begins. Unfortunately, in the process, the client is likely to feel shamed and demoralized if her important goals have somehow been discredited through a biased reflective process.

• **Reflecting mechanically.** The skill of reflecting meaning is based on insightful awareness of who the client is, what the client needs, and whether the timing is right for an intervention of this nature. When a coach asks clients what they mean by different messages only because the asking process is one of the things that a coach *should* do, mechanical reflections are the likely result. When coaches carry out reflection of meaning as part of a rote process of questioning or as part of a script that they have for differentiating their work from that of personal trainers, they stand the chance of inappropriately using the skill and thereby distancing themselves from their clients. Reflecting meaning involves peeling away the superficial layers of client messages and, in so doing, increases the chances that clients will feel vulnerable. When a mechanical probing process creates this increased vulnerability, clients may well be aware of being exposed to a coach who does not seem to have a well-guided rationale for opening up these deeper levels of data and relating them to the client's agenda.

• **Probing too deeply.** As noted earlier in the discussion of reflection of meaning, this type of inquiry gets beneath the surface. How deep it needs to go depends on agreements with the client and the coach's ability to justify such explorations as critical to advancing client progress. Coaches need to ask themselves exactly how much information they need to help formulate strategies for working with clients and assisting them in their processes. More is not always better. In fact, with some clients minimal meaning reflections will suffice. Going deeper may cause them to spin in indecision and uncertainty. The process may create an overlarge agenda or produce too many options to consider. Coaches need to guard against the phenomenon of "bringing up the bottom." Some clients may have struggled to find the motivation to engage a coach to help them with their work, and they may live with barely concealed dissatisfaction with their physical appearance, weight issues, or life struggles. Asking too many questions about their reasons for wanting to exercise regularly or to achieve certain health change goals may reawaken self-rejecting thoughts and feelings, which in their reinvigorated state may serve to counter the positive motivations.

Summary of Reflection of Meaning

Coaches need to be acutely sensitive to the pacing of relationships. Coaches should never pursue meaning for its own sake; they should seek it only in service of the clients' agendas. As the relationship progresses and deeper levels of trust develop, clients will likely reveal more of the details necessary for coaches to work efficiently. Clients reveal what they want you to know, and in cases when even they do not know the meanings of things, they will usually forewarn you through nonverbal messages of comfort or discomfort about whether you are welcome in this deeper realm of their being. Sometimes coaches can encourage clients to search for their deeper meanings without necessarily revealing them. The coach may not need to know what certain things mean to the client, as long as the client has this understanding. In this respect, meaning reflections do not always have to be answered overtly. Although a coach may deem it relevant for a client to explore certain issues, she can support the client in doing this privately. For instance, a coach may recommend that a client spend some time between sessions considering why her stated goals are critical for her to achieve at this particular time. In the following session the client may wish to share her reflections or may choose to keep them private.

Coaching for Insight and Discovery

In this chapter we have seen how and why coaches may use combinations of skills to deepen the coaching relationship and discover new meanings and insights with their clients. Probably evident throughout the discussions of focusing, immediacy, and reflection of meaning is that these skills do not so much represent new techniques as they do sensitive and probing applications of the basic skills of reflection, questioning, and summarizing. It might also be apparent that as skill level develops, so do the risk and responsibility that coaches assume within the relationship. Through traditional fitness assessments, an advisor may note that a client has a 30% body fat composition, and the advisor may immediately proceed with the client's overt compliance to design an exercise program to reduce that percentage to a healthier level. Without considering the additional details and information gathered

through a lifestyle fitness coaching process, the likelihood for success of the fitness advisor's unilateral prescription may be modest.

Because certain additional information is deemed important and because the quality of the relationship between coach and client provides the vehicle for identifying valid and attainable goals, these more probing skills assume importance. Although the coaching profession is increasingly well known, clients in a health fitness context may yet need to learn of the nature of the work with coaches and the depth of some of the issues that they may need to explore before they can codetermine and successfully pursue **ecologically valid goals.**

Influencing Clients in Change Processes

eight

*"You gain strength, courage,
and confidence
by every experience
in which you really stop to
look fear in the face."*

Eleanor Roosevelt

Lacking an adequate information base, coach and client will probably create a poor plan of action. Without planning and action, clients may spin in self-analysis until they either become demoralized or quit. Balancing data gathering, rapport building, and action strategies would likely be simpler if it were always a linear process, but it rarely is. How many clients have you met who enter a change process with great expectations and exuding confidence? After a few months of implementing their plans, they may have advanced some, slipped back once or twice, and occasionally taken brief detours. Knowing how to address clients' shifts in energy and direction as well as make adjustments in goals and implementation strategies relies on skills reviewed in earlier chapters along with skills that we will discuss in this chapter.

In this chapter, we will examine what have traditionally been referred to as influencing skills (Cormier & Nurius, 2003; Ivey & Ivey, 2003; Ivey, Ivey, & Simek-Dowing, 1987; Ivey, Ivey, & Simek-Morgan, 1997), although some theorists prefer such terms as *empowerment* (Shebib, 2003), *helping skills for positive action and behavior change* (Brammer & MacDonald, 1999), *action skills* (Kottler, 2000), or *challenging and solution skills* (Young, 2001).

Unfortunately, the coaching literature seems less systematic in its panoply of skills. Here, we may find skills grouped into categories of listening and learning (Whitworth et al., 1998; Williams & Davis, 2002), although when we move beyond basic listening techniques, we find relatively little consistency about what skills might be core elements of a coach's advanced communication methodology. For instance, one approach (Martin, 2001) borrows heavily from skills used in neurolinguistic programming (Grinder & Bandler, 1976; O'Connor & Seymour, 1990), and another (cf. Neenan & Dryden, 2002) liberally samples skills from cognitive behavioral theories (Beck, 1976; Beck, 1995; Ellis, 1994; Lazarus, 1999).

Skills described in the coaching literature can, for the most part, be subsumed under more common skill areas identified throughout most of the 20th century in the literature of counseling, psychotherapy, and helping relations. As noted earlier, what distinguishes coaching is not so much the unique language or jargon of its technology but the nature of its clientele and the degree of emphasis it places on various skill applications. As we move into discussions of action-oriented, influencing skill

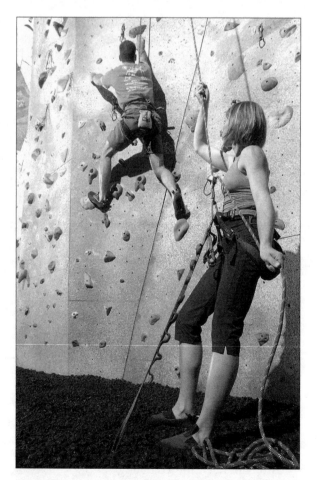

Lifestyle fitness coaches can influence their clients by challenging them and working with them to find solutions.

processes, we are to a large degree emphasizing the central skill areas of coaching.

This chapter will review seven major skill areas. Some will focus more on structuring agendas, whereas others will emphasize ways of influencing clients to change behaviors, examine ineffective patterns or strategies, or renew motivation to pursue their visions. Under the general rubric of influencing skills, we can identify at least two major categories, a modification of Young's (2001) categories as they apply to coaching. Wherever possible, the skill set described in the coaching literature will be integrated into these more traditional categories.

The first category is labeled *challenging skills*, and it is thought to incorporate skills of feedback, confrontation, self-disclosure, and interpretations. The second category contains *solution skills*, which include instructions, information, and advice or suggestions.

Challenging Skills

The concept of challenge as used in this skill set is embedded in a context of empathy, support, and trust. Although challenging includes the concept of confrontation, none of the behaviors associated with these skills represent oppositional or antagonistic action. They serve to foster not only client goal attainment but also the positive quality of the coaching relationship.

Feedback

Allowing oneself to be transparent to others has been associated with positive mental health (Jourard, 1964, 1968). Moreover, when clients confide in their coaches, a variety of health benefits is likely to accrue (Pennebaker, 1990). In chapter 6 we discussed the Johari Window (Luft, 1969) and its relevance to the coaching process. One of the principal ways of increasing client awareness about behaviors and for motivating clients toward desired change is through the skill of giving **feedback.** Feedback is the process of providing clients with specific data on how coaches and others see them.

Purposes of Feedback

Certain kinds of feedback are easier to give than others. Praise, as a form of feedback, may be relatively pleasant to deliver and joyful to receive. What we refer to as criticism, even though it may be positively framed as constructive criticism, is more challenging. The term *feedback* is associated with the field of physics and electronics in which information is fed into a system to correct processes directed toward achieving certain outcomes (Brammer & MacDonald, 1999). Indeed, with the advent of technology, most systems have built-in auto-regulating feedback devices so that when undesirable deviations from ideal performance standards occur, a self-correcting process begins.

In the realm of human behavior, feedback may be sporadic and poorly done. Consider job performance evaluations. A manager may ignore important behaviors for a long time before she one day suddenly confronts an employee with overwhelming evidence of ineffective performance and places the person on probation or fires him. The need for timely and effective feedback processes is critical to success in most endeavors.

• **Feedback serves to motivate behavior toward goal attainment.** As Skinner (1938) demonstrated in his classic works, giving people positive reinforcement following targeted behaviors tended to increase the likelihood that they would continue to engage in those behaviors. Praise or compliments exemplify positive reinforcement in a social context, whereas nonsocial forms may be awards, prizes, job promotions, or meeting personally defined goals. To provide feedback, certain criteria or benchmarks for behavior are needed. Time may be a criterion for performing some tasks like running races, whereas quality measures may be the standard for judging performance in activities like dance or diving. When clients are working toward goals through adherence to certain processes, intermittent feedback about the successes of their efforts can be highly motivating. For instance, although a client may ultimately wish to lose 30 pounds (14 kilograms), significant weight reduction is unlikely to occur in the initial weeks of a training program. Giving this client positive feedback about adhering to agreements and actions may motivate him to continue in lieu of direct evidence (weight loss) that the client is seeking.

• **Feedback functions as an error-correction process.** On some highways, ribbed strips on the shoulders vibrate the vehicle and make loud noise when a driver inadvertently veers out of the lane. This kind of feedback provides a mechanism for error correction, causing the driver to steer back into his lane and pay better attention to his driving. When clients engage in programs with coaches, they will often need feedback about how well they are doing in relation to their stated objectives. Some feedback processes can be codetermined so that coaches do not take the role of judges or police

who report infractions back to the client. Unilaterally monitored systems of feedback generally result in tension between coach and client, especially when progress is slow or nonlinear. Feedback processes need to be part of the coaching relationship, and whenever possible the schedule and structure should involve both parties in establishing criteria, gathering data, and discussing feedback.

• **Feedback enables coaches and clients to solve problems jointly.** When goals are unclear or experimental processes are used to achieve some goal, feedback may be that the goal was not reached or that the process was ineffective. Clients may commit themselves fully to a new behavior, and results may be disappointing not because the client failed to engage the process adequately but because the process was inappropriate to the goal that it was attempting to address. An example of this might be the use of the nicotine patch as a method directed toward smoking cessation. A person may religiously apply the patch, but this process alone is unlikely to produce the desired result. Situations of this sort call for review and reflection in which feedback discussions inform coach and client of the successes or failures of processes, and guide them toward solutions that are more productive.

• **Feedback deepens understanding and promotes learning.** At times, we cannot know what will hinder us from goal attainment until we engage action and encounter the obstacles hidden within or lurking outside. Predicting the future is hard, and it is difficult to see around the corners of change processes when they direct us toward places we have never been before. Reaching one's goal is not just about grabbing the brass ring; it is also about learning along the way and incorporating new skills that may have multiple applications in our lives. When we encounter what we might interpret as failure, in truth we may have simply discovered something new that we need to know or to learn. Like Thomas Edison, who viewed each failure to invent a functioning light bulb as the successful discovery of yet another way not to do it, we can view failure as an exciting way to learn. Such an approach allows us to zigzag along uncharted routes where learning adventures abound and where the goal, although getting ever closer, is no more valuable than learning and growth on the path of progress.

Guidelines for Feedback

You are standing at the checkout line at a grocery store when someone cuts in front of you and starts placing his items on the counter. Is this a good time for feedback? A car veers into your lane while you are driving on the highway. Do you beep your horn? Someone steps on your toe in a dance class. Do you say anything? A sweaty person you are following in a weight room circuit fails to wipe off the exercise equipment each time she finishes. Should you comment, and if so, when? Some situations require immediate feedback; others can wait.

Especially in coaching relationships, we must give great consideration to the timing and content of feedback to clients. Theorists converge on a set of reasonable guidelines for providing feedback in helping relationships (Brammer & MacDonald, 1999; D. Johnson, 2003; Ivey & Ivey, 2003; Young, 2001). Let us explore these guidelines with the perspective of coaching in mind.

• **Feedback is most effective when the client solicits it or, at a minimum, when its expression has the client's full consent.** Coaches are not always able to await clients' invitations to give them feedback on their behaviors. Structurally, feedback processes should be built in to the ongoing coaching relationship at regular intervals so they do not occur without notice or in response to some felt sense of urgency. When someone asks for feedback, he is more likely to accept responsibility for the information he hears, even though he may not agree with its content. When feedback is imposed without consent, clients may feel emotionally unprepared and consequently may resist input even when it is valid.

• **Feedback should acknowledge client strengths and assets.** In many perspectives of human behavior, we can acknowledge that people's intentions may be good even when their behavior is problematic. People may do things that displease or disappoint us, even though their intentions were exactly the opposite. For example, a friend may buy a gift for us that is either distasteful or insensitive to our identity. The person may have wanted to please us but instead did something that unintentionally caused discomfort. Of course, in many instances actions are intentionally harmful. In coaching relationships, however, clients may try, try, and try yet never succeed. Or they may have excuses for every occasion. Somewhere in the mix of problematic behaviors and good intentions, coaches need to search for the client's assets. Sometimes just showing up is the strength that a client manifests, even when she neglects the agreed upon actions. Coaches need to acknowledge clients' strengths and assets in a process of providing feedback, especially when the feedback addresses problematic or dysfunctional patterns.

• **Feedback should focus on what the client can control and change.** There are things we can change, and things we can't. We have control over some elements of our lives, but many other elements are well beyond our influence. A client may be able to change his weight, but he cannot change his height. He may be able to change his eating habits, but he cannot change his genetic composition. If you say someone is smart or lazy or kind or generous or wild, you usually infer these character assessments from actions or verbal behaviors. In providing feedback to clients, you may indeed be indirectly addressing their more or less immutable character, but you do so with a far greater chance for positive influence when you describe behaviors that the client perceives he can control or change. Coaches need to construct feedback messages around issues that are changeable, that are relevant to the client's goals, and about which the client has the possibility of comprehending as under his control.

• **Feedback should be concrete and specific.** Following on the previous point, feedback messages need to include as much detail as possible in terms of publicly verifiable times, places, events, happenings, words, or deeds. Character assessments such as "You just don't seem motivated" are poorly constructed and potentially damaging feedback. The coach can offer far more valuable feedback by documenting instances that represent the client's lack of motivation and describing them to the client in a manner that avoids labeling yet clearly delineates the facts. Some examples of poorly phrased and well-phrased feedback appear in "Examples of Feedback Messages" on the next page.

• **Feedback should not include judgment.** Coaches may be motivated to give clients feedback because they personally are feeling some sense of disappointment or failure regarding their clients. Indeed, when coaches invest themselves heavily in relationships with clients, they tend to take client behaviors personally. When coaches' emotions become caught up in feedback to clients, their words may unintentionally sound judgmental. Through nonverbal messages to clients, coaches may convey feelings of disapproval or rejection. Clients may be highly sensitive and reactive to these messages. Although at times it may be difficult, coaches need to avoid words that are evaluative, such as *good, bad, right,* or *wrong.* At times a coach may understandably have a load of frustration that he would happily deposit on his noncompliant client, yet doing this would likely have an adverse effect on both client and coach. When a coach cannot easily contain his feelings and judgments, he may wish to seek super-

Examples of Feedback Messages

Compare the examples of poorly phrased feedback with well-phrased feedback to appreciate the effective use of feedback as a coaching skill.

Poorly phrased feedback	Well-phrased feedback
You're always late for appointments. You just don't seem committed.	I have noted that in each of our last four meetings you have been between 10 and 20 minutes late. This seems to be a pattern that I'd like to discuss with you.
I think you're fantastic. You're just off the charts. You are one great athlete!	I am so pleased with your results. Your last races were 29.22, 29.41, 29.10, and 29.05. I think those performances are outstanding.
I know you're trying hard, but you're just not doing enough to reach your goals.	I can see by your record that you have made every training session you said you would, and that's really good to see. What concerns me, though, is what you do when you are here. Can we go over the entries you made on your chart for the number of sets and repetitions you did on the different machines during the last 2 weeks?
I can tell that you're going to succeed. You show every indication of being a success story.	I feel very hopeful about you. Here are the data I see that tell me you're likely to reach your goals: You have made every training session you scheduled, plus you added an additional one each week . . . (and so on).

visory assistance or speak with colleagues who can help defuse the excess emotional charge through compassionate and empathic listening.

• **Clients should have an opportunity to confirm what they understand from the feedback and to respond to it.** Too often, when coaches provide feedback, both parties are operating in states of heightened emotionality. Although emotions can motivate us to attend more to the content of messages, they can also cause us to distort messages, to overemphasize certain themes, or to misconstrue meanings intended by the speaker. A good practice to incorporate in feedback discussions is the paraphrasing of messages received by both parties before discussing them. If this does not occur, the ensuing discussion of perceived messages may become skewed and contentious because the client thought he heard something that the coach had either not said or not meant in the way in which the client interpreted it. A secondary advantage of agreeing to have the client paraphrase the coach's input before engaging in a discussion is that in the process of paraphrasing, the client may release some of the emotional charge that he may have been building up during the coach's feedback. Essentially, this practice slows things down.

• **Feedback should be presented in the client's frame of reference.** Especially when providing technical feedback, coaches need to word their remarks in a language that the client will readily comprehend. Moreover, when coaches are working with clients from distinctly different backgrounds, they need to be sensitive to the norms for providing feedback to clients with different cultural heritages or value structures.

• **Feedback should be limited in scope.** Coaches should deliver feedback in small, coherent doses and assiduously protect it from efforts to generalize, expand, or piggyback on the identified themes of feedback. A common experience in situations in which feedback is provided is that one of the parties will try to capitalize on the conversation by broadening the agenda. "Well, since I'm telling you about this, I might as well tell you about that." Alternatively, the recipient of feedback may use this opening in a defensive manner as a channel for voicing previously unexpressed complaints. Contracting for feedback boundaries may serve to control processes that could easily snowball into an all-out defensive argument. In agreeing to a feedback dialogue, coach and client need to delineate terms so that they will address only an identified agenda and thoroughly debrief it. They will acknowledge other issues arising during the feedback and schedule them for some future time.

• **Feedback takes time. Allow for it.** Giving someone praise does not take much time. These joyful expressions are not what most of these guidelines refer to. Feedback involving behavior that has deviated from its intended path or interactions that diminish the working relationship will likely take more than a minute, especially when one cares about the welfare of the person receiving the feedback. In this respect coaches should not offer feedback toward the end of a session unless it is highly contained and unlikely to evoke defensiveness or emotional reactivity.

Steps in Feedback

The guidelines just discussed provide general parameters for feedback. The following steps briefly describe the specific process of providing feedback:

Step 1—Deciding on the Content and Timing of Feedback Coaches and clients might agree to periodic feedback discussions in which identified content will frame the discussions and in which both parties bear responsibility for bringing to the discussion their observations and data. When emergent issues in the relationship or issues concerning client performance initiate feedback, coaches will need to delineate exactly what parameters they believe are necessary and appropriate for the feedback discussion. Moreover, they will need to think strategically about when best to engage the client in this feedback discussion.

Step 2—Framing the Feedback in Clear and Limited Units Even with praise, human beings seem to have a limited capacity to absorb feedback effectively. For this reason, coaches should organize feedback to address the most critical issues in a timely manner and in portions that the client can digest. Coaches need to guard against overwhelming clients with too much feedback.

Step 3—Negotiating With the Client for Time and Agreement to Pursue the Feedback As noted in the section on guidelines, the coach must make sure that the client is fully in accord with the decision to partake in a feedback discussion. To make this decision intelligently, the client will need to know the parameters of the feedback, which likely includes the nature of the topic to be covered. Further, the client needs to understand that although this feedback may bring to mind complaints that

she might have with the coach, she needs to limit the present discussion to an agreed upon agenda. The parties should establish at this time a tentative date for future feedback discussions arising from this agenda.

Step 4—Describing Feedback in a Supportive, Factual, Concrete, and Nonjudgmental Manner Following the guidelines in the previous section, the coach needs to express whatever he has to say in a supportive manner. This principle usually implies that within the feedback messages, the coach will acknowledge accomplishments, strengths, or assets that the client has brought to the process of the working alliance. In terms of detailing the feedback, it needs to be specific to time, place, and event. Moreover, the coach should express it in a manner that can readily be validated. For instance, talking about information heard from a third party in a feedback session cannot be readily validated in the present meeting and therefore may provoke reactivity and defensiveness. A coach who has kept records of times or behaviors relevant to the discussion can produce these for the client to review and consider.

Step 5—Relating the Feedback to the Agreed Upon Agenda for Coaching Coaches rarely offer feedback for its own sake. It needs to serve the client's agenda. Even when clients engage in behaviors that are mildly annoying to the coach, if they are unrelated to the contracted working relationship, the coach should probably avoid them as feedback topics. For instance, a client may have an annoying speech pattern of giggling after the coach provides some instruction, or he may rarely look the coach in the eye when she is talking. This behavior may suggest some personal issues that the client may choose to address in future work, but it is unlikely to be part of the agreed upon coaching contract. Whatever feedback the coach provides becomes her responsibility to justify in relation to the coaching agenda. She can do this during the discussion or at the end. Even when the coach assumes that the client must understand how the issues in discussion relate to the coaching process, the coach should check out this assumption.

Step 6—Creating Opportunities for Client Clarifications of the Feedback Before opening the discussion to hearing the client's thoughts and feelings about the feedback, the coach will need to be sure that the meanings that the client has extracted from the coach's messages are ones that she intended to communicate. This activity most likely involves a request by the coach for the client to paraphrase what he has heard from the coach. Some clients may resist this request, and when that happens, such paraphrasing is most likely needed. One interpretation of this resistance is that some part of the feedback may have triggered the client emotionally, causing him to have a distorted understanding of the coach's communications. In fact, both coach and client can use paraphrasing or a combination of reflection of content and reflection of feeling to prevent the discussion from spiraling into argumentation and to nip potential misunderstandings in the bud. A model for understanding this communication flow is presented in figure 8.1.

Step 7—Requesting Client Response to the Feedback Once the coach is sure that the client has received the intended feedback message, he can then proceed to encourage the client to offer thoughts, feelings, or behavioral evidence relevant to the matter. The coach needs to allow the client ample opportunity to describe any reactions related to the feedback. Following this presentation, the coach should paraphrase the client's messages before offering any new input.

Step 8—Bringing the Feedback to Closure Through Mutual Agreement The discussion ends when both parties feel that they have said what they needed to say, and when both have reached new understandings about how they can work together more effectively and how the client can better direct action toward his agenda.

Uses and Abuses of Feedback

As essential as quality feedback is to promoting client progress, coaches may occasionally misuse the skill of feedback by providing too much or too little, by offering poorly constructed or unnecessary feedback, or providing ill-timed feedback. Examining problematic applications of this skill may produce deeper understanding of the appropriate use of feedback.

- **Unloading complaints.** Coaches must carefully formulate feedback within the parameters of the coaching relationship and its legitimate agendas. When coaches feel irritated by clients, when personality clashes occur, or when countertransference issues arise in unconscious ways, coaches may use feedback to criticize clients or vent feelings to them. Examining the theme of feedback according to its association with the professional relationship will help guide coaches in their use of this skill.

- **Stepping over the line.** In chapter 3 we considered helpers who were motivated by the desire to be lifestyle converters (Cormier & Nurius, 2003), that is, to perform a total makeover of clients so that they conform to the coach's vision of health and fitness. Unlike the coach who unloads complaints, the first misuse of feedback, here the coach may have a positive relationship with the client and view him as an ideal candidate for conversion. Clients may be highly dependent on the coach, or they may have generalized the expertise that the coach has demonstrated in the health and fitness domain to other life arenas. As a result they may be susceptible to the coach's influence attempts, which extend beyond the contracted boundaries.

- **Increasing client dependency.** According to the seminal thinking of Skinner (1938), the use of rewards and punishments has highly predictable consequences. We know, for instance, that one of the problems of punishment as a behavior control

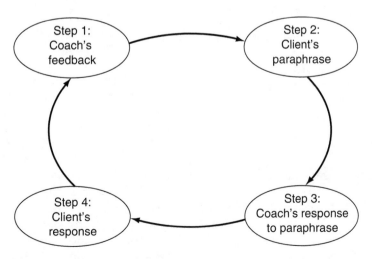

Figure 8.1 Model for information flow in feedback dialogues.

strategy is that the recipient has great difficulty separating the punishment from the punisher. For instance, a parent who punishes a child, even in a humane and appropriate manner, will nonetheless run the risk of generating negative feelings from the child. Similarly, when coaches reward someone, especially with words of praise and compliments, the recipient has difficulty distinguishing the praise from the person providing the praise. In this regard, people come to value the source of praise and may begin to behave in ways largely intended to please that person and thereby experience new gratifications. When clients have few sources or experiences of praise in their lives, they may become highly reliant on a coach who is generous in her compliments to boost client self-confidence and self-esteem. Ultimately, we all need to learn how to be the sources of our own rewards, to become capable of appropriately assessing our behaviors, and to be generous in the provision of self-rewards. We have to learn to pat ourselves on the back when we deserve it rather than wait for the grandstand and the marching band to signal our successes. The more factual and data-based the positive feedback is, the more likely it is that clients will experience it as justified and originating in their own behaviors rather than resulting from a coach's subjective feelings.

• **Feedback as argumentation.** There are many paths to health and fitness. Sometimes clients need to experience their own trial-and-error process, and they may be resistant to the voice of authority telling them what to do. In the lingo of social science, they may be **counterdependent** (Bennis & Shepard, 1956), meaning that they become oppositional when others, especially those in perceived roles of authority, try to influence them. Coaches and clients can become caught in a vicious cycle of trying to prove who is right. Clients can experience feedback as the coach's attempt to control their behaviors. Ironically, although clients pay coaches to tell them what to do, this embedded pattern of resistance may emerge when coaches do so. If coaches play the game, they will assume the role of all-knowing authority and use feedback to convince clients about the errors of their ways.

Summary of Feedback

Using the skill of feedback generally requires that coach and client accumulate certain shared experiences and data concerning the client's engagement with the coaching agenda. Coaches need to frame feedback consistently within the purposes and structure of the coaching relationship, not around

their needs to educate, inform, or counsel the client about matters that may be relevant to the client's lifestyle or behaviors but for which no working agreement was articulated. This guideline may sound highly restrictive, yet the working alliance of coach and client must continue to focus strongly on what the client said he wanted to achieve and what the coach agreed to do to help him in this regard. Although other agendas may arise, before the coach can legitimately provide feedback, the original contract must be revised through discussion and negotiated agreement.

Confrontation

The term **confrontation** may sound harsh, as if it involves conflict and emotionally charged encounters. For some, the word strongly suggests hostility. Indeed, these outcomes are possible, but they are not the predominant meaning of confrontation as a coaching skill. The essence of confrontation is one of bringing to conscious awareness discrepancies in the messages that clients communicate during the coaching process. Such actions require delicacy and extreme sensitivity to the client's readiness to address incongruities. Confrontation has been referred to as *articulating* in some of the coaching literature (Whitworth et al., 1998, p. 40), with the suggestion that the coach, in responding to all the client's verbal and nonverbal messages, may need to present the hard truth.

Another expression that has been used as a substitute for confrontation is *challenging* (Brammer & MacDonald, 1999; Ivey & Ivey, 2003). The coach challenges certain aspects of the client's communications. In common usage within the health and fitness field, however, challenging a person is more likely to be associated with efforts to motivate, raise the bar, or engage the individual in a competitive venture. One way in which confrontation and challenging have meanings that are more congruent is in the case in which a coach challenges a client positively by noting the discrepancy between the client's potential and actual behavior. In so doing, this challenging confrontation may serve to motivate the client to perform at higher levels (Gladding, 2000).

Using confrontation effectively may be one of the more difficult applications of coaching skills (Kottler, 2000). Confrontation is based on observations of client messages, behaviors, and self-reports. When coaches note significant discrepancies or inconsistencies, they may choose to describe in nonjudgmental ways the evidence as they experience it (Hackney & Cormier, 2001).

Purposes of Confrontation

Confrontation is a skill that coaches use to direct clients to examine aspects of their thinking, emotions, or behavior of which they otherwise might not be aware (Shebib, 2003). According to Gilliland and James (1998), when helpers use confrontation in a careful and empathic manner, it can serve to build trust with clients rather than breach rapport. These authors further assert that "confronting client excuses, explanations, or rationalizations is necessary to facilitate client movement toward responsible behavior" (p. 283).

When helpers use confrontation skills, their purpose needs to be clearly aligned with the goals of the working alliance. Evidence suggests that confrontation can help clients "see more clearly what is happening, what the consequences are, and how they can assume responsibility for taking action to change in ways that can lead to a more effective life and better and fairer relationships with others" (Tamminen & Smaby, 1981, p. 42). In fact, the failure to confront clients on important issues may be detrimental to the coaching relationship.

In summarizing the purposes of confrontation, the following are major themes suggesting the application of this skill:

• **Exploring other ways of perceiving.** Through confrontation clients may learn to see themselves or issues they are addressing differently (Cormier & Nurius, 2003). Egan (1998) associates this purpose with helping the client gain greater awareness of blind spots. Clients may be missing certain pieces of information about their functioning or thought processes, and through a coach's confrontation the client may become more cognizant of his way of being in the world. As Cormier and Nurius (2003) also suggest, confrontation may include dealing with client distortions whereby clients' interpretations of their experiences may pass through faulty filters resulting in problematic behaviors. Clients with body-image problems may choose goals or behave in ways based on distorted perceptions of themselves. Other clients may have inaccurate views of the effects of exercise. They may believe that certain activities are inherently dangerous for them or, conversely, they may have unrealistically optimistic perceptions of how exercise can counter the effects of negative habits (e.g., smoking, excessive alcohol consumption, or poor diet).

• **Identifying discrepancies.** Most theorists (Cormier & Nurius, 2003; Gladding, 2000; Ivey & Ivey, 2003; Kottler, 2000; Shebib, 2003) consider the identification of discrepancies as paramount to the application of confrontation. Clients' words may differ from their actions, their words may differ from other words, or they may show inconsistency in actions. Argyris' (1970; Argyris & Schon, 1974) studies of human behavior suggest that people tend to be inconsistent and that we continue unwittingly in our inconsistent ways partly because of lack of feedback. He describes this in terms of differences between our **espoused theories of action** (what we say we do) and our **theories-in-use** (what we actually do). We espouse certain beliefs and values, yet our actions often fail to represent what we espouse. In his view, healthy people respond appropriately to evidence that confronts them with their inconsistencies. They take action to bring behaviors in line with their values and beliefs. Coaching relationships are premised on the assumption that people who seek coaches rather than counselors or psychotherapists are both able and willing to function in mature, responsible, and mentally healthy ways. Confronting coaching clients with incongruities, discrepancies, distortions, or other forms of inconsistency may be difficult, yet if the coach is skillful, results should be positive.

Types of Confrontation

To understand the skill of confrontation better, it may help to examine different types of mixed messages and how coaches might respond to them (Cormier & Nurius, 2003; Egan, 1998; Hackney & Cormier, 2001; Ivey & Ivey, 2003; Kottler, 2000; Shebib, 2003).

Inconsistent Verbal and Nonverbal Messages The client describes certain reactions or feelings, yet nonverbal messages suggest other messages.

• **Example 1.** A client tells a coach that he is enjoying a particular exercise routine that the coach has suggested, but he is showing obvious signs of discomfort.

> **Coach's confrontation:** "I hear your words that you're enjoying what you're doing, yet your facial expression looks pained."

• **Example 2.** A client describes his job as challenging and fun, yet the more he talks about it the more anxious he appears (e.g., biting lips, furrowing brow, clenching fists).

> **Coach's confrontation:** "You say that your job is fun and challenging, but the more you talk about it, the more I see tightness in your face and your fists clenching."

Inconsistencies Between Two or More Verbal Messages The clients says one thing at one time and a makes a contradictory or inconsistent statement at another.

- **Example 1.** Earlier in the session, the client reports that she always follows through on what she says she will do, and later she describes how she continues to let herself down by not completing what she has started.

  > **Coach's confrontation:** "I'm hearing that you feel disappointed about letting yourself down, though earlier I recall your saying that you 'always do what you say you will.' Can you help me understand these two messages?"

- **Example 2.** In the first session, the client says that his family totally supports his new commitment to be fit and healthy, and in the third session, he expresses how his wife has been complaining about the time he spends at the gym.

  > **Coach's confrontation:** "When we began our work, I remember you saying that your family 'totally supports' your training, and now I'm hearing that your wife is complaining about the time you spend here. Can you tell me more about this?"

Inconsistencies Between What the Client Describes and Circumstances A client voices certain thoughts, wishes, or aspirations, yet her circumstances are either insurmountable obstacles or conditions that contradict her words.

- **Example 1.** A client says that she is unable to train while she is traveling but also informs the coach that every hotel where she stays has state-of-the-art fitness centers.

  > **Coach's confrontation:** "I may be missing something that I hope you can help me with. You say you don't have the means to exercise when you travel, yet you said all the hotels where you stay have great fitness centers."

- **Example 2.** A client says that he has to reduce his coaching commitment because it is too expensive, yet he has just described going for a weekly massage and is considering expensive cosmetic surgery.

  > **Coach's confrontation:** "So, you want to reduce our frequency of meeting because of costs. Can you tell me how this fits with what you told me about getting a weekly massage and perhaps having cosmetic surgery? From

what you've just said, your desire to cut back on coaching may not only be about cost. I'd appreciate understanding more about how you feel and what you're thinking."

Inconsistencies Between Words and Actions What the client says differs significantly from how the client acts.

- **Example 1.** A client says that he simply doesn't have time to do the full workouts that he agreed to do, but the coach has seen him spending at least an hour each training day sitting in the lounge talking with other members.

  > **Coach's confrontation:** "May I check out something that I've been observing? [Pause for agreement.] You just told me that you don't have enough time on your training days to do the full workouts that we developed together, yet each day that you have been here training during the last 2 weeks, I've noticed you sitting in the lounge before or during your training talking with other members. Can you help me understand how this fits with what you've described?"

- **Example 2.** A client labels herself as clumsy and awkward, but the coach sees her in a highly choreographed group fitness class following the routine better than most of her classmates.

  > **Coach's confrontation:** "Jane, you describe yourself as clumsy and awkward, yet I happened by the group fitness room yesterday and noticed you in Ben's class. His choreography is very difficult, but you seemed to follow him better than anyone else in that room. What do you think about what I'm saying?"

Inconsistencies Between Two or More Nonverbal Messages The client exhibits two contradictory or opposite nonverbal communications.

- **Example 1.** A client smiles and laughs as she describes an important incident, but her hands are tightly clenched and her arms are rigid.

  > **Coach's confrontation:** "I'm feeling a bit confused right now. I see you smiling and hear you laughing, but I'm also aware that your hands are clenched into fists. Would you be willing to talk to me about what you're experiencing?"

- **Example 2.** A client massages a previously injured calf muscle while grinning at his coach after a tough training period.

Coach's confrontation: "I'm aware of you smiling at me, and I also see you rubbing that calf muscle you injured a while back. Is there something happening that I should know about?"

Inconsistencies Between Client Reports and Those of a Significant Other The client may describe a situation or behavior, but another observer provides a different and contradictory report.

- **Example 1.** A client has been working with a personal trainer as part of the coaching process. He reports that he met with the trainer three times in the past week, but the trainer had been ill except for one day during the past week.

   Coach's confrontation: "Ed, something doesn't fit here. You just said that you trained with Jenny three times last week, but I believe she was out sick most of the week, except Monday. Can you clear this up for me, please?"

- **Example 2.** A client has agreed to work with a nutritionist as part of her program. She reports that she is following the diet exactly, but the nutritionist's report to the coach, which the client agreed to, shows poor adherence, and the client is gaining weight rather than losing it, as she had desired.

   Coach's confrontation: "Marilyn, we agreed that Ellen [the nutritionist] would give me weekly reports on your progress, and the report I have here says that you haven't been following the plan, but you just told me you were. Can we talk about this a bit more?"

Steps in Confrontation

Pointing out discrepancies to clients is no doubt easier when their self-perceptions are less favorable than objective evidence indicates. Such confrontations may serve to build client self-esteem and increase rapport between the coach and client. For instance, indicating that a person's actual running performance is much better than she perceives it to be is likely to generate positive feelings in the client. In some of the examples described above, however, the use of confrontation may mark the beginning of the end of the relationship. More optimistically, even in difficult confrontations, the relationship may become more honest and genuine because of the confrontation. When applying the skill of confrontation, coaches may wish to follow the structure suggested in the following section. These steps have

been modified from a number of sources for the role of lifestyle fitness coach (Cormier & Nurius, 2003; Ivey & Ivey, 2003; Kottler, 2000; Shebib, 2003).

Step 1—Gathering Information The role of the coach is not to police the client's behavior, yet the job does require awareness and sensitivity. Although the coach is not responsible for following up on a client, it is reasonable, especially with a team approach, for allied professionals to communicate with each other, with the client's permission. If a coach's place of business is a health fitness center where clients train, the coach may naturally observe clients without functioning in a surveillance mode. More typically, information suggesting discrepancies or inconsistencies will surface within the coaching session.

Step 2—Determination of Relevancy and Timing The coach who has information about inconsistencies or incongruities does not necessarily have to communicate this information to the client. The first criterion to apply is whether the matter is relevant to the coaching relationship or its agenda. The second criterion is whether the relationship has been sufficiently well established to allow the use of confrontation, especially when the client may be emotionally reactive. In some of the examples provided earlier, the coach reacted immediately to the evidence of incongruity. This approach will not always be appropriate. The coach may gather information and, either when the inconsistency occurs again or when it seems timely to discuss the information, she may use confrontation.

Step 3—Formulating a Nonjudgmental Message With Specific Data Messages about inconsistencies may be difficult for clients to digest. To ease the process, whatever wording the coach uses in specifying the details of mixed client messages must in no way imply judgment, blame, or guilt. Moreover, the more objective, factual, and nonemotional the coach's message is, the easier it will be for clients to hear. You may have noted in some of the earlier examples that the coach's message simply stated the discrepant pieces of information without a conclusion but did include an invitation to discussion.

Step 4—Requesting Client Permission When Appropriate Coaches may assume that they have chosen a good time to bring up a confrontational message, but they cannot be certain. In addition, clients may be aware of their own inconsistencies and simply not want to address them. Enlisting the client's commitment to the process by requesting permission to discuss the topic is helpful in many cases. When clients accept responsibility for the discussion, they are less likely to terminate the discussion abruptly. This approach may require that the coach headline the topic so that the client has a clear idea about the nature of the discussion to which she is agreeing.

Step 5—Encouraging Client Discussion The use of confrontation, like the use of feedback, takes time. In some instances, when the confrontation serves to deepen the discussion, the client may only need to acknowledge the discrepancy and integrate this awareness in the continuation of the discussion. For instance, when a client tells the coach that her experience was positive but looks pained in describing it, the client may simply take this confrontation, acknowledge it, and express more fully her feelings about the experience. When the confrontation involves important dynamics in the relationship, such as the case in which the client wants to reduce coaching for financial reasons yet is spending considerable money in other ways, the coach may need to encourage the client to talk. The coach must be sure to handle defensive reactions constructively. Coaching dialogue 8.1 on the next page offers an example of such an exchange.

Step 6—Emphasizing the Relevance of the Issue to the Goals of Coaching How does the confrontation relate to the goals of coaching or the enhancement of the coaching relationship itself? If the coach is uncertain about the client's understanding of the coach's reasons for confronting mixed messages, the coach must highlight its relevance. Of course, if the client denies, discredits, or refuses to address the matter, achieving this objective is unlikely. In these instances, the coach may have to address the more salient matter of how to proceed in the face of such client responses to confrontation.

Step 7—Codetermining the Implications of Confrontation for the Future When the issues addressed in the confrontation warrant, the concluding segment of the discussion should concern not only implications for the goals of coaching but also how this information might affect future ways of working together. For instance, if a client unilaterally decides to reduce the number of sessions contracted for in the coaching relationship, will it be possible for this client to have the necessary support, advice, instruction, and guidance to reach goals originally contracted for? If a client falsely reports information about program adherence and the coach confronts him with this fact, how does the relationship proceed to reestablish trust?

Uses and Abuses of Confrontation

When clients show evidence of critical inconsistencies, responsible coaching likely entails confronting the client with pertinent evidence. Although the coach's intention will generally be to improve the climate of the relationship and to facilitate the client's goal attainment, confrontation can backfire. Clients may prefer to avoid the truth, to hide out, and to attempt to engage the coach in a process of collusion. Like the story of the emperor's new clothes, some clients may find it easier to have the coach pretend along with them rather than live in the truth. Yet, the use of confrontation is not always warranted, even when clients communicate mixed messages. We have identified some cases when this would be true. The following section summarizes problematic applications of the skill of confrontation:

• **Confronting matters peripheral to the coaching agenda.** What is the client's legitimate agenda? Does the client have a hidden agenda? The same questions apply to the coach. When the coach implicitly broadens the agreed upon agenda by confronting matters that have at best indirect relevance to the client's goals, there is reason for concern. Confrontation can be an engaging process, and clients may gain valuable insights through a process that sensitively brings to light discrepancies in their thoughts, feelings, or actions. A coach may be highly skillful, and her evidence may be entirely accurate, yet unless the issues relate to the contract, the coach is out of bounds. Imagine, for example, that a client brags about having eliminated all sweets from his diet, but the coach sees him walking into the gym eating an ice cream cone. If this behavior is not part of the contract, the coach should probably ignore it.

• **Confronting issues with insufficient information or detail.** Some approaches to coaching recommend "speaking from your gut," or, as the technique is described, "blurting out" whatever the coach's intuition happens to be (Whitworth et al., 1998). Indeed, at times a coach may speak from hunches, and the effect can be entirely beneficial. But coaching is not about being charismatic or enigmatic. Even when speaking from some felt sense, the coach should have articulated to herself what the data are that formed her impressions. You may have had the experience of a person saying something similar to the following: "I have a real sense about you . . . I just know that you are feeling [fill in the blank]." When queried about this sense, the speaker may be unable to produce any verifying data, even as he continues to assert that his sense is correct.

Coaching Dialogue 8.1   Confrontation As Value Clarification

Read the following dialogue to understand how a coach pieces together discrepant communications and employs the skill of confrontation to help a client acknowledge what she is experiencing.

Background Information

The client is a 46-year-old woman who has been involved in a coaching process for 3 months with weekly meetings and occasional telephone sessions. Her original goals were to work on her self-esteem and energy level through regular exercise and to achieve reasonable performance goals in her training. Through discussions with her coach, she determined that improving her body image through well-guided exercise participation would probably make her feel better about herself. She had exercised sporadically throughout her life but mostly experienced exercise as unpleasant and uncomfortable. At the beginning of this session, she mentions to her coach that she wants to reduce her coaching sessions for financial reasons. A while later in the session, she mentions that she has started going for weekly massages. Shortly afterward, she talks to the coach about scheduling elective cosmetic surgery.

Dialogue

Coach: "Dorothy, I've been hearing some things from you today that I believe would be important for us to discuss a bit further. Would that be OK with you?"

Client: "Uh, sure, I guess . . . What do you mean?"

Coach: "It's hard to headline it without getting into it, but it pertains to some of your comments about cutting back on coaching. I imagine it will take about 10 minutes for both of us to look at the issues, and it will help me in knowing what directions we're heading in."

Client: "OK, I guess."

Coach: "Sounds like you're still a bit uncertain."

Client: "No, no, it's OK. Sure, go ahead. I'm just a bit scattered today."

Coach: "I want you to feel as much in charge of this discussion as I am, so let's take it step by step, and you can let me know if you're still OK with it as we go along."

Client: "Yeah, great."

Coach: "You mentioned that you found our work together really important, yet you wanted to cut back our sessions to once every 3 weeks because of the cost factor."

Client: "Yeah, that's right. I simply can't afford it on a weekly basis."

Coach: "I can understand that. Doing this kind of work is a considerable investment, and I have appreciated your commitment not only to our sessions but to your training as well."

Client: "Thanks, yeah, it's real good . . . although exercising regularly is still hard for me."

Coach: "Uh-huh . . . Yes, I realize that, and I have also seen steady improvement in your performance."

Client: "That's true. My times are getting better, and that pleases me to no end."

Coach: "Great! [pauses] . . . You also mentioned going for weekly massages starting a couple weeks ago, and scheduling some optional surgery next month."

Client: [Slightly defensive] "What are you getting at?"

Coach: "I'm sorry if my words may have sounded in any way critical—not my intention . . . I did want to look at your comment that you couldn't afford our sessions, along with your

(continued)

159

(continued)

mentioning these new expenses. Can you help me understand how this all fits together for you?"

Client: "Well, I like getting a regular massage. It feels good, especially with the kind of stressful job I have."

Coach: "I couldn't agree with you more. A good massage can be real important in reducing stress."

Client: "Yeah, well, I know that costs money, too, but I need it."

Coach: "I would imagine you do. No doubt, that's why you've decided to do it. Makes sense to me."

Client: "OK, so this surgery thing is definitely going to cost a lot of money, and I really need to budget for that."

Coach: "Uh-huh. Elective surgery is expensive."

Client: [Defensively] "Why do you say 'elective'? I really need to do this."

Coach: "So, you believe you need to do this, and my saying 'elective' doesn't land well."

Client: "No, it doesn't. All this training has helped, but I need something that's guaranteed to make me feel better about myself—right now!"

Coach: "So, the training is working, but your feeling better about yourself simply isn't happening fast enough—and surgery will give you a guaranteed, fast change. Is this it?"

Client: "Yes, well, maybe . . . I'm not entirely sure, but I think so, and like I told you, training is hard for me."

Coach: "For sure, I know that becoming regular about training, and enjoying it, takes time, and right now it's hard for you."

Client: "Maybe I'm just doing my old thing."

Coach: "What 'old thing' is that?"

Client: "You know. I talked about it in the beginning. If I don't see results right away, I find some quick fix. [Pauses.] I think I'm doing that again."

Coach: "So, the surgery may be a quick fix?"

Client: "Yeah, I think so . . . Maybe I shouldn't act so impulsively. Maybe I need to think this through some more."

Coach: "Well, you seem to be slowing it down right now and thinking about it some more. And I want to add that whatever you do is your choice. You're in charge. From my point of view, I needed to understand better what was happening . . . Not that I was judging. I simply heard some things that didn't fit together without some additional details, and I needed to get that information from you.

Client: "You had every right to ask . . . and I thank you for bringing it up."

Coach: "You're welcome . . . and I thank you for allowing the space for the discussion. We've spent about 10 minutes, as I thought we might, so I'd like to ask you how you'd like to continue our session from here?"

When clients are vulnerable or impressionable, such undocumented confrontations are troublesome. They serve to increase the mysterious powers of the coach and may either distance the client or, conversely, deepen client dependency. Coaching is not a guessing game. Whenever coaches confront clients, they need to be able to document their impressions publicly, and in doing so, empower the client to validate or invalidate the information.

• **Stacking confrontational messages.** A client's tolerance for confrontational messages may vary depending on the nature of the material. Usually, the process of confronting discrepant messages involves some emotional charge. Clients may initially be defensive, but through the coach's skillful communications, this reactivity may diminish. If the coach continues to be confrontational, however, the client may feel attacked. The concept of saving face plays into the use of confrontation. Coaches need to do whatever possible to support client confidence and self-esteem. When use of a particular skill begins to erode a client's sense of competency and esteem, the coach should curtail its use. Failure to do so may have negative consequences for all involved.

• **Confrontation as a control strategy.** Clients generally do better when they discover their own inconsistencies rather than have them repeatedly identified by coaches. This argument is not in support of containing all confrontational messages but is rather a general perspective about the dynamics of the relationship. When clients hear themselves verbalizing different thoughts or feelings, they increase the chances of catching themselves delivering discrepant messages. The active listening skills reviewed in chapter 6 provide coaches with nonconfrontational ways of helping clients hear themselves. In many respects, a delicately delivered confrontation might sound like a simple reflection of content or a summarizing response. The client, in this case, may not even realize that the coach is confronting him. Instead, he gets to discover, through the coach's paraphrasing, how his messages may be incongruent. The use of confrontation as a control strategy refers to cases in which coaches jump on discrepant messages through direct confrontations and in this manner attempt to bolster their expertise and prove how much clients need their help. If information is a source of power (French & Raven, 1959), coaches can increase their power over clients by seeming to have extraordinary awareness of the client's thoughts, feelings, and actions. Such behavior will likely backfire in the long run. Although some clients will develop dependencies on the coach, others will recognize the

strategy for what it is. In either case, the coach will have failed to empower the client to become autonomous, need fulfilling, and personally successful.

• **Confronting too deeply.** We discussed this final issue earlier. Although coaches may be aware of deeper issues that, if confronted, could help the client achieve fundamental and lasting changes, the possibility also exists that through such confrontations clients will have far more to deal with than they had originally bargained for. To some degree, this is a dilemma. As noted in chapter 4, malpractice may be demonstrated in cases in which the professional fails to use a technique that would have been more beneficial to the client. But this form of malpractice must nonetheless be referenced to what it was the client has contracted with the coach to achieve. In life or death matters, the coach may undertake an intervention that has not been specifically negotiated because without doing so, a client may perish. More typically, the coach will rarely invoke this justification for choosing a deeper intervention without discussion. The way out of this dilemma may be straightforward. If the coach has ample reason to consider bringing to the client's awareness through confrontation issues that may otherwise remain unknown to the client, the coach can open discussions concerning renegotiation of the original client agreement.

Summary of Confrontation

The use of confrontation in the coaching relationship must be well reasoned, and when relevance, timing, and other factors strongly support it, coaches should not avoid using confrontation. Skillful confrontations can motivate clients to change and help them develop insight about how they function (Shebib, 2003). Conversely, inappropriate use of confrontation can be destructive. Blending the skill of confrontation with other skills will generally lead to more beneficial responses from clients. Giving clients ample opportunity to integrate information from the confrontation, paraphrasing client reactions, and demonstrating empathy for whatever clients may be experiencing in this process will foster a more productive working alliance. As valuable as confrontation can be to the coaching process, it never is an end in itself.

Self-Disclosure

Many clients want to know about their coaches (Hendrick, 1988). Questions regarding whether coaches should share, what they might share, when they would share, and for what purposes they might self-disclose require considerable exploration.

The purposes, styles, and intentions of **self-disclosure** in nonprofessional relationships are likely to be different from those of the skill of self-disclosure used by coaches in professional relationships. Sidney Jourard (1958, 1964) did much of the original work on self-disclosure. As he defined it, self-disclosure was about individuals making themselves known to one another through revealing personal information. His research illustrated the benefits of self-disclosure, including the fact that such behaviors tended to establish trust in relationships.

D. Johnson (2003, p. 46) has also provided a useful analysis of self-disclosure within an interpersonal, nonprofessional context; he defines it as "revealing to another person how you perceive and are reacting to the present situation and giving any information about yourself and your past that is relevant to an understanding of your perceptions and reactions to the present." In this perspective, self-disclosure has certain characteristics that are hypothesized to benefit interpersonal relations. Johnson emphasizes that to be most beneficial self-disclosure should be structured to

- focus on present reality rather than history,
- include references to feelings as well as facts,
- cover a wide range of topics,
- have depth in terms of personal revelations, and
- be reciprocal, especially in the formative stages of a relationship.

These specifications for beneficial self-disclosure in nonprofessional relationships stand in sharp distinction to the emerging wisdom about self-disclosure as a skill in professional helping relationships. For the most part, the use of self-disclosure as a professional skill refers to "a conscious, intentional technique" by which the helper strategically shares personal information with the client to achieve a specific benefit to the relationship or for the client (Simone, McCarthy, & Skay, 1998, p. 174).

Caution abounds regarding the use of self-disclosure in a professional context. Opinion varies concerning whether or not it is helpful to create a sense of shared experience with the client through the helper's use of self-disclosure (Wachtel, 1993; Watkins, 1990). Within the realm of counseling and psychotherapy, disciples of more orthodox approaches strongly discourage helper self-disclosures (Roazen, 1974), whereas other schools advocate the use of self-disclosure so long as it benefits the client and the helping relationship (Evans, 1979). Some research indicates that clients experience helpers' self-disclosures as extremely valuable (Knox, Hess, Petersen, & Hill, 1997), whereas other investigations urge helpers to be circumspect in their application of self-disclosure (Donley, Horan, & DeShong, 1990).

Human experience has many commonalities. But when professionals attempt to match their self-disclosures to a client's framework, there is much room for error (Hendrick, 1988). For this reason, the use of self-disclosure is thought to be a risky strategy (Watkins, 1990). Common sense alone suggests that coaches are unlikely to have relevant personal experiences to share with all their clients. Perhaps on occasion the coach may be able to capitalize on some similarity in experiences to bring benefit to the client, but this is unlikely to occur frequently. In some instances, a client may perceive a self-disclosing helper as more caring than one who discloses little (Capuzzi & Gross, 2001). Helpers who disclose too much, however, may be perceived as lacking in discretion and being untrustworthy (Levin & Gergen, 1969). Moreover, too much self-disclosure may result in client perceptions that the coach is preoccupied and needs help (Cozby, 1973).

Unlike personal relationships in which, as D. Johnson (2003) and Jourard (1958, 1964, 1968) suggest, people should engage in self-disclosure from the outset of relationships that they wish to nurture, professional relationships normally do not include self-disclosure in the earliest stages of the relationship because the helper knows so little about the client (Farrell, 2001). Coaches may indeed put themselves at risk by disclosing personal information to clients who may be poorly suited to the coaching process.

When a coach decides to disclose personal information, it must be relevant to the client's concerns and should in no way burden the client (Egan, 1998) or distract the client from her own issues (Sexton, Whiston, Bleuer, & Walz, 1997).

Although opinion is mixed about the use of self-disclosure in counseling and psychotherapy, the literature on coaching takes a more favorable view of self-disclosure, no doubt because of the assumption that coaching clients are inherently more stable and emotionally healthier than clinical clients (Martin, 2001; Whitworth et al., 1998; Williams & Davis, 2002). Although this makes good sense, such beliefs remain assumptions until they have been verified on an individual basis.

Purposes of Self-Disclosure

What might justify the use of self-disclosure in the coaching process? Theorists have suggested a number of purposes:

- **Modeling behavior.** For the coaching process to advance, clients must reveal to their coaches essential details of their histories and experiences. Coaches who engage in appropriate self-disclosures may model styles of interaction for clients and thereby support them in revealing relevant information to their coaches (McCarthy, 1982).

- **Increasing trust and augmenting the working alliance.** Because the roles of client and coach differ considerably, clients may feel threatened by perceived status differences or the unidirectional nature of questioning and disclosures. When coaches share appropriate details and information, clients may come to see them as more human and less distant, as more trustworthy and authentic (Egan, 1998; Helms & Cook, 1999).

- **Developing new perspectives.** Effective coaches are not likely to chime in with self-disclosures of personal success experiences in response to a client's description of some victory. Coaches tend to apply self-disclosure when clients' stories contain messages of confusion, uncertainty, defeat, or even despair. The coach may strategically self-disclose as a means of instilling hope or clarity, or perhaps as a way of encouraging the client to develop new perspectives about specific events or dilemmas (Egan, 1998). The coach's story must be true and must have sufficient content and process overlap with the client's story so that the client can recognize his own experience, although in a different light. The coach's intention should never be to match experiences either to show identification with the client or to compete with him. In friendship relationships, one person may describe a particular kind of experience and the other joins in with a similar report. The purpose is one of connection, demonstration of similarity, and perhaps identification; it is not intentionally helpful or therapeutic. The purpose of sharing in coaching is to motivate or to enable the client to achieve new awareness.

- **Increasing client self-acceptance.** Clients may think that they are the only ones confronting particular issues, or they may somehow view themselves in a one-down position in relation to their coaches because they have revealed intimate life details that may not be complimentary. Coaches may strategically share some of their own disappointments, failures, or other unsettling life events as a way of balancing the power in the relationship and helping clients be more self-accepting. Through appropriately matched self-disclosures, coaches communicate to clients that they too experience difficulties and that, indeed, they have strong feelings about issues (Hackney & Cormier, 2001).

Types of Self-Disclosure

Not all self-disclosures carry the same weight or meaning. We can distinguish a few different types of self-disclosure:

- **Professional information.** It is appropriate, if not necessary, for coaches to disclose to their clients the nature of their training and credentialing. Clients may need reassurance that their coaches are qualified to provide the kinds of services for which clients are engaging them. Coaches can share this information in a straightforward manner through brief professional resumes.

- **Personal information.** As Helms and Cook (1999) point out, different cultures have specific norms about sharing information. For some cultural groups, coaches would not be expected to reveal personal details such as age, marital status, number of children, and so on. People of other groups, however, would expect coaches to share some details about family of origin. Coaches need to be aware of the potential meanings to clients of certain biographical information. A client who asks how old the coach is may be asking, in an indirect manner, whether she can trust the coach because the coach appears to be younger than she is.

- **Content congruent stories.** In personal relationships, a story about buying a house is matched by a story of similar content. Endings and details may differ, but the essential content is similar. A content element of the teller's story constitutes the thread of connection to the next speaker's story. More commonly, we may think of social conversations in which a person uses some aspect of the speaker's remarks with which to launch into a personal revelation. People share stories and disclose personal information, and the intended benefits include a pleasant passage of time and a felt sense of commonality. When coaches have stories that have similar content to those of their clients, they will choose to share them consciously and for strategic reasons, assuming that the stories will positively affect the working alliance or their clients' capacities to address their goals successfully.

- **Thematic stories.** Embedded in each story is a theme—one of victory or defeat, of hope or despair, of love or loss. Coaches are unlikely to have stories with content that always corresponds well to their clients' stories, but they may have had experiences with similar themes. For instance, if a client tells a story about being discouraged and not being able to find the personal resolve to overcome obstacles confronting her, the coach may speak about a personal experience containing the same themes or dynamics.

From your own experience, either in casual conversations or in professional interactions, you have no doubt disclosed many details about your life and stories of your experiences. Learning activity 8.1 provides you with an opportunity to review the intentions and purposes served by these disclosures.

Steps in Self-Disclosure

The literature on helping and counseling (Cormier & Nurius, 2003; Ivey & Ivey, 2003) helps describe the process by which coaches decide whether to self-disclose and then how they might formulate a message of self-disclosure. The steps outlined below apply primarily to the stories coaches tell (content congruent or thematic stories) rather than to professional or personal details.

Step 1—Evaluating the Reasons If the purposes of self-disclosure are to increase trust, build rapport, provide new perspectives, or increase client self-

acceptance, does the coach have sufficient reason to believe that a specific self-disclosure will accomplish one or more of these purposes?

Step 2—Assessing Client Readiness How ready is the client to have the coach reveal personal stories? Simone, McCarthy, and Skay (1998) provide some evaluative questions that coaches may wish to answer in determining client readiness:

- Will the coach's story take the focus away from the client's experiences?
- Will the boundaries of the coaching relationship remain intact?
- Might the coach's seeming vulnerability disturb the client?
- Will the client see the coach as less capable because of the self-disclosure?

Step 3—Timing Another aspect of client readiness is timing, although timing also refers to the available time in a session and the placement of the self-disclosure message within the session. Because self-disclosure is to serve one or more coaching purposes, will enough time be available in the session for the client to respond to and integrate the coach's message?

Step 4—Formulating the Story How the coach tells the story is pivotal. Its details must clearly match either the themes or the content of the

Learning Activity 8.1　Appreciating the Functions of Self-Disclosure in Life and Work

Self-disclosure serves different purposes at different times and in different contexts. Most likely, in personal relationships an intention is to deepen the relationship or to share intimacies that friends and family members might appreciate. At work, self-disclosures might occur less frequently and with more of a strategic intent.

Recall some recent experiences in which you told a detailed story of a life experience to someone with whom you have a personal relationship. What was your intention in telling this story? What effect did it have on the other person? How did you feel after telling your story?

Now, recall another experience in a professional or work context when you told someone a story about your life, knowing that you wanted to make a particular point with the story. What was your intention here? What effect did it have on the other person? How did you feel after telling your story?

You may wish to recall other occasions when you disclosed details of your life to others and the outcomes were mixed or problematic. What was it about these instances that seemed to trouble you? Was it how the other person reacted? Was it your concern about how the person would perceive you? Did anything change in your relationship with this person as a result?

The more you explore ways in which you have used self-disclosure in the past, the more insight you will gain about its appropriateness and applications to professional work as a coach.

client's experiences, and the client must construe its embedded messages in a way that serves the coach's intended purposes.

Step 5—Intervening with Awareness Telling the story in the coaching process occurs with awareness of the here-and-now communications of the client as the story is being told. Nonverbal cues will often reveal whether the client is receiving the coach's self-disclosure in a positive, neutral, or potentially negative way. Coaches should not be so committed to telling their stories that they cannot refocus the session on the client if client reactions warrant immediate attention. For instance, a client tells a story without fully experiencing her own emotions, but as the coach tells a similar tale, the client begins to cry. Most likely, the appropriate coaching response is to pause and inquire about the client's immediate experience.

Step 6—Refocus on the Client At the conclusion of the self-disclosure, the coach will somehow bring the focus back to the client. Although the client may probe for additional details about the coach's experience, the coach should reply only if these requested details continue to serve the coaching purposes. Otherwise, the coach might frame a question to the client such as "I wanted to share this story with you because I hoped that in some way it would be helpful. Does my story create any new awareness about your own experiences?"

Uses and Abuses of Self-Disclosure

By following the steps outlined earlier, coaches who offer a well-formed and appropriate self-disclosure will likely be serving the purposes of coaching. When coaches share their experiences without carefully attending to their reasoning and the client's readiness, problems may occur. The following issues should serve as a cautionary review regarding the use of self-disclosure as a coaching skill (Young, 2001):

- **Incompatible themes or content.** As discussed earlier, the coach must know enough about the client and her experiences to predict with reasonable accuracy that she will perceive the story as meaningful. Sharing a story simply because it has some content connections may be unsuccessful and could serve to convey the impression to the client that the coach is acting in a manner of friendship rather than as a professional.

- **Inappropriately deepening the relationship.** When Jourard (1958, 1964) first began investigat-

ing the power of self-disclosure, he recognized that it could create a deepening spiral of intimacy in relationships. As social creatures, we are likely to match the depth of another person's story. If someone describes a frivolous, superficial happening, we do the same. If someone discusses a tragedy, we respond at a similar depth. Coaches who wish to deepen the level of self-disclosure by clients can lead the way through the telling of their own stories. As long as this serves the client and the negotiated agreement, such action is justified. But when coaches tell emotionally significant stories to lead their client along the same path without clear justification and agreement, they are operating inappropriately and with potential risk to their clients' welfare.

- **Poorly timed self-disclosure.** Have you ever had an experience in which you told a significant personal story, and no sooner had you finished than the listener initiated his version of the theme? Somewhere in this exchange, you may have felt that your story got lost. Coaches need to listen well in the silences following a client's disclosures. The occurrence of a pause does not mean that something should be said. Clients often reflect inwardly after saying something meaningful. In addition, the concept of timing relates to the purposes of this kind of intervention. Do you want the client to have your self-disclosure as the parting words that she will reflect on in the interval between sessions? Or is it important to ensure that the client has ample space to reflect with you on the meanings derived from your story?

- **Self-serving self-disclosures.** From all that has been said, it should be amply clear that client needs and the enhancement of relationship dynamics must guide the decision to use self-disclosure. For coaches to tell their stories for self-serving purposes, for instance, to bolster their self-image or reputation or even just to entertain, is rarely justified.

- **Overuse of self-disclosure.** As Cormier and Nurius (2003, p. 155) point out, "Self-disclosure is a complex skill. There are ethical issues surrounding the use of it, requiring critical thinking and judicious adaptation, perhaps more so than with any of the other listening and influencing responses." Coaches should use this skill sparingly, especially when the stories they tell are detailed and involved. They can use other skills, such as those of immediacy and feedback, to increase their transparency and sense of authenticity without telling historical stories from their lives.

Summary of Self-Disclosure

Professional helpers may use self-disclosure frequently early in their careers and again later on when they are seasoned veterans. Inexperienced helpers may attempt to reduce their own anxieties by identifying with their clients through too frequent self-disclosures (Cormier & Nurius, 2003), whereas highly experienced helpers may have accumulated so much wisdom about the human condition that they want to cut to the chase by short-circuiting clients' stories through sharing their own considerable experiences. In both instances, these helpers apply self-disclosure more in response to their own needs than to those of their clients. Research does not provide unequivocal endorsement of self-disclosure as a beneficial helping skill. This result is probably due to misuses of self-disclosure more than to the nature of the skill itself. Coaches need to be highly sensitive to client issues and conditions of the relationship before choosing to self-disclose. Benefits are likely to abound from the skillful use of self-disclosure, but negative consequences will surely accrue when coaches apply the skill insensitively. Learning activity 8.2 offers some opportunities to explore how you would approach self-disclosure in practice settings.

D. Johnson (2003) offers sage advice that would apply well to coaches who choose to use self-disclosure in their approaches to clients. First, he indicates that self-disclosure requires a high degree of self-awareness. Translated into coaching process, the implication is that coaches need to understand what their own needs and issues are and how they might be relating to the client in the moment. Second, self-disclosure relies on a strong sense of self-acceptance. Coaches who risk exposing their own vulnerabilities or stories through self-disclosure need to have accepted their own behaviors and imperfections, particularly as they might represent them in the stories they tell. The third point is that coaches must have no conscious needs for approval, reward, or acceptance from the client related to their self-disclosures. If coaches expose certain vulnerabilities in their self-disclosure and clients react negatively, having expectations for acceptance or approval might cause coaches to respond defensively or critically. Clearly, such responses would be counterproductive.

Interpretations

The skill of **interpretation** is one of the oldest approaches in the helping professions (Clark,

---

Learning Activity 8.2   Using Self-Disclosure in Coaching

Consider each of the following client scenarios and formulate a response that may begin with an acknowledgement of the client's issues through the use of reflection of content or reflection of feeling, and then continue by using a self-disclosure based on your life experiences. Base your self-disclosure on thematic similarity or content similarity.

- **Client A:** Jeff has been a coaching client for over a year. He has recently sustained a temporarily disabling injury from a biking accident. His doctor indicated that he would recover full function of his fractured wrist in about 6 months. Jeff is discouraged and feels that all his work has been for naught. Moreover, he believes that he was getting all the intended benefits from his program and that nothing else will have much value for him.

- **Client B:** Marge is in her 3rd week of coaching. She is eager to see results but doubts that she will ever achieve her goals. She has started many projects in her life but rarely follows through. She wonders aloud whether she has any reason to believe that things might turn out differently this time.

- **Client C:** Edna has never asked anyone for help in her life. She has always given herself generously to others but is uncomfortable having the coach focus attention completely on her. She knows that she cannot make the changes without help, but she feels that she should be able to.

- **Client D:** David is afraid of trying new things. He wants to stretch himself, to explore his interests and capabilities, and to stop being so cautious. At this moment, he is being critical of himself and is unwilling to accept any longer that he has fears. Yet, the less he acknowledges his fears, the more paralyzed he feels about moving forward in his program.

1995), and one of the most widely misunderstood. Within the emerging field of coaching, the term *interpretation* continues to be widely used (Neenan & Dryden, 2002; Whitworth et al., 1998; Williams & Davis, 2002), although it is often associated with such other concepts as reframing and the use of metaphors. There are multiple types and levels of interpretation. It is not an esoteric skill that would be inappropriate for lifestyle fitness coaching; indeed, practitioners apply it so commonly that most might not be cognizant of when they are interpreting client messages.

Interpretation is often associated with the highly complex and arcane works of psychoanalysis (Freud, 1964). Within various offshoots of the Freudian tradition, interpretation is considered "a sophisticated and complex skill in which intellectual knowledge of psychodynamic theory is integrated with clinical data about the client" (Ivey, Ivey, & Simek-Morgan, 1997, p. 248). But psychodynamic practitioners are not the only ones to use interpretation. According to Frank and Frank (1993), virtually all professional helpers interpret their clients' behaviors according to the theoretical frameworks in which they were educated.

Young (2001, p. 336) says that interpretation "consists of encouraging the client to look at the problem in the context of the theoretical orientation of the practitioner. Once the helper explains the reason for the problem, a client develops insight and is then better able to change. . . . Insight may occur suddenly ('aha') or it may dawn gradually. Once insight occurs, that learning may be applied to other situations." This definition, however, is far too narrow to encompass the wide range of verbal responses by coaches that we could readily describe as interpretations.

Ivey and colleagues broadened the narrow framework created by psychodynamic theorists by describing interpretation as "the renaming of client experience from an alternative frame of reference or worldview" (Ivey, Ivey, & Simek-Morgan, 1997, p. 248). A client tells the coach a story, and the coach puts the client's words into her own language or experiences and feeds that back to the client with the intention of creating some greater awareness or even behavior change (Brammer & MacDonald, 1999).

In a more recent work, Ivey and Ivey (2003) have gone even further in adapting the concept of interpretation to the everyday use of helpers, coaches, counselors, and other professionals. The concept is now referred to as interpretation/reframing. In this somewhat different perspective, they describe how clients tell their stories and how helpers employing the skill of interpretation/reframing enable clients "to look at the problem or concern from a new perspective" (p. 311).

Another useful way of appreciating the skill of interpretation comes from the coaching literature. Whitworth and colleagues (1998) think of interpretation as a kind of hunch or intuition that a coach has about the situation a client is experiencing. In this view, interpretation is not a judgment or even something definite. Coaches develop a sense about what is going on and in their own words, using their own meanings, try to communicate their hunches to their clients. Borrowing more from the concept of reframing, Williams and Davis (2002) indicate that what coaches do is to "find other words or descriptors for something that appears to be a challenge, problem, or deficiency in the client's view. You place the behavior or perception, as articulated by the client, in a new context or frame. This allows the client to see whatever the situation or concern is in a new way. Rather than viewing the problem as a weakness, it can be seen as an opportunity for learning" (pp. 107-108).

Types of Interpretation

Examining some types of interpretation might facilitate understanding. Ideally, this analysis will remove any remaining beliefs that this skill belongs more to counseling and psychotherapy than to coaching. Coaching dialogue 8.2 illustrates the different types of interpretation in the context of a specific coaching encounter. To some degree, the following types of interpretation might also be seen as varying along a continuum of depth, that is, type A, adding implied messages, is probably less involved than type B, connecting messages, and so on.

Type A—Adding Implied Messages In Egan's (1998) terminology, interpretation would be seen as advanced accurate empathy, in which the coach would incorporate in reflections or paraphrases any messages that the client might imply but not put into words. A client may look sad or elated when describing an experience but never label her feelings. If the coach were to reflect the content of the client's messages and add the unspoken element of feelings, this would be a low-level interpretation. What justifies the labeling of this message as an interpretation is that the coach, not the client, brings to the situation the framework for understanding feelings from nonverbal messages.

Type B—Connecting Messages and Adding Implications or Conclusions When the coach brings together different messages that a client has delivered within a session or over time, the skill involved is likely to be that of summarizing. But when the coach summarizes a number of client messages and then adds something that may be implied or even something that the coach infers (a hunch) from the information, this action employs the skill of interpretation. It may seem like splitting hairs, but the distinction between reflecting actual messages and adding something that has been unspoken can have major consequences for the relationship and the client. Coaches may think that what they are sensing in a situation must be obvious to the client as well. Possibly it is, yet making the implicit explicit can be important. When it is not evident, the coach will have brought to consciousness something in the client's blind area that may foster movement toward goal attainment.

Type C—Reframing This form of interpretation has sometimes been described as looking on the bright side of things (Whitworth et al., 1998). But it is more than this. When clients are struggling with issues, they may be unaware of the strengths that they are exhibiting or the potential for growth inherent in their dilemmas. Walking in a fog, one may not realize what lies just beyond the range of vision. To someone less involved in the situation, possibilities may abound, whereas to the client the situation seems hopeless. Reframing is a way of taking what the client is describing and presenting an alternative and usually more adaptive view for the client to consider. Through this process, the client gains an opportunity to step outside the situation that he perceives and appreciate it through another's eyes.

As noted, reframing generally provides perspectives with greater potentiality and hopefulness, although this is not necessarily so. A reframe may present the dangers or negative implications of a client's scenario with the intention of alerting the client to unforeseen consequences that, with the new perspective, he may avoid.

Type D—Metaphorical Interpretations Metaphors may be simple or complex. "You seem to be rising above it all now and seeing it for what it truly is" is a metaphorical expression of rising above a situation to gain perspective. This simple metaphor captures in visual imagery some aspect of what the client may be experiencing; however, the description comes from the coach rather than from the client. Metaphors that are more complex may take the form of stories that the coach tells to capture certain dynamics of what the client has been expressing. Fables and fairy tales are elegant metaphors from which we usually draw some moral. Coaches may use metaphorical descriptions of mythical characters so that clients may begin to identify and eventually realize that the story is a parallel of their lives as reflected in the coach's tale.

Type E—Theory-Based Interpretations When a coach has a particular theory that informs her actions with clients, interpreting a client's thoughts, feelings, or behaviors within this framework can provide the client with an entirely new way of understanding. Chapter 5 described the transtheoretical model (Prochaska, Norcross, & DiClemente, 1995), one of the more frequently applied theories in health fitness settings. When coaches describe

Coaching Dialogue 8.2   Types of Interpretation

Explore the different types of interpretation that a coach might offer in response to messages that he has heard over the course of different sessions. Notice how interpretations can vary in depth and potentially in effect on the client.

Background Information

Jenna, a 27-year-old recreational athlete, has been working with a coach for over 6 months on a multifaceted program to build confidence and compete successfully in an amateur tennis association. She performs well in practice but invariably makes errors in competition that she almost never does in practice sessions. The coach has worked with her using sport-focusing training and mental imagery practice, along with guiding other aspects of a cross-training program and adherence to sleep and nutritional commitments determined through consultations with a doctor and a nutritionist. In recent sessions, the client has made these remarks, which the coach has noted carefully.

Client comment A: "Even at work I seem to clutch whenever I feel someone is watching . . . I don't like people looking over my shoulder."

Client comment B: "I want to win so bad that I make stupid mistakes because I'm trying too hard."

Client comment C: " I hate competition . . ."

In this session, the client is upset about a recent loss against an opponent whom she always defeats in practice.

Client comment D: "Darn it. She's such a loser . . . I threw the game away . . . She can't play anywhere near the level of tennis I play, yet she trounced me yesterday . . . Maybe I'm the loser."

Types of Interpretation

Type A—Adding Implied Messages

Coach: "Jenna, it sounds as if you're feeling quite frustrated with yourself . . . like you're a 'loser' and someone determined to defeat herself."

Type B—Connecting Messages and Adding Implication or Conclusion

Coach: "Jenna, I can really hear how disappointed you feel with yourself, and I sense from other things you've said—like about work and about 'trying too hard'—that when the spotlight shines on you in competition, you 'clutch' and 'make stupid mistakes.' There seems to be something in this about not being able to perform well when it counts the most."

Type C—Reframing

Coach: "Jenna, I hear you . . . how disappointed you feel with yourself . . . like you set yourself up for failure. Yet, maybe there's another message in this. I remember you telling me one time that you 'hate competition.' Perhaps some part of you is trying to get through to you that how you are engaging in this game doesn't work for you. You do well in practice because you're having fun. As soon as you define the situation as competition, the fun exits—and this overaggressive, angry competitor that you really don't want to be comes roaring out."

Type D—Metaphorical Interpretation

Coach: "Jenna, ouch . . . Seems like you're really hurting and upset about this. I have this image of you tying your shoes together before you go out on the tennis court and saying to everyone watching, 'Look at me . . . I'm going to make it as difficult as I can for myself to win . . . Reminds me of that children's story *The Little Engine That Could* except you're saying, 'I know I can't, I know I can't, I know I can't.'"

Type E—Theory-Based Interpretation

Coach: "Jenna, I can see how upset you are and how you're blaming yourself for all this. I wonder if you'd be willing to look at some of this with me. [Pause for agreement.] Things you've said to me over the past few weeks make me wonder whether this all might be about a fear of success. You know that your inherent skills are far better than what you demonstrate when you're competing . . . and you've also said that you 'hate competition,' yet you continue to place yourself in the limelight of these kinds of events . . . So you do what you don't like or even 'hate' under conditions that you normally find upsetting, that is, having people watch you, and then, no surprise, you fail, almost like you set it up to happen that way. I guess the unknown in this little theory of mine is what would it mean to you if you were to be successful at something that you wanted so badly. Does any of this make sense to you? I may be way off with this, but I sure would like to know what you might be taking from what I'm saying."

their clients' behaviors in such frameworks, they are using the skill of interpretation. Similarly, if coaches use certain inventories or profiling tests to understand their clients, and they communicate meanings that they extract from these measures to their clients, they are using theory-based interpretation.

Purposes of Interpretation

Interpretation serves a number of purposes that resemble those of other coaching skills such as reflection of meaning, summarizing, and immediacy, yet the distinction to bear in mind is that the coach intentionally addresses these purposes by providing the input. With other skills, the coach functions in ways to bring about new awareness or change by having clients discover for themselves certain meanings, implications, or solutions; here, the coach provides this kind of input.

- **Developing insight and new perspectives.** When coaches reframe client experiences or reflect unspoken dimensions of client messages, clients may have insights about reasons that they behave as they do or they may be able to understand themselves in a new light. Such insights and perspectives are not ends in themselves; they must always serve the coaching agenda.

- **Discovering hidden skills and opportunities.** When in decades past women returned to work after raising their families, they often confronted the difficult task of putting together a credible resume of skills and experiences. Not having held a salaried position for many years, they tended to view themselves as unskilled and therefore unemployable. Only through reframing the tasks that mothers do in raising children and managing homes were they able to understand the talents that they had been nurturing and perfecting over many years of unpaid employment. The skill of interpretation allows coaches to open windows for clients on the experiences they have had so that they can recognize latent talents, unacknowledged successes, and hidden possibilities for growth and action. Interpretation serves the growth and development agenda of clients by breaking through clients' self-defined limitations and restricted worldviews.

- **Generating energy for change.** When clients realize some kind of breakthrough or insight as a result of an interpretation, they will typically discover new reserves of energy that they can use to foster their chosen change agendas.

- **Building the relationship.** Insightful coaches who are able to propel the relationship forward

through skillful interpretations provide their clients a great service. Although interpretation involves a degree of risk, when it is successful, clients are likely to express more trust in their coaches and to feel more comfortable in exploring other issues that may be impeding progress.

Steps in Interpretation

Interpretation relies on the prior establishment of sufficient rapport to permit the coach to attempt to influence the client and to sustain the potential negative effects of a misguided or incorrect interpretation. Coaches may apply brief or simple interpretations straightforwardly, as in the case of reflections of content or summarizing. They must construct and implement deep-level interpretations with great sensitivity. The following steps have been suggested in discussions of interpretation within the helping professions (Brammer & MacDonald, 1999; Cormier & Nurius, 2003; Ivey & Ivey, 2003) and are reframed here for coaching roles.

Step 1—Ensuring the Sufficiency of Rapport and Trust To judge the likelihood of success of an interpretation, the coach must sufficiently appreciate the way in which the client responds to situations, how she describes matters, her level of openness to new ideas, and her receptivity to the coach.

Step 2—Comprehending Implicit Client Meanings In more traditional forms of helping, interpretations may be formulated over a long period without being expressed. That is, a helper may continue to gather data and organize it into meaningful themes over the course of the relationship. Whatever themes are present in a client's thoughts, feelings, or behaviors will continue to repeat themselves in a variety of ways. An attentive coach will note these patterns and through the accrual of information will begin to develop hypotheses or insights about the client.

Step 3—Formulating a Structure for Interpreting Meanings When the coach decides to use the skill of interpretation, she might use any number of strategies. She can offer simple images or metaphors. She can use a process of reframing. Or she might tell a story. With each strategy, the depth of the intervention could differ and, therefore, the relationship will need to be sufficiently established to support the chosen strategy.

Step 4—Timing the Intervention In long-term coaching relationships, the amount of information that coaches may have about their clients and the degree of rapport established will likely allow for the repeated use of certain interpretive messages, as ways of reminding a client about some of their patterns. For instance, a client who generally seems to be walking on eggshells in all realms of life might benefit from hearing a reminder from the coach whenever the coach hears the pattern emerge in client messages. When a coach is to deliver a meaningful interpretation for the first time, however, he may need to ensure that the client will be receptive to such messages and that sufficient time remains in the session to discuss the client's thoughts and feelings about the interpretation.

Step 5—Delivering the Interpretation For straightforward and simple interpretations, the coach may blend the message, in the form of an image or metaphor or observation, into a paraphrase, summary, or reflection. When the interpretation is more lengthy and involved, the coach may choose to request the client's agreement to providing this kind of information.

Step 6—Assessing the Effect As the coach is delivering the interpretation, her awareness should focus on the client. If the interpretation is lengthy, the coach may wish to suspend delivery of her message if she notes any indications of client resistance to or discomfort with hearing what she is saying. Following the interpretation, the coach will work with the client to understand whether it seemed reasonable and accurate and, if so, what meanings or implications the client might draw from the coach's message.

Step 7—Exploring the Client's Associations When interpretations are lengthy and complex, coaches may encourage clients to connect the relevant aspects of the interpretation to as many domains of their thoughts, feelings, and behaviors as justified within the parameters of the coaching relationship. Bearing in mind that people manifest certain degrees of consistency across domains of their lives, coaches will need to guard the boundaries of their professional relationships by helping clients shape implications of interpretations within the legitimate realm of their contracts.

Uses and Abuses of Interpretation

We have seen how interpretations can foster understanding, the development of new perspectives, the pursuit of new directions, and the enhancement of the working alliance. We also have acknowledged that because the coach is offering something unspoken by the client—framed in the coach's world-

view—a degree of risk accompanies this strategy. The preceding sections have suggested some of the more obvious misuses of interpretation. The following points highlight problematic aspects of employing the skill of interpretation.

- **Interpreting matters peripheral to the coaching agenda.** A client may manifest certain behaviors or even attitudes that could interfere with some realms of his functioning, but if the coaching contract does not extend to these domains, the coach must either broaden the scope of the contract or allow these matters to go without comment.

- **Interpreting with insufficient information or detail.** Some presentations on coaching (Whitworth et al., 1998) encourage coaches to verbalize their hunches and intuitions. Perhaps they can do this once the coaching relationship is on solid ground. Even then, however, it may be risky. Clients in the early stages of the relationship may have a heightened level of dependency on the coach, which should diminish as coaching progresses toward its conclusion. As such, what coaches express as hunches, clients may value too highly. They may attribute degrees of insight and power to the coach that are unwarranted, and they may accept inaccurate or faulty interpretations. Coaches need to document to themselves the rationale underlying interpretations before verbalizing them to clients.

- **Interpreting too deeply.** The role of lifestyle fitness coach does not encompass the wide range of cognitive, emotional, and behavioral ramifications of a client's lifestyle that would be appropriate to counselors and psychotherapists. Although a coach may be exceptionally insightful, she must always judge the decision to share these insights according to the criteria of the relationship's agenda.

- **Poorly timed interpretations.** Well-formed interpretations are generally based on sound evidence gathered over time. Although highly experienced coaches may be able to identify core themes affecting client progress early in the coaching process, they may need to wait for the relationship to develop before they can use this information effectively in an interpretation. Brown and Srebalus (2003) argue that the use of interpretation is most likely to be appropriate after the accomplishment of all the initial tasks of relationship building, contracting, and the development of understandings.

- **Interpretation as an end in itself.** The use of interpretation as a coaching skill is never an isolated event. The coach must always frame it within the purposes of the relationship. Coaches may have exquisite intuitions about clients, they may create impressive images of how clients function, or they may have wonderful stories carrying inspirational messages. As long as they relate to the agreed upon agenda, they are acting appropriately; otherwise, they need to remain within the coach's internal processes.

• **Being attached to an interpretation.** Coaches can be completely correct about their interpretations, but if the client resists strongly, the timing is obviously not right for the client to receive the message and deal with its implications. Coaches should guard against trying to convince clients of the accuracy of their interpretations, especially through amassing more and more evidence that may seem irrefutable.

• **Being mysterious.** Offering clients interpretations of their thoughts, feelings, or behaviors is not about being psychic. A hunch or an intuition or some visual image of the client comes from somewhere. The coach needs to be able to articulate the bases of her interpretations rather than imply to clients that they should trust her inner wisdom.

Summary of Interpretation

Interpretations can transport clients to new levels of awareness and functioning. They can also create distance between coach and client, either by elevating the status and power of the coach or by causing confusion and mistrust in the relationship. Interpretations are of different types, some of which are quite commonplace in most relationships, as when a listener fills in the blanks in a speaker's communication. Interpretations need not be tied to theory, but they will always represent input from the coach that may have been implied by the client but never spoken. They are likely to be helpful in instances when the coach catches a client in some repetitive and unproductive cycle of thought or behavior. Interpretations in these instances can help clients think outside the box and thereby develop new perspectives and fresh energy with which to address their agendas.

Solution Skills

This category of influencing skills mostly involves messages from coaches that provide guidance, direction, advice, or opinions to clients based on the wisdom and expertise that coaches have gathered through education, training, and professional practice. When offered by a lifestyle fitness coach, these highly influential skills are likely to be perceived as legitimate, appropriate, and even expected. Just as someone walking into a group fitness class will expect the instructor to lead the class rather than ask participants what they want to do, clients working with lifestyle fitness coaches may expect directives concerning sport and fitness activities. In this respect, the coach must use some kind of assessment, matching, or discussion involving client experiences and background to determine the degree to which different sports or activities are appropriate for clients.

Before examining similarities and differences among instructions, information, and advice or suggestions, we should mention some special considerations about this category for lifestyle fitness coaches. A gradual evolution of roles has occurred within the fitness industry from such highly directive ones as sport coach and instructor to more collaborative roles as advisors and personal trainers. When considering the concepts of direction and control, certain questions arise: Who gives direction? Who has legitimate authority within a relationship? Looking at this in the context of health fitness professionals and their clients, we can define a direction and control continuum such as that depicted in figure 8.2. The role of lifestyle fitness coach would most likely occupy a place close to the center, that is, with client and lifestyle fitness coach providing more or less equal direction. Personal trainers might be somewhat left of center, whereas athletic coaches and group fitness instructors would tend to fall to the far left of the continuum.

Although the role of lifestyle fitness coach bears some relationship to other roles within the fitness industry, its emphasis on collaborative, bidirectional processes is far more embedded in its patterns of interaction. This circumstance creates a dilemma for coaches when they give instructions to clients, because this type of communication is stylistically linked to unidirectional decision making and control. The degree to which instructions, information, and advice or suggestions represent communication strategies of coaches will determine the extent to which clients see themselves as responsible collaborators or passive recipients of the coach's influencing messages.

Let us examine the three skills in this category to understand ways in which coaches might best use them. We will begin with brief descriptions and purposes of each, and then consider steps for application and uses and abuses for the three forms of solution skills because considerable overlap exists among them.

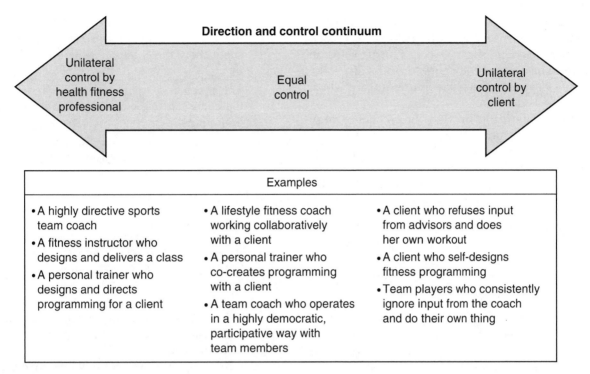

Figure 8.2 Direction and control continuum of health fitness professionals.

Instructions

In the health fitness world, clients often require instruction. They do not know how to perform certain exercises, or they are unaware of proper form and technique. If instructors instruct, what do coaches do? The answer depends on the range of work for which coaches have contracted with their clients. Some coaches may serve in a few different capacities, partly as guide, partly as support, partly as resource, and partly as instructor or personal trainer. Other coaches will define their involvement in different ways. For example, they may implement the actual training components in a team approach with a personal trainer or other kinds of sport experts (e.g., a tennis instructor).

Instructions indicate to a client what he should do, in terms of thoughts, feelings, or behaviors (Ivey & Ivey, 2003). Examples include the following:

Thoughts

"Think about it this way . . ."

"Stop imagining that."

"Focus your mind on the ball."

"Imagine your opponent as someone who is going to help you win."

"Listen to your inner voice."

Feelings

"Feel what's happening inside your body right now."

"Sense the energy in your center radiating out through your arms and legs."

"Feel light, easy, and joyful in your movements."

"Smile inwardly just as you are about to begin."

Actions

"Do that again."

"Hold your arm this way."

"Lower your center and relax your breath."

"Breathe in to a count of 10 and then slowly release your breath to a count of 10."

Instruction will take on different faces when coaches engage in dialogues with clients versus when they work with them on the floor in fitness facilities. In actual training programs or sport coaching, instruction will take the form of verbal messages describing how to perform physical actions and sometimes nonverbal messages, including hands-on postural corrections. Within coaching dialogues, instruction might take the form of mental imagery exercises, sport focus training, or clear reinforcements for action (e.g., "Continue doing exactly what you have been doing!"). A coach might use guided imagery to help a client overcome performance anxiety in sports or to facilitate the client's visioning of positive futures toward which she can direct action.

When operating on the floor, coaches may be expected to provide strong, clear instruction, whereas in a private coaching dialogue, the permission to use instruction may need to be negotiated. The following example may clarify this latter application:

Coach: "So, it seems that when you are on the court, you're not sure what happens, but you suddenly become aware of a shakiness in your knees and something like fear in your stomach. Is that what you're saying?"

Client: "Exactly . . . but I don't know how I go from feeling so calm when I'm sitting on the bench to feeling so anxious when I'm out on the court."

Coach: "Would you be willing to try something with me? Maybe we can get some more information about this."

Client: "Sure, anything that will help."

Coach: "I'm going to ask you right now to close your eyes. [Pause until client closes eyes.] Now, imagine you are sitting on the bench about to go out on the court. Tell me how you're feeling."

This interaction, which relies heavily on the use of instruction, is the beginning of a **behavior rehearsal strategy** (Suinn, 1986) and demonstrates how the coach enlists the client's permission and collaboration at the beginning of the process.

Presumably, a coach who is also serving in the role of personal trainer would have discussed the activities and obtained the client's general statement of permission to train before taking the client on the floor.

Shebib (2003) and Young (2001) concur that providing instruction will be appropriate and can enable the client to move forward under certain conditions. These conditions include the following:

- The coach has expert knowledge or training related to the client's agenda.
- The coach has extensive experience in helping clients with the specific approaches being used.

- The coach is fully aware of the limitations of the approach and appropriately advises the client about the potential benefits and liabilities.
- The coach has adequate understanding of the client's history, needs, capabilities, and limitations.
- The coach is able to adapt instructions to fit the client and the circumstances.

Information

According to Young (2001, p. 220), "Information giving is the supplying of data or facts to help a client reach his or her goal." Information might include ideas about how to accomplish something, or the coach may use information to correct erroneous ideas. Young notes that helpers should provide information sparingly because too much information can overload the client, and the client will likely ignore it.

Health fitness professionals rely heavily on the use of information as a strategy for guiding and motivating change processes. Clients may put themselves unnecessarily at risk out of ignorance, and coaches and trainers can help them become aware of the consequences of their actions by offering information. How professionals convey information may take a multitude of forms, from verbal descriptions to readings, videos, or even Web sites. As Cormier and Nurius (2003, p. 146) suggest, giving clients information is generally appropriate when "the need for information is directly related to the client's concerns and goals, and when the presentation and discussion of information are used to help the client achieve these goals." These authors recommend that helpers determine whether to use information by asking and answering three questions: What does the client need to know? When does the client need this information? How can I deliver it to achieve optimal results?

Information is not necessarily unbiased or value-free. When informing clients about options or activities, coaches will often present their own knowledge base about a topic or refer the client to certain resources, including magazines, journals, books, videos, or Web sites. None of these may be definitive, but they may be representative of a segment of available knowledge. As an increasingly diverse population engages the world of health and fitness, coaches must describe more caveats, according to the particular backgrounds, capabilities, limitations, needs, and interests of clients. For instance, although clients may think of yoga as a low-risk activity, certain postures could be harmful to pregnant women. Coaches can use information to persuade clients to engage in certain actions, in which cases it is wise to ensure that the data are accurate and representative.

Information becomes an important strategy for increasing client understanding and awareness. Yet, according to the transtheoretical model (Prochaska, Norcross, & DiClemente, 1995) reviewed in chapter 5, a client's stage of change in relation to a particular behavior determines whether information needs to be more or less factual or dramatic. For instance, getting someone to move from precontemplation to contemplation about a behavior such as smoking cessation would likely require graphic and perhaps disturbing information concerning the long-term consequences of this behavior. On the other hand, a client who is in the action stage of smoking cessation may require more sanguine information regarding relapse prevention.

Using information is not generally a neutral act but rather one that attempts to influence thoughts, feelings, or behaviors in particular directions (Ivey & Ivey, 2003). Clients negotiate with their coaches about specific agendas, and within the boundaries of these agendas, coaches should provide relevant and unbiased information.

Advice or Suggestions

Of the three skills reviewed in this category, giving advice or suggestions is most problematic, and likely to be the most commonly used (Brammer & Mac-Donald, 1999; D. Johnson, 2003). Considered from the perspective of relationships with friends and family, advice is one of the most common responses that people give each other (D. Johnson, 2003).

According to Shebib (2003), North American society conditions people to seek advice from experts. Novice helpers are especially vulnerable to the expectation that they should provide expert advice on how clients might manage their lives and solve their problems. Yet, as Kleinke (1994, p. 9) notes about advice giving in therapy, "Clients can get all the advice they want from acquaintances, friends, and family members. They hardly need to pay a therapist to tell them what to do." Brammer and MacDonald (1999, p. 94) offer an even stronger rebuttal to advice giving. In their view, advice giving "reflects the arrogance of helpers who assume they are so all-knowing that they can advise other persons on a course of action."

Research and professional opinion on the use of advice are sometimes at odds. Research has found

that clients value receiving advice from their helpers, and they seem to benefit as well (Murphy, Cramer, & Lillie, 1984). Yet some theorists argue that clients do not really want their helpers' advice, but rather they want assistance in understanding and managing their problems so that they can eventually solve them on their own (Oldfield, 1983). Shebib (2003, p. 16) joins forces with this position by commenting that "Clients often seek advice even when they know what to do to manage their problems. Seeking advice can be a way of expressing dependency or transferring responsibility for decisions and outcomes to someone else."

A more positive way of framing this issue comes from the work of Compton and Galaway (1984, p. 73) who conclude that the wisdom of helpers "lies less in the substantive areas of knowing what is best for the client and more in the process area of assisting clients to develop alternatives for themselves, make decisions among the alternatives, and implement decisions."

Yet the fact remains that giving advice and suggestions is not only a common form of professional help (whether it is helpful or not is another matter) but also one of the forms most expected by clients. To clarify this matter, we might identify conditions under which advice giving would be appropriate. Borrowing from arguments by Young (2001), Shebib (2003), and Brammer and MacDonald (1999), the following applications would seem acceptable in coaching relationships:

- Offering suggestions to enable clients to be aware of unforeseen consequences of their actions
- Providing advice when clients may be at risk of harm or injury
- Recommending courses of action that the client may not know about or might have overlooked
- Advising clients based on expert information, research, or valid information
- Providing clients with strategies for dealing with issues instead of offering solutions
- Suggesting processes of communication that might help clients deal more effectively with matters related to their agendas
- Making recommendations based on extensive experience with and knowledge about an issue

Most professionals consider it entirely inappropriate to offer clients advice for dealing with major individual choice questions, including decisions about careers, families, or other relationship matters (Shebib, 2003; Young, 2001). Other instances when giving advice might be contraindicated include cases in which giving advice unduly reinforces client dependency, when the outcome cannot be known yet the client is seeking reassurance, or when the client may be gathering opinions for use in arguments or actions involving other people (Young, 2001). Another instance in which giving advice can be problematic was initially described in works by Eric Berne (1961, 1964), founder of transactional analysis. He characterized the behavior of "help-rejecting complainers" in a communication pattern called "Why don't you . . . Yes, but . . ." In this transactional "game" a person achieves some kind of psychic gain by seeking advice only to reject it when it is offered. Continuing to offer advice and suggestions to clients who continually criticize them or fail to put them into action is generally unwise.

Advice giving is considered problematic because it tends to foster dependency, as well as remove responsibility from the client and place it inappropriately on the coach's shoulders. Even when it is useful and the client accepts it, advice serves mostly to increase the helper's self-esteem and undermine that of the client (Shebib, 2003). Typically, clients do not follow the advice that they receive because they often seek it disingenuously. By falling into the trap, helpers may incur the wrath of their clients (Brammer & MacDonald, 1999).

D. Johnson (2003) argues that giving advice builds barriers in relationships and results in defensiveness, rejection, resistance, termination of exploration, and indecision. Moreover, the advice that a coach gives may communicate more about the coach's values, needs, and perspectives than it does about the client's issues.

The following ways of giving advice, however, are considered more acceptable (Cormier & Nurius, 2003; Shebib, 2003; Young, 2001):

- Outlining the risks as well as the benefits of a recommended action
- Presenting advice as an alternative and encouraging the client to generate other possibilities
- Inviting response and discussion rather than offering advice categorically

Young's (2001, p. 218) remark probably summarizes the matter most eloquently: "What we need to remember is that while a client may appear to be asking for advice, he or she is really looking for opportunities to think aloud, to be understood, and to explore the options."

Shebib (2003) offers some creative alternatives to giving advice. To draw out the client's intrinsic wisdom, the coach might ask the following questions, adapted for the role of lifestyle fitness coach, in lieu of giving advice:

- What are your ideas about this?
- How might you approach this situation?
- Have you had any thoughts that merit deeper exploration?
- If I were to give you advice, what do you think it would be?
- What might your best friend suggest to you?
- What do you think your options are?

Steps in Instruction, Information, or Advice or Suggestion

Some types of instruction require little contemplation before being communicated to clients. Likewise, clients may request information about topics, and coaches may easily respond to such requests. When it comes to giving advice or suggestion, coaches will need to give careful consideration before responding to client requests for such input. The following steps, reflected in part in other procedures for the helping professions (Cormier & Nurius, 2003; Ivey & Ivey, 2003; Shebib, 2003), may be applicable to instances in which coaches are considering giving advice, providing instruction, or offering information.

Step 1—Assessing the Need What is it that the coach perceives the client needs most in this instance? Is it information? Is it the coach's opinion? Is it instruction? Or is it a need to resolve her own issues with the coach's guidance? Although some within the coaching field optimistically believe that clients have all the resources they need to resolve their own problems (Martin, 2001; Whitworth et al., 1998; Williams & Davis, 2002), clients may not have all the information they need, nor might they have mastered the requisite skills. Certainly, coaches can provide appropriate instruction and information that is well aligned with the client's agenda.

Step 2—Determining the Strategy Although we are considering information, instruction, and advice or suggestion, other communication skills may achieve the same ends. If clients need to discover their own answers, the coach might use such skills as reflection of meaning, summarizing, feedback, or immediacy with more positive long-term effect on client self-efficacy and self-determination. When it is a matter of providing instruction, information, or advice, coaches may have good reason to choose one over the other. Depending on the quality of trust and rapport in the coaching relationship, coaches may decide to be highly influential by adding their own weight to clients' deliberations. This action would imply offering advice rather than giving information. Comparisons of these three approaches appear in coaching dialogue 8.3

Coaching Dialogue 8.3 Uses of Instruction, Information, and Advice or Suggestion

This section describes three scenarios in which it might be appropriate for the coach to provide instruction, information, or advice. The risk and benefits accompanying each of the three coaching messages can be estimated by imagining how the fictional clients might respond to the kind of input that the coach is providing. You will recognize in some instances that the input the coach is providing may have a low probability of success or may not match the implied needs of the client.

Scenario A

A 62-year-old engineer wants to deal with certain inflexibilities he experiences in his movements. He also defines himself as being a rigid person and hopes that his program will help him loosen up a little. Through coaching, he has determined to support his desired objectives with novel (for him) activities like stability ball classes, Pilates work, and yoga. This exchange occurs in the coach's office:

> **Client:** "I think I'm way too stiff to do these yoga exercises. Besides, I feel very strange going into these classes with mostly ladies, and my mind freezes up on me. What do you think I should do?"

Coaching Instruction

> **Coach:** "I want you to try this exercise with me. OK? [Pauses for agreement.] Start by closing your eyes and thinking of your goals. [Pause, client complies.] Say to yourself, 'I am open to change. I am challenging my old beliefs. I am becoming more flexible.' Keep those words going. Keep saying those words to yourself. Nod your head when you've got it. [Client nods.] Now, I want you to imagine yourself walking into the yoga class saying those words to yourself. Nod again, when you're doing it. [Client nods.] Now, let all of this slip from your mind and slowly open your eyes and tell me about your experience."

Coaching Information

> **Coach:** "It is normal for people to feel a bit uncomfortable when they try new things. However, by continuing to engage in new behaviors, eventually a level of comfort and familiarity develops. My experience is that it seems to take about 6 weeks of going to a new class for people to start feeling more at home."

Coaching Advice

> **Coach:** "My opinion is that you should keep doing it even if you feel uncomfortable. I believe your gains are going to far outweigh the slight discomfort you feel. I think you need to do this to accomplish your goals."

Scenario B

A 31-year-old woman who is preparing for a triathlon is working with a coach on training techniques as well as mental strategies. In this exchange, she is talking with her coach right after finishing a spinning class.

> **Client:** "Biking is my weakest . . . I also am experiencing some severe knee pain when I bike."

(continued)

(continued)

Coaching Instruction

Coach: "I want you to get back on the bike so that we can go over some basics. But first I want you to raise your seat a bit. Sit on the bike now and we'll make the adjustment."

Coaching Information

Coach: "Everyone has a weak sport and a strong sport in triathlons. A study I just read says that triathletes should not overemphasize training in their weak area to the detriment of training in their areas of strength. As for the knee, research says the angle of the knee at maximum flexion should be between 110° and 120°."

Coaching Advice

Coach: "I think you're being too hard on yourself. You're doing fine. Just ease up on yourself . . . As for your knee, I think you should check with the sports doctor at our club."

Scenario C

The client is an obese 42-year-old man who is determined to get back into shape after more than a decade of inactivity. He has shown complete adherence to the program he designed in conjunction with his coach, but his annual vacation starts next week and he is going to be staying at an all-inclusive resort.

Client: "I have been feeling so good about myself, but now with my vacation starting, I'm afraid I'll just slip back to square one."

Coaching Instruction

Coach: "I know the resort where you're staying. I've checked with the staff there by e-mail, so I know what equipment they have. Here's a list of exercises I want you to do every other day while you're on vacation. Follow this list exactly."

Coaching Information

Coach: "Vacation periods are one of the great challenges to adherence. People may have highly reliable performance while at home, but on holidays their routines can vary greatly. Research recommends that you write down a structure for exercise while on holidays before your departure."

Coaching Advice

Coach: "I think you should talk to your wife about this. My sense is that if your spouse is on board about your exercising while on vacation, it will help."

Step 3—Formulating the Message Taking into account the client's unique history, needs, agendas, and cultural heritage, coaches will organize their messages in such a way as to have maximum effect over the long term. Keeping in mind that it is the client's job to effect change, coaches should avoid manipulative or even highly persuasive ways of communicating information or providing advice. The goal is not always to provoke immediate change but perhaps only to stimulate thinking or to help clients begin to reframe their situations.

Step 4—Delivering the Message With Awareness Having a clear strategy in mind, with awareness of its varying consequences, coaches may begin to deliver their messages while maintaining keen sensitivity to client responses. As always, should clients show signs of discomfort or overt resistance (e.g., shaking head from side to side, as if saying no), coaches should discontinue the delivery and check with their clients about their immediate experiences.

Step 5—Inviting Response and Dialogue After delivering the message, the coach might conclude with an invitation to the client to comment, reflect, or otherwise respond to what was said. Even if it takes a while for the client to integrate the message, it is best that the coach pause deliberately until the client speaks.

Step 6—Evaluating Effect   Through the ensuing dialogue, the coach may become aware of the multiple meanings and values that the client has taken from the coach's communication. If it is not clear how this type of coaching message has affected the client, the coach might ask directly, "Now that we've talked about this for a while, would you be willing to summarize what you're taking away from this discussion?" Using the skill of immediacy, the coach might also want to ask the client about the potential implications of the message for the coaching relationship: "You asked me for my opinion, and I willingly gave it to you. I'm wondering now if I could ask for your opinion about something. How do you think this discussion and the opinion I gave you might affect the way we work together?"

Uses and Abuses of Instruction, Information, or Advice or Suggestion

Discussions of the three skills in this category have highlighted uses and abuses throughout. A brief summary of these points will recapitulate the major themes. The distinction between what coaches do in dialogues with clients and how they work with them on the floor is critical. Coaches can establish norms for each setting so that a style compatible with coaching remains distinct from one deemed more appropriate for training. Some clients may have difficulty separating the coach's work in these different venues, so the coach is largely responsible for reinforcing the behavioral guidelines for each setting. When coaches use instruction and information in their dialogue sessions, ideally they will be responding accurately and appropriately to clients' needs. Advice giving and suggestions will always remain risky interventions, so coaches should probably use them as a last resort, except when their use is clearly indicated, such as in emergencies or to steer clients clear of imminent danger. The following are some of the ways in which coaches might misuse these skills:

• **Providing information, instruction, or advisement on matters external to coaching.** Effective coaches may experience a degree of referred power from clients who have come to trust the legitimate advice and information that they have received. Over time, coaches may be elevated unrealistically so that clients attribute knowledge bases

to them unwarranted by the coaches' actual training and experiences. Seeing their coaches as wise, intelligent, sensitive human beings, clients may be inclined to ask them for all kinds of input. Even when clients preface their requests with statements such as "I know this isn't your area, but I wanted your opinion anyway," coaches are strongly advised to avoid the trap.

• **Providing biased or ill-conceived information, instruction, or advice.** We sometimes hesitate to make public our ignorance, especially when we personally believe that we should know the answer to a question. Coaches are often tempted to answer questions out of a feeling that they should know the answer. You will do far better to tell clients that you will check into matters about which you are uncertain or confess ignorance rather than stumble through an ill-informed response.

• **Increasing client dependency.** Wherever possible, coaches should encourage clients to be self-determining. Giving clients the tools to address their own issues empowers them. Instruction is often necessary in a sport and physical training context. Coaches may closely control information or, conversely, they may encourage clients to discover whatever information they need through personal investigation and research. Coaches need to examine carefully the effect that these skills will have on client dependency and use them sparingly when the risk of increasing client dependency is present.

• **Instruction, information, or advice as a means of control or self-enhancement.** A coach may feel satisfaction in being perceived as the expert and being able to give detailed and accurate replies to clients' questions, but this situation may serve to disempower clients. Giving information or instruction may come across as lecturing, and although coaches may enjoy the opportunity to share their wisdom, providing too much information or instruction may diminish rapport and the degree to which clients take responsibility for their own actions.

• **Poorly timed instruction, information, or advice.** As with all coaching skills, timing is key. The core messages of information, instruction, or advice may be sound, but the delivery may be ill timed.

Summary of Instruction, Information, and Advice or Suggestion

The skills of information, instruction, and advice or suggestion were categorized as solution skills because they are likely to provide methods, directions, or potential answers to client issues. New clients may perceive coaches with well-established reputations as highly competent, knowledgeable, and therefore credible. In such instances, rapport might develop easily, and coaches could use these skills successfully early in the relationship. In other cases, when coaches need to establish a basis of trust and credibility with clients, coaches should use these strongly influential skills minimally in the early stages of the relationship. In addition, when clients show signs of resistance or counter-dependence (Bennis & Shepard, 1956), requests for advice or information could be traps whereby clients deliberately test their coaches.

In situations in which lifestyle fitness coaches also serve in a hands-on capacity with clients in their training programs, they will use these skills more frequently than they do when they work more through processes of dialogue. As noted, when coaches occupy complex roles with clients, they should establish clear norms about how they operate on the floor and how they function in dialogue sessions.

Power and Responsibility in Influencing Clients

The process of coaching is best thought of as a weave of skill applications that emerges from the unique combination of who clients are, what they need, who coaches are, and what they are best able to provide. In an elegant coaching process, a natural flow of communication advances the client's agenda while nurturing and supporting his need for trustworthy connection. The skills reviewed in this chapter may take years of practice and reflection to master. Coaches must thoroughly understand the challenging skills of giving feedback, confrontation, self-disclosure, and interpretation not only for what they potentially offer clients but also for how they can adversely affect the working alliance. Through study, practice, and reflection, effective coaches acquire an exquisite sensitivity to need, situation, and timing.

In considering solution skills, you may believe that these are less complex and perhaps already within your comprehension and basis of practice competencies. You may already know how to instruct, how to give information, and how to provide advice. In your competency may lie the risk that you will use these skills too liberally. When teaching classes or instructing individual clients, your ability to direct and guide may be highly developed. But the transfer of this knowledge base to the processes of lifestyle fitness coaching is neither simple nor direct. Some of the points raised earlier warrant repetition: Clients may seem to want your advice and opinion, but often what they really need is to be heard and to work diligently to uncover their own meanings and solutions. Even in situations in which clients express deep gratitude for the opinions you give them, you may want to reflect on what you have actually done. Have you become their guru? Have you increased their dependency? Or have you shown them the path to self-efficacy and greater self-determination?

In lifestyle fitness coaching, clients normally do not resemble those who seek psychologists, social workers, or psychiatrists for more problematic issues. In the latter case, clients may have unclear goals and much uncertainty, framed within feelings of sadness, confusion, or despair. Coaching clients frequently enter the relationship with specific goals in mind. Although these goals may evolve or change over the course of the coaching relationship, one of the first processes in which coach and client engage is that of establishing agreements about the likely and reasonable goals and directions for the working alliance. The advantage of beginning the relationship with a sense of purpose and focus is that thoughts, feelings, and behaviors can readily be referenced to the client's stated agenda. In this light, skills described in this chapter become potent coaching vehicles for advancing the relationship and the client's progress toward goal attainment. Providing feedback, responding in the moment to what is happening, confronting clients about their inconsistencies, or interpreting behaviors that may impede progress make far more sense when clients have stated their commitments, agreed to an action plan, and begun to engage the work of implementing their programs.

Coaching Dialogues

SKILLS IN ACTION

*"As you move forward into your life,
You will come upon a great chasm.
Jump. It is not as wide as you think."*

Advice to a young Zuni warrior
upon initiation into adulthood

We can view coaching as a series of conversations occurring over time. Continuing involvement in the coaching process occurs in periods between conversations by reflection, planning, preparation, and action. The term *dialogue,* as recently reframed by the late quantum physicist David Bohm (Bohm & Nichol, 1996), is probably most apt in describing these conversations.

Dialogue is a conversation between two or more persons or an exchange of ideas and opinions. But not all communication is dialogue, especially in Bohm's sense of the term (Bohm & Nichol, 1996; Elinor & Gerard, 1998). Dialogue may be understood as a shared exploration toward greater understanding, connection, or possibility. Dialogue is an almost magical process whereby we move beyond static definitions of ourselves and others toward discovery of possibilities and new ways of thinking, acting, and feeling.

Understanding Coaching Dialogue

The terms *dialogue, discussion,* and *conversation* are sometimes used interchangeably, and in previous chapters these words have often substituted for one another. Now that much of the groundwork is in place for understanding what needs to occur in effective coaching relationships, we will reconsider these terms and move toward a definition of the coaching process as one of dialogue.

Conversations and discussions may lack the fluid, deeply connected quality generally believed to characterize dialogues. Conversations, and perhaps more so discussions, often look like tennis matches with participants serving their opinions and positions up to opponents and then returning their responses with more argumentation and defense. Bohm (Bohm & Nichol, 1996) noted that the word *discussion* derives from the same root word as *percussion* and *concussion,* connoting such actions as hitting, striking, and shaking.

Dialogue, in contrast, engages participants in a process of joining thoughts and feelings to create shared meanings that continue to evolve. The end points of dialogue are rarely foreseen at the outset. Criteria for dialogue include the notion that participants talk about what is truly important to them, and they listen carefully to what each other has to say. The purpose of listening is not to formulate the best defense for one's position but rather to develop deep appreciation of each other's views and experiences. Participants in dialogue have no intent to make the other person wrong; instead, the focus is on learning through mutual exploration. Finally, the two parties share the talking space, even to the degree of actively ensuring that the other person has ample opportunities to speak.

Bohm's approach to dialogue engages participants in a collective effort to understand the assumptions and beliefs underlying their individual realities (Bohm & Nichol, 1996). In this manner, dialogue enables participants to uncover blind spots and incongruities that can then be reduced or eliminated. As related to coaching, dialogue implies that both coach and client speak about what is truly important and listen to each other in earnest with the intention of generating shared understandings from which they can launch meaningful and well-guided action.

We may be able to understand dialogue more clearly by comparing it to a debate (Bohm & Nichol, 1996; Elinor & Gerard, 1998; Senge, 1994; Yankelovich, 1999). "Distinguishing Characteristics of Dialogue and Debate" summarizes distinguishing features of these two communication processes.

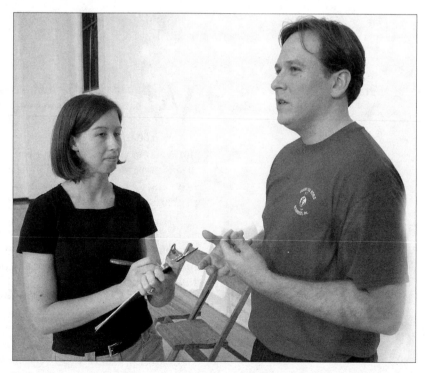

Good dialogue requires the speaker to talk about issues relevant to him and the listener to understand and appreciate the speaker's view.

Distinguishing Characteristics of Dialogue and Debate

Although it is unlikely that the coaching process would resemble a debate, appreciating the differences between dialogue and debate may enable coaches to understand relationships in which client resistance to change is high or in which clients are for some indeterminate reason opposing ideas suggested by the coach.

Dialogue	Debate
Collaborative.	Oppositional.
Goal is finding common ground.	Goal is winning.
Listens for understanding, meaning, and agreements.	Listens to find flaws and counterarguments.
Broadens and potentially changes participants' views.	Affirms each participant's own views.
Uncovers assumptions for exploration and testing.	Defends assumptions as truths.
Provokes reflection about one's own views.	Encourages critique of the other's views.
Creates possibilities of new and unforeseen opportunities and solutions.	Defends one's own solutions while devaluing the other's solutions.
Creates openness to change and willingness to admit error.	Creates closed-minded attitude and determination to be right.
Acknowledges that the other's input will improve one's own input rather than diminish it.	Defends one's input no matter what, maintaining that it is right.
Requires a temporary suspension of one's beliefs.	Requires total and unwavering investment in one's own beliefs.
Searches for basic agreements.	Searches for points of difference.
Searches for strengths in the other.	Searches for weakness and flaws in the other.
Expresses a genuine concern for the other and a desire to cocreate a trusting atmosphere.	Expresses little or no concern for the other or the relationship, only for one's own position.
Assumes that the other can provide missing pieces with which to create the best solution.	Assumes that only one answer is right and that only one person has it.
Remains open-ended.	Works toward conclusion.

The remainder of this chapter will examine dialogues between coaches and clients at various stages of the relationship. The primary purpose of these dialogues will be to illustrate the use of coaching skills and to appraise their function in moving the agenda forward and cocreating an optimal working alliance between coach and client. The previous material on the nature of dialogue should make it clear that all the skills described in earlier chapters are well suited to this collaborative coaching process. Moreover, a key element of dialogue is the possibility of discovery.

Although clients may enter the relationship with preconceived notions of how the relationship will progress, what the coach will do, and what exactly they want to achieve, these ideas may well evolve as coach and client work together from initiation to goal setting and action planning and on toward implementation and goal attainment.

In early stages of coaching, some skills, notably those most closely related to listening, will predominate. As the relationship develops, influencing skills will come into more frequent use.

Two Coaching Dialogues

We will follow two fictional clients from their initial meetings with their coaches until a reasonable point of engagement with goal-directed activities or termination. Although their histories and experiences are fictional, these clients are a composite of issues and agendas taken from real clients in coaching relationships.

Let's meet the coaches. One coach, Rachel, will work with her client in dual capacities of lifestyle fitness coach and personal trainer, and the other coach, Luke, will function solely as a lifestyle fitness coach. Both coaches may choose to refer their clients to other professionals, as they perceive the need and opportunity. The coaches developed their coaching capacities through formal training, supervised practice, and extensive reading, and both have certification as personal trainers by internationally respected organizations. Neither coach has extensive knowledge or training in other fields such as nutrition or physiotherapy.

Now, let's find out about the clients. Rachel's client Harry is a 46-year-old school administrator who works long hours in a job that returns diminishing rewards for all his commitment and efforts. He is married with two children, both of whom are in college or graduate school and living on their own. His wife, Mariah, has a thriving consulting practice and is often on the road. Harry thinks of himself as experiencing a midlife crisis, and he wants to figure out the next season of his life, which seems to imply to him a major career change. He is trim but unathletic. As a child he was timid and introspective, but he has managed to achieve a reasonable level of success in his career through his intellect and compulsive work habits.

Luke's client Kate is a recently divorced 50-year-old freelance journalist. She has traveled the globe on various assignments and has never stayed in one place long enough to grow roots. Her health habits are problematic, and though she looks fit, her cardiorespiratory functioning is poor. She is in the midst of writing a book about her experiences, and she hopes that she can change from journalist to nonfiction writer so that her life will have more stability and predictability.

Beginning: Developing the Relationship and Agenda for Coaching

In chapter 10 we will examine methods and tools for gathering and synthesizing information to guide

action programming with clients. For now, we will rely on a simpler framework. We will begin the coaching process with four orienting themes that the coach will explore with the client:

1. Who is the client? What background characteristics, attitudes, values, beliefs, and needs are relevant to explore in relation to the client's stated goals and objectives?

2. What are the goals or objectives that the client wishes to achieve through the process of coaching?

3. What expectations and understanding does the client have about coaching and the way in which the coach will help the client toward goal attainment?

4. What are the parameters within which the coaching relationship will form and according to which coach and client will create viable processes to pursue goals and objectives?

These themes may be seen as orientations embedded in the clients' sessions. Although coach and client can probably address these themes sufficiently in a lengthy (60 or more minutes) first session, they will continually explore aspects of these themes throughout the coaching relationship.

The dialogues will be presented in a way that identifies the coaching skills along with the functions that they are serving. You should first read the script of interactions between coach and client on the left side of the tables without regard for the skills and comments on the right side of the tables. After you have read the script once, you should reread it, along with the notation of skills and comments corresponding to each coaching intervention. Realize that these dialogues are not complete; rather, they provide brief segments of interaction between coach and client as demonstrations of the sequencing of skills and the effects that they generate. Take a moment now to read coaching dialogue 9.1, "Initial Session: Rachel (Coach) and Harry (Client)."

This segment of the session seems to go well. The client, Harry, is reasonably astute about his needs and issues. He appropriately seeks help from a skilled professional. His attitude is positive, and he seems highly motivated.

Throughout the dialogue, Harry responds openly and genuinely to Rachel's prompts. Had there been any indications of resistance, Rachel may have had to change her approach. For instance, consider the exchange in which Rachel puts the question back to Harry (segments 26 through 28). Although the attempt is to get Harry to take responsibility for

dialogue

Coaching Dialogue 9.1   Initial Session: Rachel (Coach) and Harry (Client)

(A few minutes into the session.)

Dialogue	Skills	Comments
1. Coach: "Harry, can you tell me about your goals or objectives for coaching? What is it that you'd like to achieve or change?"	Open questions.	Facilitates client expression without limiting the options.
2. Client: "Well, I want to start training. I want to be a lot more active than I have been."		
3. Coach: "Uh huh" (accompanied by nonverbal expressions of interest, e.g., nodding head, good eye contact, forward lean of the torso).	Minimal encourager.	Supports the client in continuing to talk.
4. Client: "And I want to do things differently than I've been doing."		
5. Coach: "Do things differently?"	Question framed as a reflection of content.	Seeks clarification of a specific point.
6. Client: "Yes. You don't know this about me, but I'm a very hard-working person . . . committed, maybe too committed to some things . . . and, unfortunately, I'm having less and less fun doing what I'm doing."		
7. Coach: "So, you're real hard-working, but you're not having as much fun these days."	Reflection of content	Facilitates continued expression without adding input.
8. Client: "Right. The reason I decided I needed a coach was that I don't know much about what's out there in the exercise world, and I thought if I went about it on my own, I'd probably pick something safe and boring, and stick to it nonetheless . . . Then I'd be doing the same here as I do at work."		
9. Coach: "You don't want to repeat the same pattern here."	Selective reflection of content.	Focuses the client on an emerging theme.
10. Client: "No, I don't! In fact, I want to break some of my old habits. You can give me the most boring task in the world, and I'll keep at it until it's done . . . I'm not a kid anymore. I'm beginning to feel my age, and I want to start having more fun."		
11. Coach: "Fun is real important to you in whatever we create for you here."	Reflection of content.	Brings together the client's emphasis on fun and references it to the goals of coaching.
12. Client: "I need to explore, to try out new things, to learn to look at myself differently, and so I need a guide to the exercise world, someone who can help me make good choices and stick with things that may be a bit on the wild or unusual side. I know I can do boring things, but I'm not sure how I react to novelty."		

(continued)

Dialogue	Skills	Comments
13. Coach: "I'm beginning to understand. You want to get involved in a variety of sport and fitness activities, to experiment, yet this may be a real challenge for you because things that are different and novel may be harder for you to stick with than something that's very basic, highly structured, and perhaps boring. Is this it?"	Immediacy and then a reflection of content, but the coach offers a slight interpretation (by adding words). Ends with closed question.	Draws together the emerging theme and by using the word challenge provides a slight interpretation that might move the client along, if correct.
14. Client: "Exactly. Believe it or not, my wife is a real daredevil. She's off to a new place every week—or so it seems. Me, I've been at the same job for 22 years, ever since I finished grad school. Sure, I've gotten lots of promotions, but it's still pretty much the same place, the same kinds of tasks, just a lot more responsibility."		
15. Coach: "You've been at the same agendas for a long time, and it seems like it's time for change. I have the results of your fitness testing that you completed when you joined the club, so I have some idea about your medical background and your physical capabilities. What else do you think I should know about you before we begin to explore the options?"	Reflection of content, information, and open question.	Acknowledges the client's message. Advances the coaching agenda by bringing in the testing data and checks for additional relevant information.
16. Client: "Hmmm. Well, I think you said some of it when you mentioned the word 'change.' I told my wife last week that I thought I was having a midlife crisis." [laughs self-consciously]		
17. Coach: "A midlife crisis?"	Question framed as reflection of content (or minimal encourager).	Seeks clarification of a specific point.
18. Client: "I don't mean anything serious . . . I just think I'm ripe for change. I've even been considering switching careers . . . But that's another story."		
19. Coach: "Tell me more about how this 'midlife crisis' fits with how you think we'll be working together."	Indirect question in the form of an instruction, that is, "Tell me . . ."	Keeps the client focused on the coaching agenda instead of supporting discussion of the broader topic of midlife crisis.
20. Client: "Well, I expect to still have a job—the same job—for a while to come, but in some way by being my own guinea pig here at the club, I am hoping to open up my thinking, loosen my mind, so to speak, to consider different alternatives. I think I've been in a rut and I believe enough in the fact that if a person changes one aspect of their lives they influence all others. So, maybe the fitness thing is my first step. It's something I've wanted to do for a long time, but each time I thought about it before, I imagined myself running on a treadmill five times a week, and that boredom coupled with the increasing boredom of my job made the whole thing a nonstarter, if you know what I mean."		
21. Coach: "I think I do. Working with me on a fitness agenda is like your pilot project to bring about change in your life, and also to do something you've wanted to do for a long time."	Immediacy followed by reflection of content and reframe (interpretation).	Captures the essence of the client's message and provides a different perspective by using the expression "pilot project" rather than reflecting "guinea pig."

Dialogue	Skills	Comments
22. Client: "Yeah, that's it, a pilot project! I like that. That's great! This is my pilot project to see how I deal with novelty and how I function according to some different kinds of rules."		
23. Coach: "Rules?"	Question framed as a minimal encourager.	Seeks clarification of a specific point.
24. Client: "Yeah, like how do I deal with the unexpected? How do I function when I don't know what's coming next? And how quickly do I learn, especially in areas like fitness where I don't think I'm very good?"		
25. Coach: "That's clearer . . . Thanks. Is there anything else you want me to know right now?"	Immediacy and open question.	Assures the client of the coach's understanding and checks for additional relevant information.
26. Client: "I'm sure things will come to mind, but that seems like a good start. Where do we go from here?"		
27. Coach: "Good question. I could ask you the same. Where would you like to go from here?"	Feedback and open question.	Confirms relevancy of the client's focus and offers the client an opportunity to be self-directing.
28. Client: "Well, I'd like to start putting something together with you."		
29. Coach: "Terrific. I have an idea of how to start. Maybe you could tell me what activities or sports come to mind with a big 'X' through them, like 'definitely not, too boring,' and then you could let me know what activities or sports seem to capture your attention."	Advice or suggestion.	Confirms the client's direction and offers a strategy for moving forward.
30. Client: "OK, but remember, I don't know that much, so don't be disappointed."		
31. Coach: "Whatever you tell me will be helpful. I imagine you have some impressions, and it would be great to know what they are."	Immediacy and suggestion.	Deals with the client's apparent anxiety and provides reassurance.

planning, the strategy could have backfired. Harry could have said, "Why are you asking me? This is your job." Had this occurred, Rachel might have used this response as a way of informing Harry about the collaborative nature of coaching. To his rebuttal, she might have responded, "Harry, you're right, it is my job—and the way in which I like to work with my clients is to keep them involved as codirectors of this whole process. Yes, I have some ideas, yet it is extremely important to me that I have your full input at every point along the way. Does this make sense to you?"

Clients may perceive coaches as so expert that they almost expect their coaches to read their minds. Harry's question, "Where do we go from here?" implies that the coach sets the direction and has a precise roadmap for the coaching process. Early

behaviors in coaching are norm setting, that is, if the coach takes on the steering function from the outset, the client will begin to expect that kind of role behavior. So, although Rachel may have taken a risk by putting the question back to Harry, by doing so she sets the pattern for a collaborative working alliance.

The second client, Kate, has a coaching relationship more complex than the one between Rachel and Harry. Take a moment now to read coaching dialogue 9.2, "Initial Session: Luke (Coach) and Kate (Client)" on page 188. In this dialogue, the client is aware of the challenges that she presents and struggles to maintain focus in the session.

Kate kids the coach (segment 8) about being able to fix all her problems, yet underlying this remark may be the unrealistic desire for the coach

dialogue

Coaching Dialogue 9.2 Initial Session: Luke (Coach) and Kate (Client)

(A few minutes into the session.)

Dialogue	Skills	Comments
1. Coach: "Kate, I would very much like to hear about your reasons for wanting to work with me. What are your goals?"	Indirect and open questions.	Facilitates client expression without limiting the options.
2. Client: "Oh boy, that's a big question. I think this is going to be a challenge for you!"		
3. Coach: "A challenge for me?"	Question framed as a reflection of content (or minimal encourager).	Seeks clarification of a specific point.
4. Client: "Yes, indeed. I need to make some big changes in my life, and getting fit is just one of them."		
5. Coach: "So, there are some big changes you want to work on—and getting fit is one of them. Can you tell me more?"	Reflection of content and open question.	Facilitates continued expression from the client without directing the content.
6. Client: "Well, I smoke, I don't eat regularly, I'm trying out a new career, I'm out of shape, I just got divorced, I don't sleep well, I've been all over the map in my life—both geographically and in my lifestyle. What else do you want to know?"		
7. Coach: "I think the biggest question for me would be what goals or expectations do you have for the work that we would do together?"	Indirect question with a focus.	Focuses the client on the specific agenda for the coaching relationship. Redirects the client from a generalized life perspective to the lifestyle fitness coaching agenda.
8. Client: "You mean you can't fix all my problems? [Laughs.] Just kidding. I guess I need to develop some stability in my life and getting fit, especially at my age, seems real important . . . and I know it's not going to be easy."		
9. Coach: "Stability and fitness—is this the agenda you want to work on with me?"	Selective reflection of content plus closed question.	Focuses the client on an emerging theme and asks for verification. Does not respond to the "kidding" remark or to the age theme.
10. Client: "Well, yes . . . I mean I don't expect you to create stability in my life. That's too much to ask . . . No, what I've been thinking is that if I can get regular about exercise, that will go a long way to helping me settle down and focus."		
11. Coach: "I'd like to know more about this connection you're making with a fitness program."	Indirect question with a focus.	Asks the client to make connection between themes. Does not respond to the "too much to ask" remark.

Dialogue	Skills	Comments
12. Client: "Here's the short version. I used to travel a lot. I just got divorced. I have been terribly inconsistent in how I lived. And I don't always take the best care of myself. It's going to be hard for me to exercise, but I believe if I can make this change, I can make others."		
13. Coach: "If you can make this change, you can make others . . . Is this mostly how you see it?"	A partial reflection of content ending with a closed question.	Attempts to identify the client's core motivation. Does not reflect all the content but chooses to focus on the client's reason for wanting to exercise.
14. Client: "Yes. I need to do something, anything, with consistency . . . That's what I need . . . But I guess I really need to exercise, too, and I'm almost dreading it."		
15. Coach: "I'd like to hear more about how you're thinking about exercise. You mentioned that you thought it would be hard, and now you say you're 'dreading it.'"	Indirect question with a focus plus selective reflection of content with a focus.	Opens exploration of the client's attitudes and feelings about exercise, and focuses the client on two expressed attitudes.
16. Client: "Well, that's one reason why I hired you. Let's face it—exercise is boring. And it's hard work. And my life has been anything but boring. Being a freelance journalist, I've lived on adrenaline most of my life—Bosnia, Afghanistan, Iraq—you name the hot spot, I've been there."		
17. Coach: "So you think it will be hard work and boring."	Selective reflection of content.	Seeks clarification of a specific point while avoiding diversion into life issues or past experiences.
18. Client: "Don't get me wrong, I'm not afraid of hard work, but I do bore easily. I could go for white-water kayaking or parasailing, but I'm no kid anymore, and I'm certainly not in any kind of shape to do those activities. I don't want to get injured—any more than I have been already!"		
19. Coach: "So far what I'm getting is that in addition to creating a consistent pattern in your life, you'd like to do something that won't be boring but that your body can handle without getting injured. Is this the sense of it?"	Summary with a minor interpretation. Ends with a closed question.	Builds on the emerging theme while adding a new theme of physical safety in exercise. Note that this slight interpretation is not entirely consistent with the client's history.
20. Client: "Yes . . . but I think there's more."		

(continued)

(continued)

Dialogue	Skills	Comments
21. Coach: "Great. Tell me."	Minimal encourager plus indirect question or directive ("Tell me").	Reinforces client expression. Indicates keen interest in hearing more.
22. Client: "Getting old . . . Do you know what I mean?"		
23. Coach: "Tell me more."	Indirect question or directive.	Seeks additional detail without making an assumption.
24. Client: "I feel old. I think my bad habits are catching up with me. I feel sluggish. My mind isn't as sharp as it used to be. And I gotta give up these cancer sticks."		
25. Coach: "You're concerned about the effects of things like smoking and other habits, and you don't feel in top condition."	Partial reflection of content.	Captures the essence of the message, without focusing on the remark about age.
26. Client: "No, but I want to . . . and I'm afraid it's too late."		
27. Coach: "So, in my way of hearing your story, it sounds as if you have strong motivation to make a solid connection to an exercise program."	Minor reframe (interpretation).	Focuses on strength in the client's fear. Chooses to avoid focusing on the client's emotion.
28. Client: "Yeah, I think you could say that. But is it too late?"		
29. Coach: "Let me answer that briefly—we can talk about it more at some other point. Exercising regularly has all kinds of benefits, including increasing energy levels, improving mental alertness, and giving you an overall feeling of well-being. And it's never too late to start. The more you get into your program, the more you will experience these benefits and more."	Information.	Selective information addressed to the client's specific concerns. Reassures client without dwelling on the underlying fears and doubts expressed by the client.
30. Client: "Well that's encouraging . . . So what do I do about the boredom?"		
31. Coach: "We will figure that out together. But before we begin considering sport and fitness options, what else would you like to tell me that will help guide our work together?"	Information about the coaching process and open question.	Provides details about how the client's question will be answered and then probes for additional information. Avoids premature focusing on program details.
32. Client: "Well, I'm not a chicken. I like challenges."		
33. Coach: "Great . . . So you like challenges. What else?"	Minimal encourager, reflection of content, and open question.	Offers support, indicates listening, and continues to probe.
34. Client: "I guess you already know this, but I keep irregular hours so it's going to be hard for me to keep to a schedule."		
35. Coach: "Hard to keep to a schedule?"	Indirect question.	Probes for details about specific issue.
36. Client: "Well, because I don't like it. It used to be because of my work, but now I'm my own boss so I guess it's just bad habits."		

Dialogue	Skills	Comments
37. Coach: "OK, so you imagine keeping to an exercise schedule will be challenging, yet your time is under your own control."	Reflection of content (implied confrontation).	Brings together attitude and reality concerning scheduling. The client may experience it as confrontation.
38. Client: "Yeah . . . I guess that's a bit contradictory . . . Oh, I guess one more thing is that I'm a bit turned off by 'gym bunnies' who do nothing but work out and look at themselves in the mirror . . . Maybe I'm a bit jealous too."		
39. Coach: "So, you have some attitudes and feelings about people who are at the gym all the time. Anything else?"	Reflection of content and open question.	Indicates listening, but the probe directs the client to new topics rather than exploration of the expressed theme.
40. Client: "No, that's mostly what comes to mind. I'm sure there will be more. So, how would you put all this together?"		
41. Coach: "You want me to summarize what I'm hearing from you so far?"	Closed question.	Serves to verify the request in case the client may actually be seeking something else.
42. Client: "Well, not really. I think what I really want to know is if you think you can work with me and help me—given all my bad habits and what I'm asking for."		
43. Coach: "I guess we're back to what you said earlier . . . You said you were going to be a challenge for me. And now that I've heard more, you sound concerned that with all your so-called bad habits I may not be able to help you."	Summary.	Brings together the early remark about challenge with concerns about likelihood of change.
44. Client: "Yes, that's it . . . but I do want to change, and I will do my best."		
45. Coach: "Terrific. That's important. This is a 50–50 deal. You do your best. I'll do my best. And together I believe we can move you closer to your goals. Does that answer your question?"	Immediacy, information, immediacy, and closed question.	Provides support and information about the process of coaching. Focuses on the coach's commitment and intention.
46. Client: "Yes, thank you. I think I was looking for reassurance and promises, but I really know it's up to me."		

to make all of her life better. Presumably, Luke has delineated his role as coach and the parameters of his work with the client either at the very beginning of the session or in a prior conversation when Kate arranged to hire him. In this segment of dialogue, Luke works to define boundaries and keep Kate focused on the legitimate domain of lifestyle fitness coaching. Although he does not reiterate what the coaching domain is, he listens carefully to her responses and asks questions to elicit what her perceptions are about how they might work together.

As the session progresses, Kate's remarks take on a more self-deprecating quality. She describes her bad habits, and she eventually seeks some kind of reassurance from Luke about whether or not there is hope for her. To some degree, segments 40 through 46 may represent the issue of responsibility. Kate asks Luke to put it all together (40), and when he questions whether this is, in fact, what she wants, she admits to her deeper agenda, which is to be reassured. Yet there is a hint here that Kate is asking Luke whether he can fix her even if she does not necessarily accept personal responsibility for all that she must do. Luke skillfully avoids the trap of responding to her request for reassurance by reflecting her remarks and by describing the 50–50 nature of the coaching relationship. In Kate's final remark (46) in this excerpt from the session, she owns her responsibility and in so doing begins to commit to the coaching process.

At different points, the coach selectively attended to client messages. For instance, he did not focus on Kate's concerns about her age. He did not follow up on her adrenaline-fueled lifestyle, her recent divorce, or her new career directions. Although he acknowledged her concerns about health habits, especially smoking, he chose not to provide information, advice, or instruction. His selective attention may be interpreted as implicit statements about his role. He was not going to discuss her relationship issues, her career concerns, or her non-exercise-related health habits at this time. Yet some of these issues may later interact with the programming that Kate and Luke develop and with Kate's adherence to the agreed-upon activities. Perhaps when these issues arise in another context, the coach may have to address them.

Dealing with Resistance: Engaging Change and Exploring Meaning

Relationships develop at different rates and in varying ways, yet sooner or later coach and client will likely encounter resistance in the process. Resistance is not necessarily bad nor is it entirely preventable (Dym, Jenks, & Sonduck, 2002); in this respect, it must be addressed rather than avoided. According to Dym and colleagues,

> resistance wears many faces. It may look like outright refusal, denial, skepticism, lethargy, incompetence, pessimism, or helplessness. At times, people resist by questioning the competence, credentials, or motives of coaches and by going into a bunker-type mode until the siege of change passes. (p. 341)

The function of resistance in the client's world is essentially to seek stability in a world characterized by change. Although change may be self-directed and is likely to be positive, it nonetheless disrupts the status quo; it propels the client from the comfort zone (McWilliams, 1991) into an unknown, unpredictable, and perhaps frightening new realm of being. The client may be seeking familiar ground because the change process has become too demanding and too stressful, or because the client lacks sufficient motivation. How interested

is the client in changing (Hepworth et al., 1997)? What may have seemed a great idea takes on new dimensions when clients engage the realities of change. Frequently, people simply do not know how wide reaching the effects of change can be. We are "human systems"—change one part of our lives and most others may be affected.

Coaches must avoid personalizing resistance. Although clients may be critical of their coaches during periods of resistance, their judgment is unlikely to be personal. Rather, clients' criticism will reflect the internal stress and discomfort that they experience and can no longer contain. The result is that they project these feelings onto situations, other individuals, or external elements.

What skills are required for dealing with resistance? Conceptually, when a client is resisting change and the coach is positioned as a person promoting or supporting change, then the client may perceive the coach as the enemy. In brief, rapport may diminish when clients steadfastly resist change. Resistance may intensify when coaches rely heavily on influencing skills. For instance, if coaches provide instruction, information, or advice, clients may demonstrate resistance by refusing to comply, by engaging in actions that defeat the coach's intentions, or by arguing with the coach. Coaches may need to rely more on skills that rebuild rapport (chapter 6) or that enable the client to increase awareness, develop insights into behavior, and deepen motivations (chapter 7). As trust and rapport redevelop, coaches may begin to use challenging and solution skills that are more advanced.

We will explore through the continuing dialogues of Rachel and Harry, and Luke and Kate how coaches might address resistance. Take a moment now to read coaching dialogue 9.3, "Dealing With Client Resistance: Rachel (Coach) and Harry (Client)."

The rich emotional ground of this dialogue was evident throughout. Feelings that the client encountered in his program triggered him, and his attempt to project blame onto the coach made it clear that he had difficulty containing his feelings or owning responsibility for them. He was in too much discomfort and therefore was unable to gain perspective of his experience. By remaining supportive of the client and not personalizing the feelings that Harry was projecting onto her, Rachel successfully steered the conversation through the rough waters to a place where Harry could begin to understand things differently.

Had Rachel at any point defended herself, the relationship might have taken a turn for the worse. For instance, Rachel knew that she had discussed

Coaching Dialogue 9.3 Dealing With Client Resistance: Rachel (Coach) and Harry (Client)

(Harry has been involved in his training for about a month. He is discussing his progress with Rachel. They are midway into the session.)

Dialogue	Skills	Comments
1. Coach: "Harry, it sounds as if your experiences with your program are less than satisfactory. Is this correct?"	Reflection of content and closed question.	Supports the client, demonstrates listening, and determines accuracy.
2. Client: "Oh no. It's going OK. " [long pause]		
3. Coach: "Earlier you mentioned that you didn't like the core training class you're taking, and now you're saying, 'It's going OK.' Can you clarify this for me, please?"	Confrontation and closed question.	Points out discrepancy between two verbal messages and asks for clarification.
4. Client: "Well, I don't have to like everything, do I? True, some of this stuff isn't my cup of tea."		
5. Coach: "Some of this stuff?"	Question framed as reflection of content.	Focuses the client on a particular aspect of the message.
6. Client: "Look, it was your idea I take this class. What did you have in mind anyway? I mean what was I supposed to get out of it?"		
7. Coach: "Sounds like you're upset with me for suggesting this class."	Reflection of unexpressed feeling plus content (interpretation).	Acknowledges the client's emotion without being defensive.
8. Client: "No, I'm not upset. I just don't get it."		
9. Coach: "Can you help me understand what the 'it' is, Harry?"	Open question with selective focus.	The client denies emotion. The coach does not pursue the point but chooses to refocus on the content.
10. Client: "Look, you knew I wasn't a great athlete to begin with and there are all these acrobats and gymnasts in this class, and well . . . I feel like a total klutz."		
11. Coach: "Hmmm. That sounds real unpleasant—feeling like a total klutz in a class."	Reflection of feeling plus content.	Acknowledges client feeling without responding to the implied blame projected onto the coach.
12. Client: "Well it is! I know I wanted to try new things but this is ridiculous . . . I mean I feel ridiculous."		
13. Coach: "I'm so sorry to hear this, Harry. What can I do to help?"	Immediacy and open question.	Genuine expression of concern for the client's feelings in the session, coupled with an offer of help.
14. Client: "Oh, it's no big thing."		

(continued)

(continued)

Dialogue	Skills	Comments
15. Coach: "Well, it sounds like a big thing, feeling ridiculous . . . and yet, I hear you minimizing your own feelings in this, like you should be able to deal with it no matter how you're feeling."	Confrontation, feedback, and minor interpretation.	Addresses the discrepancy between the client's words and emotions. Feeds back the coach's observation that it sounds like a "big thing." Interprets client behavior as one of minimizing his own feelings with the intention of increasing awareness.
16. Client: "I should, shouldn't I? I mean I got what I asked for."		
17. Coach: "You got what you asked for . . . Would you tell me, Harry, what was it that you wanted from this?"	Effort to reflect meaning through a reflection of content and open question.	Focuses on the client's experience and probes for clarification. Encourages the client to search for meaning.
18. Client: "I'm not sure anymore. I know I didn't want to do some routine workout. I wanted to break my mold, my patterns. I guess I didn't realize how doing boring things actually suits me . . . I don't feel threatened. I know I can do it . . . There's a kind of security in it, and I can actually succeed at boring, routine things, whereas most people don't."		
19. Coach: "So there's something about being safe and successful that you're not feeling with this class. Is that it?"	Continuing to probe for meaning through a reflection of content and closed question.	Identifies the core elements in the client's story that may enable the client to find deeper meaning in the experience or gain insight.
20. Client: "I guess so . . . I didn't realize that until now . . . I feel embarrassed and I think I've avoided situations in the past where I would feel embarrassed."		
21. Coach: "So, is this a situation where you are successfully experiencing an opportunity to change your pattern?"	Reframe (interpretation).	Reframes the client's experience in terms of his goals and objectives, so that he can view what he has felt as discomfort as purposeful and in line with his growth agenda.
22. Client: "Huh? Say that again. Do you mean that by being a klutz, I'm being successful?"		
23. Coach: "Sort of . . . You said you wanted to experience new things, to break the mold, to change your patterns. So part of your pattern has been to keep yourself safe by doing things you would for sure succeed at—even if they bored you to death."	Summary to explain reframe.	Helps the client understand because he is still experiencing some confusion.
24. Client: "Yeah, so far that's right."		
25. Coach: "And now, you have a goal to do things differently— you might say to do things that are unsafe, not boring, and where your success isn't so secure."	Continuing explanation of reframe.	Enables the client to understand experiences in a different perspective.
26. Client: "Right."		

Dialogue	Skills	Comments
27. Coach: "So, in this class you seem to be having the experience you wanted to have—even though it's pretty tough—and in this sense you are succeeding at achieving your goal."	Completion of reframe explanation.	The client is gaining insight as expressed in his responses to the coach, so the coach continues to explore the new perspective.
28. Client: "Wow. That's the fanciest talking I've heard in a while, but, you know, you're right . . . Yes, you're right. Why didn't I see it that way?"		
29. Coach: "I think when you're in the midst of a storm—an internal storm of feelings—it's hard to be clear about things."	Information and interpretation.	Offers support to the client, who has now begun to be self-critical. Also, interprets experience as a "storm of feelings."
30. Client: "Well you're right about that, too. I'm sorry for being upset with you before. I guess I wasn't handling my feelings too well, maybe because I didn't even allow myself to know about them . . . We set up this program together, and you explained the challenges I might encounter. I think I've been so comfortable with boredom in the past that doing something like this class overloaded my circuits."		
31. Coach: "Understandable . . . and frankly I'm glad we had a chance to talk about this. It seemed real important. I feel good about our conversation . . . but before we conclude anything here maybe we should look at what you're doing a bit closer. Maybe there are other options you can consider that won't be as upsetting."	Immediacy and advice with implied question.	Offers acceptance and support. Encourages the client to explore similar issues in the future. Keeps the topic open so that implications can be examined.
32. Client: "No, I don't think that's necessary now. You've given me a real shot in the arm . . . I needed to get outside myself to see this situation better. You're right, I am on track and I am being successful, and knowing that will help a whole lot when I take these classes. And besides, I'm really not the worst one in the class . . . I just feel that way sometimes . . . Since I've begun, I've made some real progress. There are at least a half dozen people who aren't doing nearly as well as me."		
33. Coach: "That sounds great . . . So acknowledging your feelings and getting a broader perspective of this has helped. Sounds like something that's worth keeping in mind."	Feedback, minor interpretation, and advice.	Reinforces the client's conclusions, provides perspective through a minor interpretation, and supports the client in understanding this behavior as a possible pattern worth noting.
34. Client: "You bet. I didn't realize how much I could really get out of my training. I know when we first talked, I spoke about the mind–body thing, but talking about it and experiencing it first hand are worlds apart."		

potential reactions that he might have to this class and that he willingly agreed to participate in it. She might have said, "Look Harry, I told you what you might experience and you agreed to do it. So, don't blame me." The dialogue would then have become a debate about who was right. The relationship would have suffered, and any chance of insight or understanding would have diminished.

Rachel took a calculated gamble in segments 21 through 28 by reframing what Harry was experiencing as negative and painful into a positive, goal-related success story. This approach could have backfired. By this point in the dialogue, however, Rachel had enough evidence of renewed rapport and trust along with Harry's diminishing emotional reactivity that she risked this strategy. The **reframe** is the coach's awareness of the strengths or assets evident in a client's story that the client is unable to see because of his emotionality.

Once the client accepted the reframe, the next agenda that Rachel puts to Harry is to integrate this new knowledge with his current plan (29 though 34). Are adjustments implied by this new awareness? Are there implications for how the client functions in general? Without undue emphasis, Rachel helps Harry consider these angles. His responses suggest that through the reframe he will be able to draw new energy to motivate his actions and continue on his path. In addition, Harry indicates a profound new understanding of the difference between ideas and lived experiences, and through this he may gain increased acceptance of his own emotions.

Lifestyle fitness coaching will differ significantly from other health fitness professions such as personal training partly by virtue of the depth of discussions considered legitimate. Coaching dialogue 9.4, "Dealing With Client Resistance: Luke (Coach) and Kate (Client)" on page 197, represents this difference. Take a moment now to read this dialogue.

Toward the end of this exchange, we note that Luke clarifies the boundaries of the relationship based on Kate's behaviors and remarks in the session. She becomes aware that she is behaving with Luke in a manner reminiscent of a previous intimate relationship. Technically, this illustrates the phenomenon of transference. Kate is also perceptive enough to identify this issue as inappropriate for her coaching relationship, and Luke validates this assessment by reinforcing the possibility that she find a professional counselor with whom to discuss this issue further.

Luke absorbs a great deal of emotional projection from Kate in the early segments of the exchange. He does not react defensively, nor does he attempt to correct her assertions. At the same time, his reflections in no way represent statements of agreement. For instance in segment 13, Luke says, "I know you said I've failed in my work with you . . . Are there other reasons?" He does not say, "I've failed." By continuing to reflect, Luke allows Kate the opportunity to explore her thoughts and feelings and to release some of the energy that she is experiencing. If Luke were to react to her comments, his words would no doubt fuel the conflict. By absorbing her reactions and containing his emotions, the oppositional nature of the dialogue gradually diminishes.

In segment 19 Luke decides that it is time to shift focus. He requests permission to address some of his own feelings and perceptions, ultimately in service of the relationship and the client's goals. Kate's response to his request (20) continues to reflect a somewhat hostile and aggressive pattern, so Luke (21) discloses his personal feelings and reiterates his request. The power of this use of immediacy appears in Kate's reaction (22) of dropping her hostile approach and acknowledging her behavior. This is a turning point.

As the remainder of the dialogue evolves, Kate owns more and more of her reactivity and behavior. In segment 32 Kate has a major insight, brought about in part by Luke's candid feedback and immediacy responses. Had Luke continued to reflect content and feeling, his approach would have been not only inappropriate but also unlikely to help Kate develop awareness.

Coaches do not serve as dumping grounds for client emotions. Although coaches must learn to contain their emotions long enough to understand what is happening and to time their interventions appropriately, they must respond genuinely when doing so is possible and when the likelihood of successful outcome is reasonably high. Imagine that Kate had accelerated her attack on Luke, showing no softening as a result of his caring responses. Depending on the history of the relationship, the coach would have some sense of whether Kate was capable of learning from a genuine exchange or whether her behavior suggested that the relationship was no longer viable. We all have bad days, yet even so it is not the coach's job to absorb client accusations and verbal assaults indefinitely. Had Kate continued and had Luke judged her unable to deal with his feedback, confrontations, and self-disclosures, his best option might have been to end the session with a request for Kate to reflect on what had occurred, to schedule another meeting, and to determine then whether or not the relationship would continue.

Coaching Dialogue 9.4 Dealing With Client Resistance: Luke (Coach) and Kate (Client)

(Kate has been struggling with adherence to her program for about 2 months. She is becoming increasingly frustrated and in the past week made excuses for missing all her training sessions. She and Luke are midway into the session.)

Dialogue	Skills	Comments
1. Coach: "Tell me more about what's happening with your program, Kate."	Indirect question in form of a directive.	Guides the client's discussion of a particular topic.
2. Client: "What program? I'm not doing anything!"		
3. Coach: "You're not doing anything?"	Indirect question framed as reflection of content.	Facilitates the client's discussion of message. Note that the coach avoids addressing the client's sarcastic remark.
4. Client: "What's the matter . . . You deaf? That's what I said, I'm not doing anything."		
5. Coach: "Sounds like you're real upset with me."	Reflection of unexpressed feeling (interpretation).	Focuses on the client's emotion without overstating emotion (e.g., "You sound angry") or reacting to it.
6. Client: "Noooo [said sarcastically] . . . Why would I be upset with you?"		
7. Coach: "OK, that's a good question . . . Why would you be upset with me?"	Immediacy and open question.	Acknowledges the dynamic in the relation by saying, "That's a good question," and treats the question as genuine rather than letting it stand as sarcasm.
8. Client: "You really want to know . . . Well, let's start with the fact that I've paid you over $800 in the past few months, and I'm no better off than when I started."		
9. Coach: "So that's for 'starters' . . . What else are you upset with me about?"	Partial reflection of content plus open question.	Instead of limiting input, the coach recognizes the message as a starter and probes for additional input.
10. Client: "Luke, I told you in the beginning that I was going to be a challenge. You took me on, and from the looks of things, you've failed."		
11. Coach: "You're right, I knew our work together would be challenging . . . and you're now seeing the experience as a 'failure.'"	Immediacy plus reflection of content.	Acknowledges prior conversation, gives personal experience of the relationship, and then probes for more information through reflection without owning failure.

(continued)

(continued)

Dialogue	Skills	Comments
12. Client: "Well, how else am I supposed to look at it? I started training and then I stopped and then I started again and then I stopped again. Now I'm doing nothing."		
13. Coach: "Sounds pretty disconcerting. What do you think accounts for this? I know you said I've failed in my work with you . . . Are there other reasons?"	Reflection of feeling, open questions, and reflection of content.	Validates the client's thoughts and feelings, and probes for more information. The coach does not engage in self-defensive reactivity.
14. Client: "Look Luke, I am probably not your easiest client. I've been working like crazy on my book—after all it's what allows me to pay you! So that's my priority."		
15. Coach: "So, your writing comes first . . . anything else?"	Partial reflection of content plus open question.	Focuses on relevant content and continues to probe. The coach does not address the continuing theme of Kate as difficult client.
16. Client: "Yes, as a matter of fact there is. The program you gave me is way too hard, too boring, too unrewarding, and I can't see a single change it has produced."		
17. Coach: "No changes from your program and basically it's unsatisfying."	Reflection of feeling and content.	Reinforces client expression through reflections with slight shift into feeling of content by using the word "unsatisfying."
18. Client: "I mean really, what did you expect? You knew I was hard charging, adrenaline fueled. C'mon, exercise is a big bore!"		
19. Coach: "I hear you . . . Are you open to hearing how I see things?"	Brief reflection plus closed question.	Acknowledges the client's message without details and then shifts focus through question.
20. Client: "Sure, that's what I'm paying you for."		
21. Coach: "Well, to begin, I'm feeling upset right now about the way that you're talking to me . . . It doesn't sound friendly at all, so before I continue, I need to know if you are willing to listen with an open mind."	Immediacy plus feedback and closed question.	Focuses on immediate experience through self-disclosure and feedback to client about the effect of her messages. Ends with a question to determine client receptivity.
22. Client: "Ooops. Sure, OK . . . You're right . . . I'm pretty frustrated and I'm dumping a lot of stuff on you. I'll chill out."		
23. Coach: "Truthfully, it does feel as if you're dumping a lot of stuff on me, so it would help me if we could work on whatever is going on here together—as a team rather than as opponents."	Immediacy.	The coach acknowledges his own feelings and reactions and offers suggestion for how to proceed.
24. Client: "Yeah, you're right. I'm sorry. I agree . . . Please go on."		

Dialogue	Skills	Comments
25. Coach: "OK . . . I've been aware of the challenges you face in turning around so many things in your life to make a clear commitment to your health and fitness—and to stick with it."	Feedback.	Provides feedback concerning personal awareness of client dynamics.
26. Client: "Well I haven't been doing such a good job with it, have I?"		
27. Coach: "I think it has been challenging, and you've taken some steps forward . . . and then when you're making progress, you start falling off your program, almost as if you're setting yourself up to fail. Your work on your book is on schedule, or so you say, so I'm not aware of any major changes in your life that have brought about this recent drop-off in your training."	Feedback, interpretation, and confrontation.	Continues to provide feedback and adds an interpretation of client behavior. Ends with a confrontation of discrepancy between different client messages.
28. Client: "Well, I told you it's boring."		
29. Coach: "Hmmm . . . I hear you saying today that it's boring, yet last week and the week before, you told me your program was great. And frankly, I don't understand how your program turned from 'great' to 'boring' in a week where you didn't participate in it."	Two related confrontations.	Confronts inconsistent client messages and then confronts inconsistency between verbal message and behavior.
30. Client: "Ooops. You got me there."		
31. Coach: "Kate, my intention isn't to 'get you' anywhere. I just want to help . . . And I can't quite explain what's happening . . . I do know that I have been hearing an increasing number of complaints directed at me, along with a sense that somehow I am responsible for making this happen."	Immediacy and feedback, and minor interpretation.	Focuses on the relationship and his intentions. Offers feedback of observations and then provides a minor interpretation in remark about responsibility.
32. Client: [Looking pensive] "This is beginning to sound familiar . . . I heard the same sort of messages from my ex-husband. I didn't realize I was dragging that baggage into the gym [eyes moistening] . . . Luke, I'm sorry. I think you're right. I've probably been setting it up . . . I need to think about it some more, but it sounds like I'm satisfying my adrenaline need by re-creating a bad relationship rather than focusing on my training . . . Now that's an insight!"		
33. Coach: "Sure sounds like one."	Feedback or immediacy.	Feedback to the client about her current experience serving to validate the client's messages.
34. Client: "I knew I needed a coach . . . I really didn't get it until now. It's not the program that's the problem, it's me."		
35. Coach: "You're seeing yourself as a 'problem'?"	Selective reflection of content.	Focuses the client on part of the message, supporting further exploration.
36. Client: "Well, what else could it be? I want to get fit and healthy. I have the time. And I have to admit, most times I feel OK about doing my program, but then I screw it up and blame you . . . like I'd rather have the drama than be healthy."		

(continued)

(continued)

Dialogue	Skills	Comments
37. Coach: "Kate, some of this is getting out of my depth. I understand what you're saying and I am willing to continue helping you focus on your training. I hear that you've made some great connections—insights—about what is happening for you, and I hope this will help get us back on track."	Immediacy, feedback, and information, plus reflection of content.	Focuses on current relation, addressing through feedback and information the boundaries of coaching. Also continues to support and validate client experience.
38. Client: "Yeah, you're right. I should be talking to a shrink about some of this stuff, but I do need your help with my fitness and health stuff. . . You're not going to abandon me, are you?"		
39. Coach: "No, Kate, as I said, I am willing to continue working with you on the agenda we set out a few months ago. As for some of the other things you talked about, as you say, you may want to talk to a professional counselor to work through some of your feelings about this."	Immediacy and self-disclosure plus advice framed partly as a reflection of content.	Continues to focus on relation, providing personal input about willingness to continue, while setting boundaries. Frames advice as a reflection, because the client had mentioned the idea previously.
40. Client: "Yeah, maybe I will . . . but for now, can we talk about how I can get back on track with my training?"		
41. Coach: "Absolutely. Maybe we can look at what happened this past week each time you were scheduled to train but didn't. Sound reasonable?"	Feedback, advice, and closed question.	Gives feedback to request and makes suggestion for continuing the session.
42. Client: "Yes, it does . . . And, again, Luke, I'm sorry."		
43. Coach: "Apology accepted. I'm on your side, Kate."	Immediacy.	Reflects personal experiences and affirms position in relationship.

Endings: Moving Toward Self-Direction and Completion

Although coaching relationships may last for years, eventually they will end. Of course, some end far sooner and not always with the markings of success. As Walsh (2003) notes, certain tasks may be addressed in the ending of a helping relationship, including examining what was learned or gained from the experience, acknowledging feelings about the relationship and its processes, and exploring future plans especially concerning maintenance of gains and prevention of relapse (Marlatt & Gordon, 1985).

When to end a coaching relationship depends on a variety of factors (Walsh, 2003). When coach and client establish clear goals or time limits for coaching, significant movement toward these goals or the completion of an agreed upon period of coaching will signal the ending. When progress is elusive or

when situational factors or client noncompliance thwarts development, coaches may at least temporarily call for a pause in the relationship. In addition, coaches may bring the relationship to closure because clients are unable or unwilling to respect the coach's professional boundaries. In some cases, clients choose to end either because of personal reasons, reactions to the process or the coach, or dissatisfaction with progress. In other cases, issues of greater urgency may arise in the coaching process, thereby redirecting the client's priorities.

We will consider two different types of endings, one representing success and the other manifesting mixed outcomes. Rachel's work with Harry will move toward a gratifying ending, whereas Luke will bring his work with Kate to closure. Let's begin our analysis of these two types of endings. Take a moment now to read coaching dialogue 9.5, "Progressing Toward a Successful Ending: Rachel (Coach) and Harry (Client)."

Coaching Dialogue 9.5 Progressing Toward a Successful Ending: Rachel (Coach) and Harry (Client)

(In this dialogue, Rachel and Harry will begin discussing an end to the coaching process. Harry has been working with Rachel for just over a year, and his efforts have been largely successful. Rachel and Harry have finished discussing Harry's progress and now are moving into a discussion of ending.)

Dialogue	Skills	Comments
1. Coach: "Harry, I am impressed. You have been 100% on target in all your activities for at least the past 3 months now. I imagine you feel pretty good about your efforts and your results."	Immediacy, feedback, and interpretation.	The coach reveals own feelings, documents feedback, and interprets the client's feelings as a way of showing strong support.
2. Client: "Yes, well, I don't take praise too easily, but in this case, I think I deserve it."		
3. Coach: "Seems that way to me."	Feedback.	Validates client perception.
4. Client: "Last week, I did some rock climbing with the club, and I was actually one of the better ones in the group . . . Imagine that at my age!"		
5. Coach: "You sure have come a long way."	Feedback.	Validates client self-evaluation.
6. Client: "When I began working with you, I knew that I didn't want to do some boring program, and when I think about all I'm doing now, there's nothing that looks even the slightest bit boring."		
7. Coach: "I agree . . . So where do you think you are now in all that you set out to accomplish?"	Feedback plus open question.	Supports client perception and probes for understanding.
8. Client: "Well, I'm not entirely there yet, but then again, I don't think I ever will be . . . This is going to be lifelong . . . lifelong learning."		
9. Coach: "Lifelong learning . . ."	Minimal encourager.	Encourages the client to develop a particular theme.
10. Client: "Yes, indeed. I knew things were starting to gel for me about 6 months ago when I began making plans to link up with my wife's consulting work and sign up for the 'gold watch' from my job . . . And so far, so good. My wife and I have gotten a few new contracts, and I'm actually doing some of the training work—and that's anything but boring."		
11. Coach: "So, you're relating this to your training here?"	Minor interpretation in the form of an indirect question.	Helps the client make the link between experiences in his career and in coaching.
12. Client: "Most definitely. You change one part and everything else falls in line . . . I think I mentioned that in the beginning."		
13. Coach: "You did."	Information or feedback.	Confirms client perception.

(continued)

(continued)

Dialogue	Skills	Comments
14. Client: "I knew I needed to become more active, and I figured if I used this as my experimental laboratory, I could test out some things here without too much risk . . . and if things worked, then I would be able to translate what I learned into other areas of my life, and that's exactly what happened."		
15. Coach: "Well, I would say, that's what you did. It didn't just happen . . . You made it happen."	Feedback and reframe.	Encourages the client to take ownership for changes.
16. Client: "Well, I didn't do it alone. You were a big part of this."		
17. Coach: "Thanks, Harry, I appreciate the feedback."	Immediacy.	Acknowledges client praise and demonstrates the coach's authenticity.
18. Client: "I have resisted saying, 'I'm a new man,' but I think I am . . . I'm not afraid to try new things, I look forward to challenges, I can deal with uncertainty a lot better . . . and on top of it all, I'm in fantastic shape."		
19. Coach: "Yes you are. And yes, I believe I see those changes in you . . . I'd like to go back to my earlier question and maybe say it a little differently. Where do you think we are in our coaching relationship?"	Feedback and open question.	Validates client perceptions and continues probing for the client's awareness of the process of coaching.
20. Client: "Do you mean, are we finished?"		
21. Coach: "That's a possibility. What do you think?"	Information and open question.	Confirms client perception and continues probing.
22. Client: "I can't say I haven't thought about it, but you've been so darn helpful to me and I'm not sure I can keep it going on my own."		
23. Coach: "So, you've thought about it and you have some concerns about going it alone."	Reflection of content.	Supports the client's discussion and expansion of topic.
24. Client: "Well, yes . . . I think I can do it, but I'm not 100% sure."		
25. Coach: "And you want to be 100% sure before you end?"	Indirect question framed as reflection of content.	Encourages the client to examine message.
26. Client: "Hmmm, maybe not. Nothing is 100% certain anyway, but I would like to have some better ideas about the what-ifs and how to stay on track by myself."		
27. Coach: "That sounds reasonable . . . So you'd like for us to do some planning for contingencies and also discuss ways in which you can train on your own."	Feedback and reflection of content.	Validates the client's suggestion and encourages further discussion.
28. Client: "Exactly. So how can we do this?"		
29. Coach: "Well, I have some ideas and I think we need to do a bit of analysis of what works for you, what doesn't, what kinds of factors put you at risk, and what helps you move forward."	Advice and information.	Provides direction to the client.
30. Client: "That sounds good."		

Dialogue	Skills	Comments
31. Coach: "We're running out of time for today, so perhaps we could outline some tasks that you could work on between now and our next meeting."	Information and advice.	Frames the session and provides direction.
32. Client: "OK, Rachel, I've got my pen and notepad ready. Let me have it."		
33. Coach: "All right, Harry, here's the first thing to write down: 'I, Harry, am in charge of me so even when I'm working with Rachel, I still have to take responsibility, and that usually means I come up with my ideas first.'"	Instruction.	Provides direction to the client in a humorous way.
34. Client: "Cute! You got me on that one, Rachel. See how quickly I slip. So, as I was saying, here are some of my ideas about what I need to be thinking about this coming week."		
35. Coach: "Great."	Feedback or minimal encourager.	Supports and validates the client.

A happy ending—and working toward ensuring its continuity. The dialogue between Rachel and Harry is the kind of ending that most coaches would like to have with their clients. Harry has lived up to his agreements, and Rachel has supported and guided his goal attainment. Moreover, rather than reinforce dependency, Rachel helped Harry become more self-directing. The exchange noted in segments 20 through 22 illustrates this point. Without raising the question of ending, Rachel encourages Harry to consider where they are in their work together (note segments 7 and 19, in particular). When he remarks, "Do you mean, are we finished?" Rachel could have responded that she had no such intention in her remarks. Rather, she allows Harry's inference, for as he notes in segment 22, he has been thinking about ending.

What is interesting in this dialogue is that we can see ending as a process rather than as an event. The topic has arisen, the client and coach have identified some of the gains of the coaching process, yet the client has other tasks to accomplish. Rachel engages this stage of the relationship in a manner similar to all others—as codirected. In the playful exchange at the end of the dialogue, she acts as if she is taking full direction only to remind Harry of his coresponsibility in this process and ultimately his complete responsibility for himself (segments 31 through 34). The quality of the dialogue between Rachel and Harry exemplifies the solidity of the work they have done together and the collaborative way in which they have engaged the various dimensions of coaching.

Although coaching dialogue 9.6, "When the Coach Ends the Relationship: Luke (Coach) and

Kate (Client)," is not high in emotion, it nonetheless is a milestone in the relationship. Take a moment now to read this dialogue.

Kate seems to have breached the contract, although she seems reluctant at first to admit to this. She appears willing to pretend that she is continuing to work toward her goal, while being unwilling to commit the necessary time and energy to its realization. Luke acts wisely and professionally in identifying the underlying dynamic. Without blaming or accusing, he softly guides Kate toward awareness of the situation, the inconsistencies in her messages, and the practicalities required for a viable coaching relationship. Although the end has been called, Luke correctly suggests that there is yet work to be done. Kate did not consider the whole experience a failure. Rather, she saw some benefit and progress. In the remainder of this session or perhaps in a follow-up meeting that the parties clearly identify as closure, Kate and Luke will identify learnings and highlight implications for the future. Ideally, Kate will come to value the lessons gained from this experience and, as she noted, approach future engagements in ways that generate greater success.

Effective Dialogue and the Need for Practice

The dialogues in this chapter served a number of purposes. First, they illustrated the kinds of dialogues that lifestyle fitness coaches might have with clients. In so doing, they suggested differences from the types of conversations that other

Coaching Dialogue 9.6 When the Coach Ends the Relationship: Luke (Coach) and Kate (Client)

(In this dialogue, Luke and Kate will reach a point where it becomes eminently clear that what Kate needs, Luke cannot provide. Although her original intent was to make a solid connection with fitness and in so doing create some stability and structure in her world, too many conflicting needs and agendas have arisen for her to make progress toward this goal. Luke and Kate are now in the 4th month of the coaching relationship. Following the previous dialogue, in which Kate realized that she was setting up the relationship for failure and projecting feelings onto Luke, she reconnected with her goal and her program for almost a month. Then a similar pattern began to emerge. Kate has just finished giving her excuses for not adhering to her program when the following dialogue takes place.)

Dialogue	Skills	Comments
1. Coach: "Kate, I'm struck by the similarity between what you've described about this past week and where we were about 2 months ago. Your adherence has been steadily declining, and this past week, you haven't made any of your sessions. What do you think is going on?"	Feedback and open question.	Guides the client to explore identified issue.
2. Client: "Well, I told you before, I have a hard time exercising—and I have other priorities."		
3. Coach: "I think I understand . . . But would you please say more?"	Immediacy and open question.	Encourages client exploration.
4. Client: "Well, you know about my book and you know I have this love–hate thing with my program."		
5. Coach: "Yes, I'm aware of these things. Is there anything else?"	Immediacy and open question.	Supports the client and encourages further exploration.
6. Client: "Yeah, well, you might say so." [pauses mysteriously]		
7. Coach: "Please go on."	Directive or instruction.	Supports the client's exploration.
8. Client: "Well, I met someone, and things are looking good."		
9. Coach: "You mean, you've met someone whom you're beginning a relationship with?"	Reflection of content with a minor interpretation.	Demonstrates listening, clarifies meaning, and encourages further discussion.
10. Client: "Yeah, you might say that . . . You know, relationships take time, and I don't want to blow it again this time."		
11. Coach: "Unh hunh . . . So this is real important to you, and you don't want to jeopardize it . . . What do you imagine are the implications, if any, for what we're doing here?"	Reflection of content plus open question.	Acknowledges the client's needs and concerns and returns the focus to the coaching relation.
12. Client: "You know, you've gotta have priorities, and right now my relationship is my priority."		
13. Coach: "And so, exactly how do you think this will affect our work together?"	Open question.	Focuses the client on the coaching relation.
14. Client: "Don't get me wrong. I plan to continue working with you. I just don't know how reliable I can be to all of this."		
15. Coach: "So your relationship is your priority, and you are imagining that you won't be able to be keep to your training commitments."	Reflection of content.	Acknowledges the client's messages without criticism.

Dialogue	Skills	Comments
16. Client: "Unh hunh . . .yeah . . . I hope that's OK with you. I mean I am getting something out of our work together. I'm in a bit better shape and even though I'm not entirely committed, doing something is certainly better than doing nothing. Wouldn't you agree?"		
17. Coach: "Yes, I do agree . . . and I'm glad to hear that what we've done here has had some benefit . . . Kate, I need to have you be even clearer with me. When you say, you may not be able to be reliable, do you have any sense of how this translates into your program activities?"	Feedback, immediacy, and open question.	Acknowledges the client's experience and the coach's own response. Refocuses on the coaching agenda.
18. Client: "I don't know . . . I really can't say . . . Maybe the whole thing just doesn't seem as important to me right now."		
19. Coach: "So, on the one hand you're saying you want to continue working with me, and on the other you're not sure how important what we're doing is to you."	Confrontation.	Points out discrepancy in client messages.
20. Client: "Sounds strange, doesn't it?"		
21. Coach: "Frankly, it does. If you and I aren't working on increasing your adherence to your program and shaping activities to meet your needs, then what do you imagine we are or will be doing?"	Feedback and confrontation through questioning.	The coach acknowledges his own reaction and then confronts implied discrepancy between the client's wants and the legitimate agenda of coaching.
22. Client: "Now that's a very good question . . . I really don't know."		
23. Coach: "I don't want to make guesses, but it sounds to me that you're not strongly motivated to work with me on your program, and that you don't really have a sense of what we would be doing together."	A focus on meaning through what appears to be a reflection of content.	Encourages the client to probe deeper for the meaning in her messages.
24. Client: "Yeah, strange, huh?"		
25. Coach: "My sense is that we may be at a point where we need to consider stopping our work together—at least until you figure out whether you want to commit to the work again."	Interpretation and advice.	Suggests meaning of client messages through an interpretation and then adds a suggestion about the process.
26. Client: "Yeah, maybe you're right . . . It costs a lot of money anyhow."		
27. Coach: "Yes, it does cost a lot of money, and from my perspective, what may be even more important is that you would be involved in a process unlikely to succeed."	Feedback and information (interpretation).	Acknowledges the client's message and then provides his expert knowledge about how continuing might affect the client.
28. Client: "You mean because I wouldn't be working on it."		
29. Coach: "Yes, because you wouldn't be working on it . . . because it requires lots of time and attention that right now you don't seem committed to."	Feedback and reflection of content.	Elaborates the client's message and offers perspective of what it takes versus what the client is willing to commit.

(continued)

(continued)

Dialogue	Skills	Comments
30. Client: "What can I say? But you're right."		
31. Coach: "I'm glad we talked about this because otherwise I think it might have become pretty discouraging for both of us."	Immediacy.	Expresses personal opinion and softly informs the client about his best guesses regarding continuing in the current manner.
32. Client: "Yeah, I was beginning to feel that way . . . So what happens next?"		
33. Coach: "Well, as you said earlier, it hasn't been all for nothing. There have been some steps forward, and some things you may have learned."	Reflection of content and minor interpretation.	Changes meaning of the client's earlier statement from "getting something out of" to "some things you may have learned."
34. Client: "That's definitely true."		
35. Coach: "So, perhaps we could spend some time identifying exactly what you did get out of our work together and what you might be able to take with you into any future plans you make. Sound reasonable?"	Advice and closed question.	Offers direction for proceeding.
36. Client: "Yup, it does . . . and I don't want you to think that any of this is your fault. I've really gotten a great deal out of this whole coaching thing."		
37. Coach: "Thanks Kate. I'm not thinking about any of this as anyone's fault. For me, it's an experience from which both of us can learn, and in that respect, we still have some work to do—to make clear what you learned."	Immediacy (self-disclosure), reframing, and advice.	Provides his viewpoint, reframes the client's perspective from fault finding to learning, and provides direction for the next steps.
38. Client: [Pausing thoughtfully] "Yes, I do want to give some time to understanding what I've learned from this so I can do it better next time."		

health fitness professionals might have with their clients. Second, they gave some sense of the stages of relationship and the relative prevalence of different types of coaching skills at different stages. Third, they allowed for the dissection of specific skills and thereby demonstrated the nonmechanical interweaving of skills along with the coach's use of timing. Fourth, these dialogues highlighted some of the inherent challenges of the coaching role in containing emotions and guarding against reacting defensively, whether justified or not. Finally, they pointed out the importance of endings as opportunities for integration, enhanced understanding, and solidifying gains.

Mastering the skills of coaching requires effort in reading, reflecting, practicing, and opening oneself to constructive feedback from clients, peers, and supervisors. You might have chosen different strategies or paths at various points in the dialogues. The words spoken, the skills used, and the flow of dialogue represent only one pattern from a myriad of possibilities. You should honor your unique style, your way of communicating, how you phrase your concerns, and other aspects of how you develop professional relationships, rather than abandon them in an attempt to graft someone else's style onto yourself. Any artificiality you might have identified in the dialogues may be as much an implicit awareness of your own approach as a sense of the necessary limitations in communicating multidimensional human behavior in scripted dialogues. A reflective exercise that you may want to undertake at this point is to imagine how you might have handled the same situations. Learning activity 9.1 provides guidelines for you to work collaboratively with another person in exploring how you might have responded to these clients. What would you have done? How would you have phrased your responses? Through such reflective efforts you will learn far more than you would through passively ingesting these exchanges as if they were the only words that a coach could have spoken.

Learning Activity 9.1   Exploring Your Approach to Coaching Kate and Harry

In learning more about your own style, you may wish to role-play dialogues with the clients you have just met in chapter 9, namely, Kate and Harry. To do this, you will need to recruit the assistance of a colleague or someone who is engaged in learning about coaching. Once you have identified someone who is willing and able to role-play these clients, ask this person to read all the material in this chapter with particular emphasis on the dialogues. If the person has little interest in learning about coaching, his or her primary task will be to get a clear sense of the two clients.

The next step is to set up a space where you can tape-record or video-record your role plays. If your "client" is not familiar with the field of lifestyle fitness coaching, spend some time familiarizing this person with the roles and responsibilities of both coach and client, along with the legitimate parameters of the coaching relationship.

Now you should be ready to get into role. Remember that your task is not to replicate the interactions scripted in chapter 9, but to see how you would deal with clients like Kate and Harry. Remind your "client" to stay in role and to try to represent the characters and dynamics of Harry and Kate as accurately as possible.

You may choose to do one of the interviews and stop to review it before proceeding with the second. After completing both interviews, you should not only review the tapes but also ask your "client" for feedback about how she or he felt during different parts of the interviews. With the other person's permission, save this tape and review it at some point in the near future so that it can continue to serve as a guide to learning.

Assessments and Guides for Coaching

"Isn't it just possible that somewhere along the line the boundary between who you are and your *ideas* about who you are got blurred?"

Richard Carson

As a lifestyle fitness coach you will make your decision to work with a particular client based on certain characteristics of the client as well as your perceived degree of fit with the client and what she or he desires. For instance, age may be a relevant criterion when the discrepancy is large or when you as a coach do not have sufficient awareness of issues confronting certain age groups. Consider a 25-year-old coach agreeing to work with a 75-year-old woman. Perhaps in the role of personal trainer, a health fitness professional who has studied biomechanical needs and concerns of seniors may feel capable of devising a training program that respects the competencies and restrictions of a 75-year-old woman. In a coaching relationship, however, that age difference may create a credibility gap too large to bridge. Advice, interpretations, reframes, and other skill applications may meet with greater resistance when the age difference between coach and client is almost half a century.

What Coaches Need to Know

Beyond what may be immediately apparent, what other information would help you accelerate the process of understanding your client and developing appropriate programming? Clearly, information about physical health and functioning is essential. You may want to have clients visit their family doctors and undergo evaluation by means of stress tests, strength and flexibility measures, body-composition assessments, and pulmonary capacity measures (ACSM, 2000). Because of the risks of physical activity, relying on client self-reports about physical capacities may be unwise. Instead, coaches may want to gather indicators that are more objective.

Although coaches may work in a group practice consisting of allied health professionals (Benefits, 2001; Durrett, 2002) and thereby have ready access to colleagues for professional consultation, coaches who are trained and experienced in specific physical challenges might be best qualified to address the needs of certain clients. For instance, coaches who are highly knowledgeable about severe cardiac conditions should normally be the ones who work with

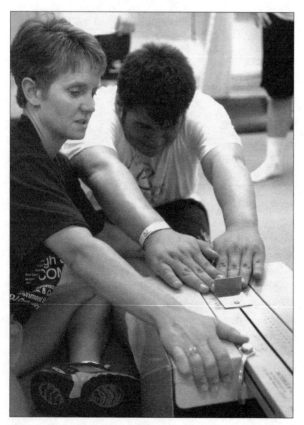

The successful lifestyle fitness coach will use a variety of assessments in order to understand his client and develop an appropriate exercise program.

clients following surgical interventions. Learning on the job is not always the best strategy.

Beyond obtaining the necessary physical indicators, what else is important? Such client characteristics as age, sex, ethnicity, and health habits may be critical. Some coaches will have preferences or unique talents for working with particular groups. Female clients may prefer female coaches, and some coaches may prefer to work only with same-sex clients. Ethnicity becomes relevant in terms of coaches' cultural awareness and sensitivity. Being concerned about ethnocentrism may not be enough. To work effectively with clients of particular ethnic origins, coaches may need to have considerable knowledge and experience with the relevant cultural group.

Questions about lifestyle and health habits also seem pertinent. A client's eating habits, sleep patterns, and other lifestyle behaviors may not be immediately apparent, so coaches may wish to investigate these matters through questions or other means such as inventories and questionnaires. Dilemmas may arise when a coach commits to working with a client only to discover some months later that this client has a serious substance abuse problem or eating disorder. Imagine realizing that a client is an alcoholic or a cocaine addict during the course of working together. Some of the client's previously inexplicable behavior patterns may become more understandable when such evidence emerges, yet the coach may then be in a quandary of whether to continue or to refer.

Coaches may readily assess more common health issues such as smoking or unbalanced eating patterns at the outset, and they may request that clients work with other professionals on these matters in parallel processes or, depending on their qualifications, may incorporate those health concerns into their overall strategies for assisting those clients.

What About Mental Health?

As much of the coaching literature suggests (Martin, 2001; Whitworth et al., 1998; Williams & Davis, 2002), clients who hire coaches are thought to have sufficient mental health and emotional stability to identify life improvement goals rationally and to work toward attaining them in a reasonably straightforward manner. But the question of psychological normalcy has always been somewhat of an enigma. Moreover, if a coach can work with someone with a serious physical disorder, what is the justification for automatically eliminating clients who have psychological disorders?

Coaches are not likely to administer batteries of psychological tests to new clients to determine their degree of mental health. For one, most coaches would not be authorized to use such measures, but perhaps more important, the legitimacy of such actions could be seriously challenged. Ultimately, this kind of discussion reverts to one about roles and boundaries. Coaches can work with clients who have psychological difficulties so long as (a) they are willing to do so, (b) they have sufficient knowledge of mental disorders to know what challenges they may face and how they will need to behave in their own and their clients' best interests, and (c) they have professional backup either in terms of referral sources or clients' involvement in therapy.

The actual prevalence of various psychological conditions is hard to guage. However, estimates suggest that roughly 50% of the population will experience a psychiatric disorder at least once in a lifetime (Epidemiology, 1994). For instance, psychological depression considered severe enough to interfere with normal life functioning occurs to one out of every six (approximately 16%) people over the course of a lifetime. Having such a disorder does not mean that the person is depressed for life, but rather that for a time, depression considerably affects the person's functioning. Anxiety disorders are also common. Approximately 12% of the North American population may be described as suffering from anxiety related problems at any given time. More disabling problems such as bipolar disorders and schizophrenia are infrequent, occurring in the population at rates of approximately 1.3% and 0.3%, respectively (Durand & Barlow, 1997).

Perhaps more to the point, we know that, as M. Scott Peck (1978, p. 15) so clearly states, "Life is difficult." Denying this reality is perhaps more of a problem than accepting life for what it is. As Peck notes, "Most do not fully see this truth that life is difficult. Instead they moan more or less incessantly, noisily or subtly, about the enormity of their problems, their burdens, and their difficulties as if life were generally easy, as if life *should* be easy" (p. 15). Most of us encounter daily stresses and strains, occasionally feel confused, and may even have blue days periodically. The fact that drugs like Prozac, Paxil, Zoloft, and Ativan are at least as well or better known than Celebrex, Fosamax, Zantax, Coumadin, and other medications for common physical problems reflects the high incidence of emotional and psychological adjustment issues in modern society.

This discussion is not to justify some type of psychological screening process for coaching clients, but rather to "depathologize" today's more or less normal psychological challenges and to advise you that some of your clients will likely be dealing concurrently with life adjustment issues as they engage in health and exercise change processes with you.

Assessment for What Purpose?

Coaches must have a legitimate rationale for gathering information from clients. The knowledge gained must serve some purpose. Possible reasons for gathering information from clients include the following:

• **Evaluations of physical and health concerns.** Essential to the work of lifestyle fitness coaches, this category of information would comprise medical history including diseases, injuries, and emerging health concerns; measures of physical capacities and functioning; body composition; and health habits, among others.

• **Evaluations of client agendas.** Although clients' initial statements of coaching agendas are likely to evolve, these objectives may be more or less appropriate to the work that lifestyle fitness coaches do or that a particular coach is trained for or feels comfortable addressing. Clients may have expectations of coaching or of the coach that may change through initial discussions because of misconceptions or unrealistic objectives (e.g., losing 30 pounds [14 kilograms] in 1 month), yet as long as coach and client eventually determine an initial agenda that is within the coach's professional boundaries, the relationship can proceed. When the agenda remains outside coaching competencies or professional boundaries, the relationship should not continue.

• **Evaluations of coach–client match.** As mentioned earlier, both coaches and clients are likely to have preferences, styles, and characteristics that are more or less suited to one another. This is not so much a matter of competency as it is of comfort and preference. Some people seem to develop rapport almost instantly, whereas others simply do not seem to click. Although coaches can apply skills to develop rapport and trust, sometimes the effort to do so is hard to justify; the client might do better to work with another coach. Are specific variables available that coaches can use to perform reliable assessments of compatibility? Evaluations of compatibility are likely to be unique to coach and client. Some coaches may have rules or explicit preferences, whereas others will assess compatibility on an intuitive basis.

• **Evaluations of client interests, motivations, styles, needs, and personality.** Much of the initial effort in a coaching relationship will go toward determining who clients are, how they function, what they prefer, what motivates them, and other personal attributes that serve to shape and form not only the working alliance but more critically the viable agendas that coaching will address. This category of information is rather broad, and different coaches will choose to emphasize different client dimensions because of either personal style or perceived efficacy. Questionnaires contained on the CD-ROM accompanying this book provide a unique methodology for obtaining client data concerning these matters. Let's begin to explore this helpful tool for lifestyle fitness coaching.

MAPS—A Model of Sport and Fitness Matching for Lifestyle Fitness Coaches

In the 20th century, thousands of studies of sports' effects on personal and mental functioning created foundations for health fitness professionals to advocate potential costs and benefits of active lifestyles. Studies have shown that exercise promotes self-confidence and self-esteem. It tends to improve mood states and can even alleviate chronic depression (Griest et al., 1979). Exercisers feel less anxious for hours after they exercise, and sustained commitment to physical training can sometimes mitigate a person's chronic anxiety. Some reports show that people who exercise regularly are more sexually active than those who don't (Frauman, 1982). Other investigators have described positive effects of exercise on intelligence and memory. In an overall perspective, exercise researchers conclude that people who exercise regularly show significant improvements across a wide range of cognitive functioning and mental health measures (Leith, 1994).

As sport and exercise trends evolve in the 21st century, people will have ever more options for participation. This fact leads to two major considerations: First, how will people find their way through this increasingly complex maze of sport and fitness opportunities? Second, are some choices inherently better for people than others? To say this differently, are there client characteristics relevant to coaching that could serve to align clients with more satisfying and beneficial sport and fitness programs? Moreover, because sport and exercise programs have been shown to affect psychological variables, would clients who are seeking particular kinds of changes be better advised to engage in certain activities rather than others?

These considerations underlie the development of a matching model intended to facilitate client decision making regarding sport and fitness pro-

gramming. The assessment tool associated with this model is the MAPS Inventory, which stands for *Matching Activity and Personal Styles*. Details of the model, the MAPS Inventory, and the principles underlying its usage will appear in the sections that follow, and more technical information is available elsewhere (Gavin, 2004). A CD-ROM accompanying this book provides a means for helping clients develop profiles of personal style and related exercise options, along with other useful information for guiding program development.

Logic of MAPS

A number of important social and psychological themes related to activity involvement (cf. Buckworth & Dishman, 2002; Gill, 2000; LeUnes & Nation, 2002; Weinberg & Gould, 2003) have been reframed within the context of lifestyle fitness coaching and its clientele. In discussing these themes, we must clarify two points at the outset. First, the themes are not exclusive. Other concepts appear in the literature, but the ones represented seemed most pertinent to lifestyle fitness coaching (Gavin, 1988, 2004; Gavin & Lister, 2001). Second, these themes refer not only to the characteristics of participants but also to physical activities and sports. For instance, we can define a sport as competitive in terms of being structured so that someone wins and someone loses, just as we can characterize players themselves as competitive or not. The interesting possibility here in terms of the interaction of person and environment is that a competitive person can engage in a noncompetitive activity but do so with an orientation toward winning (e.g., being the best in a group fitness class). Conversely, a noncompetitive person can play tennis without a care of winning or losing.

Seven themes are relevant to the MAPS Inventory:

1. **Social dimensions of sport and exercise.** People exercise either alone or with others. Activities sometimes bring people together to a shared time–space event or location, but interaction is optional. Running alone on wooded trails and swimming long distances in open waters are choices of solitary involvement, whereas going to a gym to take a class with dozens of strangers may provide social opportunities without the necessity of interaction. By contrast, playing a team sport is necessarily social. Activities themselves may require certain degrees of verbal and nonverbal social interaction, and participants may engage in these activities more or less according to their design. People may seek social interaction as part of their activities, or they may intentionally

avoid it (Dishman, Sallis, & Orenstein, 1985; Sallis & Owen, 1999; Willis & Campbell, 1992). Even when someone is running alone, that person may be having rich internal thoughts about social interactions or, conversely, may be watching the passing scenery.

2. **Competitive, collaborative, and individualistic options in sport and exercise.** The theme of competition has been widely explored in the field of sport and physical activity (Martens, 1977; Orlick, 1978). An activity can be designed with competitive, collaborative, or individualistic orientations, and participants can enter these pursuits with varying degrees of these same orientations. For instance, a person playing basketball can relate to teammates either individualistically or collaboratively, whereas in relation to an opposing team this player may manifest more or less competitive behavior. Options available in modern fitness centers allow people to choose which orientations they want to experience in their activities. Again, we may need to acknowledge internal thought processes. A person can be engaged in a seemingly individualistic activity such as running on a treadmill while keeping a watchful eye on those around him and implicitly competing with them by increasing his speed as he sees others increase theirs.

3. **Mental focus required either for participation or to enhance performance.** The terms *focus*, *concentration*, and *attention* are often applied in sport contexts. Nideffer and associates (1976, 1985; Nideffer & Sagal, 2001) have done much to advance theory and practice in this area. Their work suggests two dimensions of attentional focus: width (broad versus narrow) and direction (internal versus external). A basketball player preparing to take a foul shot exemplifies a narrow focus, whereas the same player running down court will be attending to a number of elements at the same time. The player looking at the basket before taking a foul shot manifests an external focus, whereas her concentration on breathing would be an internal focus. Another framework for aspects of this theme appears in works on associative attentional strategies (monitoring feelings and body functions, such as breathing and muscle tension) versus dissociative attentional strategies (tuning out or distracting oneself). Advantages and disadvantages have been found for each of these strategies when applied to different sports (Masters & Ogles, 1998). In the realm of recreational fitness activities, participants may desire opportunities to focus their minds on something other than pressing life concerns, or they may wish to allow their minds to wander at will while their bodies exercise. Some people watch TV, listen to music, or talk while

exercising; others concentrate either deliberately or because their sports demand it.

4. **Degrees of control or spontaneity inherent in different activities.** Some sports require precise control of movements and even thought processes (Murphy & Martin, 2002; Weinberg & Gould, 2003), whereas others allow participants to be less exact or controlled. Another concept that has been advanced in recent years is that of flow, which has been described as a holistic sensation of being totally involved and functioning effortlessly (Jackson & Csikszentmihalyi, 1999). In literature related to movement, researchers have used concepts of control and spontaneity to describe not only how people move but also corresponding psychological states of mind (Gavin, 1988; Lamb & Watson, 1994; North, 1972). Moreover, researchers within the field of psychology have widely explored the need for control over one's own behavior (Durand & Barlow, 1997). Engaging in activities that are mostly predictable and under participants' control may have certain psychological benefits, whereas partaking in activities that are less predictable or controllable may have different implications. Contrast, for instance, the experiences of taking an improvisational dance class versus training on a rowing machine. Or consider engaging in a highly structured group fitness class as compared with playing volleyball.

5. **Risk taking or thrill seeking in sport and fitness pursuits.** Different sports and fitness pursuits carry with them varying kinds and degrees of risk. Participation in high-risk sports has been associated with a trait known as sensation seeking (Zuckerman, 1984; Farley, 1986). The study of risk taking, in general, has long been a theme in psychology (Byrnes, Miller, & Schafer, 1999), and research has noted correlations with various personal characteristics such as sex and age. One may think of risk taking as both a psychological characteristic of individuals and as inherent in certain activities. Different sports have been catalogued according to the degree of physical risk that they present to participants (LeUnes & Nation, 2002). Psychological risk may also accompany activity participation. Some people may experience high degrees of self-consciousness or even embarrassment when they participate in various types of exercise programs. This circumstance may be partly related to gender biases about fitness whereby men who train in weight rooms are totally acceptable whereas males who take dance classes may run counter to gender stereotyping. Performance anxieties may present another dimension of risk for participants. Because they do not want to be seen as weak, incompetent,

or unsuccessful, some people may choose activities in which such risks are less apparent.

6. **Aggression.** We may occasionally consider aggression an admirable trait, but for the most part we think of it negatively. As LeUnes and Nation (2002, p. 188) note, "Aggression is the infliction of an aversive stimulus on an unwilling victim with the intent to do harm and with the expectation that the act will be successful." Further distinctions have been made within the realm of sport among three terms: hostile aggression, in which the intention is to harm or cause pain; instrumental aggression, in which the intent is to promote a winning effort although harm or injury to others may occur; and sport assertiveness, in which there is a legitimate use of force and unusual expenditures of effort and energy according to game rules to promote the possibility of winning (LeUnes & Nation, 2002; Silva, 1979). Aggression as it pertains to lifestyle fitness coaching represents more the sense of sport assertiveness than it does hostile aggression. Within the broader field of psychology, aggression has generally been interpreted as "any form of behavior directed toward the goal of harming or injuring another living being who is motivated to avoid such treatment" (Baron & Richardson, 1994, p. 7). But in some earlier works in psychology (Perls, 1947), aggression was considered a normal and instrumental process required by humans to survive and overcome obstacles. In the late 20th century, terms like *assertiveness* came into vogue as ways of expressing the positive face of aggression (Rakos, 1991). Although aggression with the intent to harm may rarely be justified, aggression to win or overcome obstacles may be considered more or less acceptable. Certainly, within the context of business, being aggressive tends to be a valued trait. In the fitness world, activities like weight training require a certain degree of aggression (or sport assertiveness) to move barbells up and down. From this perspective, a tai chi class may require far less aggressive energy than a weight-training experience does. Similarly, being a lineman on a football team calls for more aggressive action than does being a principal dancer in a ballet troupe. From an individual perspective, some people characteristically behave more aggressively than others do. Whether this is due to instincts (Gill, 2000), frustration (Dollard, Doob, Miller, Mowrer, & Sears, 1939), or social learning (Bandura, 1977) cannot be readily determined. Evidence does suggest, however, that expressing aggression in sport not only fails to lower it but may in fact cause it to increase (Arms, Russell, & Sandilands, 1979; Gill, 2000).

7. **Motivation—intrinsic and extrinsic.** Motivation can be defined simply as the direction and intensity of a person's effort (Sage, 1977). We may be able to understand why people direct energy toward the attainment of certain objectives and how much energy they devote to these purposes by distinguishing between **intrinsic** and **extrinsic motivations**. Intrinsically motivated acts are those in which individuals engage in behaviors for the satisfaction, pleasure, excitement, fun, or sense of mastery that they experience in the process. Extrinsically motivated actions, by contrast, are undertaken as means to ends, in which the ends are valued far more than the activities themselves. A person may be intrinsically motivated in some actions and extrinsically motivated in others. The type of motivation that a person experiences may be as much a function of the specific action or task as it is a function of the person. In the sport and fitness realm, people may be motivated to exercise solely for extrinsic reasons, such as to manage weight, look good, or remain healthy. They may experience little or no satisfaction in the process of exercising itself. Intrinsic and extrinsic motivations constitute a continuum that ranges from a total lack of motivation through extrinsically generated motivation to intrinsic motivation (Weinberg & Gould, 2003). In a value sense, intrinsic motivation is often seen as the preferred type of motivation in terms of satisfactions derived and the likelihood of behavior persistence. Moreover, although some would argue that the more (types of) motivations an individual has to support particular actions, the better, others believe that extrinsic motivations can serve to diminish an individual's intrinsic motivational base (Ryan & Deci, 2000; Vallerand & Losier, 1999).

As suggested throughout these descriptions, both individuals and physical activities can be described according to the seven themes. This makes it possible to consider the idea of matching individuals to sport and fitness programs. For instance, if someone is highly social but dislikes competitive activities, social dance classes might be a better match than competitive racket sports. If all seven themes are considered, profiles of individuals can be created and compared to profiles that characterize various sport and exercise programs. Knowing a client's profile would allow a coach to understand at least two things: the nature and degree of the challenges that the client might experience when pursuing different activities, and in a corresponding sense, the meaning and value of such challenges for the client in relation to goals that she is pursuing.

To summarize, the logic of MAPS derives from the following considerations: First, sport and fitness participation affects participants not only in the physical domain but also across a wide range of nonphysical dimensions. Second, the literature of sport and exercise psychology points to a number of recurrent themes that seem to have importance for characterizing both activities and individual participants. We cannot successfully argue that physical activity can affect all dimensions of human life, but it is reasonable to assume that participation will affect some dimensions more strongly than it does others. Third, if physical activities and individual participants can be identified along a similar set of characteristics, then it becomes possible to evaluate the degree to which different activities match the profiles of individuals. This argument is similar to one underlying significant theories of career guidance (Holland, 1985). Finally, if people understand their own profiles and the profiles of different activities, they may appreciate why some activities suit them better than others and how different activities might benefit them.

Principles of Matching Using MAPS

In working with clients, lifestyle fitness coaches should be aware of at least two considerations for using and interpreting results involving the MAPS Inventory. People who are unaccustomed to exercising regularly are likely to experience additional challenges to adherence when they engage in activities that require them to behave differently from their customary patterns or styles (Gavin, 1988). In this regard, inactive clients who are beginning to exercise may achieve more by involving themselves in sport and fitness programs that have a relatively high degree of similarity to their personal profiles.

When clients have been active for more than a year and seem to have a solid connection to fitness participation, similarity of personal and activity profiles may be less critical. In fact, clients may decide to challenge habitual behavioral patterns through choosing programs that are decidedly different on specific dimensions. For instance, an active person who is overly cautious may wish to develop more comfort in challenging or risky contexts by consciously choosing more adventurous sports and recreations.

Assume for the moment that any number of sports and activities can be compared with a client's individual profile. Learning activity 10.1 offers an opportunity for you to consider ways of matching activities to a client's profile.

Working with novice versus experienced exercisers suggests the possibility of different strate-

Learning Activity 10.1   Matching Client Patterns With Sports and Fitness

Imagine a 35-year-old female client who shows the following inclinations or patterns. Based on your awareness of different sport and fitness options, what activities might match her profile? Which ones would not? In the case of activities that match some but not all of her patterns, what challenges to participation might she experience were she to engage in these activities?

1. A preference for solitary activities rather than group-based programs or team sports
2. A desire to have control and predictability in her life as well as in fitness programs
3. A pattern of relying on extrinsic motivations, especially in fitness and exercise
4. A low level of assertiveness and a dislike of activities that require aggressive actions or energy
5. An avoidance of competitive pursuits and a preference for collaborative ventures
6. A preference for multitasking or being involved in many things at the same time and a strong desire to distract herself while exercising
7. A cautious and risk-avoidant lifestyle

In thinking through your answers to these questions, you might reflect on two other issues: First, is she currently involved in an exercise program? Second, of the patterns or styles that she manifests, does she desire to change any of them?

gies for matching. Two principles underlie these strategies:

- **Principle 1—Strategic matching.** When people do not have well-ingrained exercise habits, their activities should roughly match their personal preferences or styles. For example, matching a man who is social and competitive with activities that are social and that allow for competitive possibilities stands a better chance of encouraging adherence than having him engage in noncompetitive, nonsocial activities. A second scenario arises from situations in which people feel satisfied with how they function in life and have no great motivation to change. Here too, the best approach would be to identify programs with characteristics that match personal styles.

- **Principle 2—Strategic mismatching.** A person who exercises regularly and is interested in self-development in areas that are affected by activity participation may want to choose sports and exercise programs in a strategic manner to provide exposure and practice in areas of desired development. Imagine a man who has difficulty being assertive and thriving in a competitive work environment. If he wishes to change these patterns, a number of options are available, including counseling, workshops, and reading. He can reinforce whatever strategies he learns about by reading or psycho-educational processes through in vivo experiences in sports and exercise (see chapter 2). With the assistance of a lifestyle fitness coach, this person can consciously participate in activities that encourage assertiveness and have a competitive dimension. If we look at this as a process of behavior shaping (Bandura, 1977), this individual can be gradually introduced to activities that incorporate these elements. Coaches may help clients like this identify activities that have low to moderate levels of exposure to these dimensions and over time increase both the intensity and involvement in these types of activities.

Seven Personal Style Dimensions of the MAPS Inventory

Terminology in psychology can be tricky. Different scientists may use the same words but apply different meanings. In discussions of the seven themes found in the literature of sport and exercise psychology, meanings for such terms as *aggression, control, motivation,* or *risk taking* vary somewhat depending on how they have been conceived and measured. To match clients' profiles to those of different physical

activities and sports, consistent definitions of terms were necessary. Once defined, measurements for these terms or constructs then had to be developed (Gavin, 2004).

You may wish to complete the MAPS Inventory on the accompanying CD-ROM before going any further. The MAPS Inventory has five sections. The first (Self-Description) measures the seven dimensions of your general or personal style in life. The second (Activity Style) measures the same seven dimensions, but in reference to how you prefer to engage in sport and physical activity. The third section (Activity Interest Level) asks you to express your interest in participating in 50 different sports and physical activities. The fourth section (Reasons for Exercising) asks you to indicate whether you feel motivated by 20 different types of motives. The final section (Background Information) gathers information about background factors, including interest and prior participation in physical activity. Chapter 11 explains these sections in detail.

Using the seven themes from the literature as a means of pointing to relevant issues for people involved in sport and exercise, the following personal style dimensions are defined in a manner that allows for characterizations of both individuals and activities (Gavin, 1988, 2004; Gavin & Lister, 2001). These seven dimensions provide indications of both personal and interpersonal behaviors.

Dimension 1—Sociability

Social (interactive)–nonsocial (noninteractive): This dimension assesses the degree to which the individual or activity is characterized by social or interactive engagements that include active involvement of others (not their mere presence) and verbal and nonverbal interactions, as contrasted with behaviors or activities that do not involve others and are essentially noninteractive.

- **To assess the person:** Does the person spend time with others to achieve goals or satisfy personal needs, or does he tend to be alone more of the time? Does he actively seek social experiences, or does he prefer recreations that are more solitary? Does he like working in groups or working alone? Does he pursue opportunities to talk with others and share ideas, or does he prefer to contemplate privately? Because answers to these questions may not be absolute, the percentage of time that individuals spend in interaction or alone might provide better indications of degrees of sociability. This dimension bears some resemblance to the trait of introversion–extroversion (Eysenck & Eysenck, 1968).

• **To assess the activity:** Does a sport or fitness program require active verbal or nonverbal interactions (in group processes or in achieving outcomes) between participants to achieve some end or to satisfy some need, or do participants essentially engage in solitary actions without explicit social involvement?

Dimension 2–Spontaneity

Spontaneous (intuitive)—controlled (analytical): This dimension evaluates the degree to which the individual or an activity is characterized by flexible, intuitively guided, or spontaneous behaviors as compared with ones that are more programmed, inflexible, controlled, or analytically guided.

• **To assess the person:** Does the person tend to be highly analytical, logical, and structured, exhibiting repetitive behavior patterns or highly controlled behaviors or is she more spontaneous and unpredictable, suggesting high levels of intuitively guided thought and flexibility in action? Spontaneity and control have much to do with how people formulate action plans. A controlled person may spend a fair amount of time analyzing the pros and cons, and is more likely to produce upon request detailed explanations for choices and actions. A sense of restraint and self-management often accompanies this approach to action. Two other words that may be associated with the adjectives *spontaneous* and *controlled* are *intuitive* and *analytical.* Although not synonymous with the first pair of words, this second pair, *intuitive* and *analytical,* can be thought of as inside representations of spontaneous or controlled behaviors. Control often comes as the result of thought and analysis. On the other hand, when people act spontaneously, there is likely to be a "feels right," intuitive, sixth sense about the action.

• **To assess the activity:** Does the sport or fitness program require participants to follow inflexible patterns or structures, to move in programmed ways, to be bound by logical, rational processes, or does it call for novel, nonprogrammed, or spontaneous movements that may be either self-initiated or reactive to those of other participants?

Dimension 3–Motivation

Internally motivated–externally motivated: This dimension assesses the degree to which individuals or requirements for participation in an activity depend on drive, effort, or energy expenditure originating within the person (intrinsic) rather than rely on factors external to the person to motivate action (extrinsic).

• **To assess the person:** Is the person self-motivating, self-directed, and inclined to persist, to endure difficulty and discomfort, or does he require situational support and rely on external factors to provide incentives and motives for action? Intrinsic motivation relates to the degree to which one operates with clear, personally determined, and internalized intentions, and pursues them tenaciously. It implies an inner drive in the face of adversity and an ability to go it alone. High levels of intrinsic motivation are present when people make clear decisions and use a kind of internal gyroscope to keep themselves pointed toward their goal, no matter how hard the wind is blowing. In contrast, some people require high levels of emotional, physical, material, or structural support or reward to maintain momentum in a chosen direction. In essence, their motivation derives from external sources, appraisals, or rewards. These individuals may lack clarity about their objectives, and the needs, interests, or goals of others may easily influence them. People who are extrinsically motivated to perform certain actions may have trouble sticking with things that they find unpleasant or demanding unless rewards or desired outcomes are readily forthcoming. They may seek the support of friends or the promise of immediate rewards. Or they may depend on attractive or conducive environmental factors (e.g., music, pleasant distractions, facilities) to encourage their investments of time and effort.

• **To assess the activity:** Does the sport or fitness program provide extrinsic motivation for involvement by virtue of rewards, social and emotional support, time structures, or environmental qualities such as ambience, music, or facilities, or does it rely almost exclusively on participants' personal drive or intrinsic motivation to expend effort in initiating and continuing action?

Dimension 4–Aggressiveness

Aggressive (forceful)–nonaggressive (nonforceful): This dimension concerns the degree to which the individual or the requirements for participation in an activity can be characterized by forceful actions, strong expressions, and persistent attempts to dominate or master others or situations.

• **To assess the person:** Aggression does not always involve action directed toward another person. Aggression can occur in activities like pushing a stalled car or chopping wood. It may involve effort to overcome obstacles. In this context, we conceive of aggression as a generally positive response in which a person applies force to dominate or master. The underlying intention is not to cause harm or inflict injury but rather to assert oneself verbally or physically to achieve one's goals. Aggressive behavior may occur only when repeated attempts to reach one's objectives are thwarted (Dollard et al., 1939), or it may be a person's modus operandi. When aggressive behaviors are highly characteristic of an individual, these actions may be perceived as unfriendly or unduly forceful. How often does a person try to control and master through forceful words or action? Does she always meet force with force, or does she pursue alternative, nonaggressive options? How often does the person stand up for what she perceives to be her rights? How often is she passive when stronger action would enable her to achieve her goals?

• **To assess the activity:** Does the sport or fitness activity require participants to express forceful action to achieve mastery or dominance, or does it rely on less effortful actions? Is it characterized by strong movements and bursts of power, or by softer and more fluid actions? Does the sport or activity involve elements of confrontation with attempts to dominate or master others, or are interpersonal exchanges devoid of such elements?

Dimension 5—Competitiveness

Competitive (rivalrous)–noncompetitive (nonrivalrous): This dimension focuses on the degree to which the individual or an activity can be characterized by rivalrous interpersonal involvements in which the goals of action are to achieve conditions necessary to win.

• **To assess the person:** Does the individual exhibit competitive behaviors with the intention of emerging as best or better than others who are considered rivals, or does he avoid rivalry or situations containing elements of rivalry? Competition is such a popular term that we may confuse it with other concepts. We hear references to competition in three ways: (1) competition with oneself, (2) competition against a standard of performance, and (3) competition against another. The first two references are not as much about competition as they are about personal achievement. Competition, in its purest sense, has to do with rivalry, with the process of competing against one or more individuals who are competitors for some desired outcome. Does the person like competitive situations or not? Does the individual become anxious in situations that produce winners and losers based on some expres-

sion of skill or talent? Does he subconsciously find ways to compete no matter what the situation, or does he more often promote collaboration? Does his adrenaline flow a little faster and his performance improve when a challenger is present, or does a competitive dimension negatively affect his performance?

• **To assess the activity:** Does the activity pit participants against one another in a manner that produces winners and losers, or is the situation devoid of necessary competition between participants? Although participants may engage in an activity with a competitive attitude, a noncompetitive activity would not serve to foster this attitude by virtue of its rules of conduct, processes, or outcomes.

Dimension 6—Mental Focus

Focused (attentive)–unfocused (inattentive): This dimension concerns the degree to which the individual or the requirements for participation in an activity can be characterized by single-mindedness, consciously directed attention, and focus on specific elements of the situation as compared with the relative absence of these characteristics.

• **To assess the person:** Is the individual readily capable of focusing on the task at hand, or is she easily distracted? Does she prefer situations requiring concentration and single-mindedness, or does she enjoy daydreaming or diversifying focus? Mental focus is the ability to rivet attention in the moment, ignoring distractions and committing necessary energies to an intentional pursuit. Does the person find it easy to focus or to do only one thing without interrupting herself? Can she settle into a task and give it full attention for a prolonged period?

• **To assess the activity:** Does the sport or fitness activity require participants to concentrate, to focus their attention, and to be mentally involved, if not consumed, as compared with allowing participants to daydream, to digress mentally, and to be unfocused?

Dimension 7—Adventurousness

Adventurous (risk seeking)–cautious (risk avoiding): This dimension assesses the degree to which the individual or activity is characterized by risky, daring, or adventurous behaviors in which either psychological or physical well-being may be at stake as compared with behaviors more oriented toward feelings of security and safety.

• **To assess the person:** Life is risky. There are physical risks, emotional risks, social risks, financial risks, and risks to self-esteem. Some risks are utterly foolish, whereas others are quite calculated and conservative. Risk taking can add a sense of adventure to a person's life. It can be thrilling, or it can be terrorizing. A person might be energized by it or frightened into total paralysis. Sometimes when a person is extremely skilled at an inherently dangerous activity, he may not describe it as risky. Risk taking may be more psychological than physical. Doing something new constitutes a potential threat to self-esteem. What if the person fails? What if others are critical? What if the person looks silly? Opening the door to new choices and activities means entering the unknown. Does the individual enjoy daring adventures, or does he prefer to live in the comfort zone, avoiding new behaviors, new experiences, and novel activities? Because risk can come in a number of forms, is the person just as likely to take emotional risks as physical ones?

• **To assess the activity:** Does the sport or fitness activity require participants to take chances, to be adventurous, to be daring in action, or does it emphasize more secure and safe behavioral engagements, minimizing risks of psychological or physical harm?

Personal and Exercise Style Profiles

If you completed the questionnaires on the CD-ROM, you will have two graphic profiles of your style. One is more general, pertaining to ways in which you prefer to be in most of your daily engagements (personal style), and the other is specific to sport and exercise (exercise style). The next chapter will say more about these profiles. What is perhaps most important to realize about how you score on the seven dimensions is that scores are neither good nor bad. Your profile represents preferences and habits of action that only you can evaluate in terms of how well they function for you. No profiles are inherently wrong; they are only more or less appropriate to the needs and goals of your life. The same will be true for your clients.

One function of the personal and exercise style profiles is to permit coaches to obtain impressions of how clients function in their lives and how they prefer to engage the world of sport and fitness. Measures of this nature are suggestive rather than absolute. They provide indications rather than facts. Accordingly, they must be tentatively presented and reviewed with the intention of discovery rather than of labeling.

Another function of personal and exercise style profiles is to permit comparisons with activity profiles. Through such comparisons, clients may gain better understanding of some of their intuitive attractions to different activities as well as reasons for some of their dislikes. Before considering how one might view these comparisons, let us first understand the profiling of activities.

Profiles of Activities

An inherent feature of the MAPS Inventory is its ability to indicate similarities and dissimilarities between clients' profiles and a variety of profiles for different sports and physical activities. Client profiles are based on answers to questions contained in the accompanying MAPS CD-ROM. Activity profiles were determined through a different process, which will be described later in this chapter.

As described in chapter 2, each sport or physical activity has certain distinguishing characteristics. To some degree these characteristics are independent of participants, whereas in other respects they interact with aspects of the participants. For instance, the rules of tennis remain the same regardless of who is playing. On the other hand, the caloric consumption of an hour of tennis play will depend on how someone plays the game, as well as the person's biophysical characteristics.

In considering the profile of a specific activity, one might want to take into account what the rules are as well as how a particular individual engages in that activity. In the creation of activity profiles, however, greater emphasis was placed on the requirements for participation than on participant characteristics, because the latter would vary with each participant or client. In this respect the profiles are prototypical ways in which participants might engage in these activities, according to the nature and demands of the activities themselves.

To make this more concrete, take a few minutes to review figure 10.1. Here you will find profiles of 19 common types of activities. Each type of activity may represent a number of different sports or physical activities because graphically portraying every possibility would be difficult. For instance, one type of activity profiled is team sports. Aspects of the profile could easily be altered based on the

Fitness Personality Profile

Sports build character. What personal traits are you developing through your fitness program?

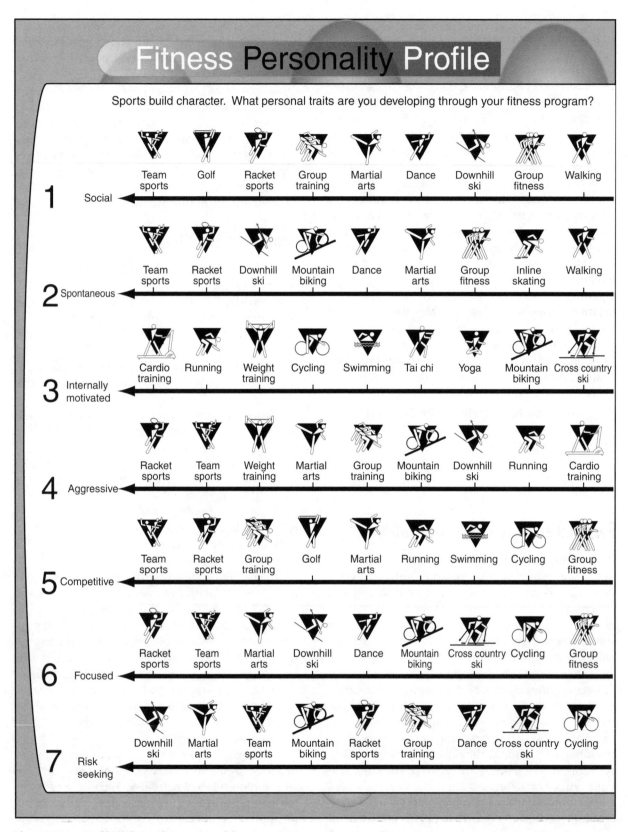

Figure 10.1 Profiles of popular sports and fitness activities on the seven dimensions.

See how seven (7) psychosocial traits are developed by different sport and exercise programs in the chart below.

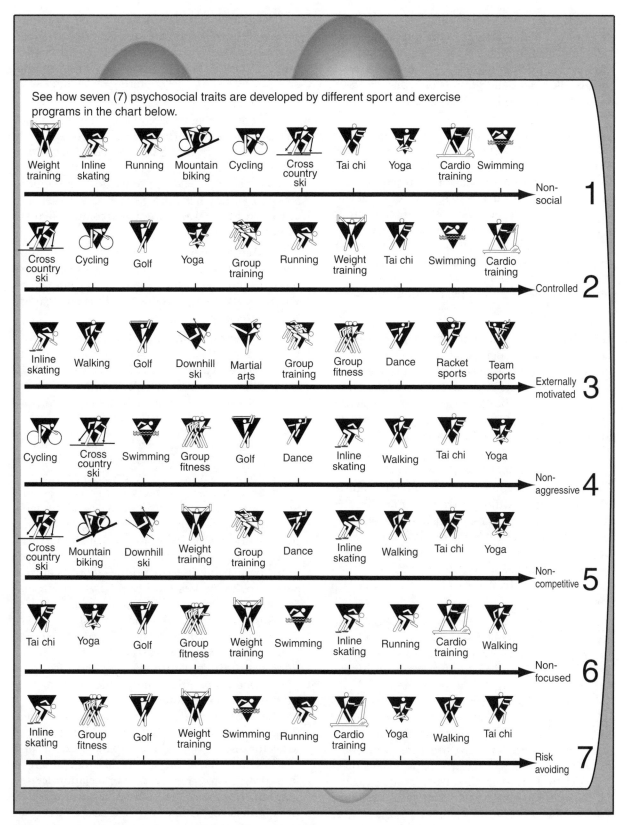

Figure 10.1 *(continued)*

exact characteristics of each team sport. Football, for example, will not have exactly the same profile as volleyball, although similarities among various team sports distinguish them, for instance, from dance. Ultimately, the profiles of types of activities shown in figure 10.1 are suggestive rather than exact.

If you were to draw a circle around a particular type of activity (as represented by its icon in figure 10.1) on each of the seven lines and then connect these circles with a zigzag line, you would have created a profile for that activity. Consider martial arts for illustrative purposes. Notice the position of the martial arts icon on each of the seven lines in figure 10.1 and attempt to decipher its meaning. Clearly, martial arts takes many forms, but for the sake of discussion, consider the popularized forms of karate as they appear throughout North America.

- **Sociability.** The martial arts icon appears more toward the social than the nonsocial side of the continuum because participants generally undertake this sport in group settings and interact physically with other participants. In this sense, people who study together are likely to talk to one another regularly, as well as interact physically.

- **Spontaneity.** Training in karate involves many precise and controlled movements, so why does its icon appear more toward the spontaneous side of the continuum? Although training may involve many ritualistic practices, partners will eventually spar with one another. Some of these interactions may be controlled, but as students become more advanced, more spontaneity is required because of the unpredictability of a partner's responses.

- **Motivation.** How different participants engage in an activity will vary considerably, but based on the nature and structure of karate training, several characterizations would seem to justify its positioning as a more externally motivated activity than as a largely internally-motivated one. Classes have a time structure, a teacher to encourage participation, and fellow students with whom participants might develop relationships. Moreover, karate training has a reward structure represented in the belt system, which leads to the achievement of black belt status. These elements combine to offer participants something more than sweat and hard work as incentives for participation. Again, note that some participants may have higher levels of intrinsic motivation, whereas others will be more oriented to the rewards, physical outcomes, and social processes of the activity.

- **Aggressiveness.** Bearing in mind that aggression is defined as forceful action often directed toward mastery or domination but without the intent to inflict harm or injury on others, martial arts can be readily described as more aggressive than nonaggressive.

- **Competitiveness.** Notice that tai chi, considered by some a martial art, is represented separately from the more typical fight-style martial arts. Competitions do not occur in tai chi or, for that matter, in some other martial arts like aikido. Competitions are quite common in karate schools, however, and advanced students are expected to compete in these events.

- **Mental focus.** If you do not pay full attention in martial arts training, you might easily be injured. Students must focus their minds in the moment on what they are doing. Karate offers little opportunity for daydreaming.

- **Adventurousness.** This dimension is about risk, both physical and psychological. Injuries in martial arts are common. Add to this the psychological challenges of competition, and its rating more toward the risk-seeking than the risk-avoiding end of the continuum is understandable.

The MAPS CD-ROM includes profiles for 50 separate activities against which client profiles can be compared. These activity profiles were developed through extensive interviews and discussions with sport and fitness professionals and students (Gavin, 2004), as well as through a logical analysis of normative requirements for participation. Within types of activities, specific forms are sometimes indistinguishable in their profiles. For instance, a step aerobics class is hard to differentiate from a low-impact aerobics class. Karate would be hard to distinguish from taekwondo. A distinction was made between contact and noncontact team sports, but within each of these categories further distinctions were difficult to make. For instance, how would one differentiate the profile of ice hockey from the profile of football?

The activity profiles are arguable, and such debate has great value. Activity profiling provides ideas for discussion and participation. Clients and coaches may review information like that presented in figure 10.1 to gain greater appreciation for the kinds of dimensions that sports and physical activities emphasize. With an eye to personal development, coaches may suggest activities to clients as ways in which to practice and reinforce behavior patterns that clients may then transfer into other arenas of their lives.

How to Compare Activity Profiles to Personal and Exercise Style Profiles

If you have completed the questionnaires in the MAPS CD-ROM, you will have found tables of activities listed in your report according to how well they match your personal and exercise style profiles. Although the next chapter will say more about the reports derived from the CD-ROM, we need to examine here how these tables were created.

Figure 10.2 compares a hypothetical personal style profile with the profile for the activity of yoga practiced in a group setting. (Yoga as practiced alone has a separate profile.) The solid line represents a hypothetical client's profile, and the broad shaded band displays the group yoga profile.

What does the band for yoga indicate? In interviews and discussions with sport and fitness professionals and students in the field, opinions varied about the profiling of activities—and rightly so. For instance, yoga classes across North America probably exhibit variation in styles. Reflecting this variation, scores on each of the seven dimensions for an activity encompass a range of numbers rather than one exact score. Consider the aggressiveness dimension as applied to yoga classes. Each of the numerous schools of yoga has a different emphasis. Moreover, Western forms of yoga include such styles as power yoga. Although the degree of forcefulness in yoga will be considerably lower than that characterizing weight training, power yoga will offer participants a more energetic and strenuous workout than more traditional forms of hatha yoga will.

If you examine the client's profile as represented by the solid line, you will note points where her score falls within the band of scores characterizing group yoga. Each of the client's seven scores has a corresponding opportunity for a match. A match is present whenever the client's score falls within the band of scores for the activity.

Matches and mismatches are equally important in understanding the implications of an activity for a particular client. When a client's score falls within the band, we may assume that the client's style is more or less compatible with the nature and required behaviors for participation in the activity. When a client's score is outside the band, the implication is that this dimension of the activity will be a stretch for the client. That is, it may challenge the client to behave in ways that differ from her normal patterns. Depending on whether the client is open to such challenges, the activity may or may not be well advised. In all, each activity can match a client's profile in seven ways. The higher the number of matches, the more congruent the activity is with the client's personal style. The profile of the hypothetical client depicted in figure 10.2 shows five matches with the activity of group yoga classes. Her profile does not match two dimensions—sociability and spontaneity. We might speculate that this client will experience some dissatisfaction because of the relative lack of opportunity for social interaction in these classes and because she seems to prefer more structure or control in her activities. But she might be able to compensate for these issues by taking a class regularly so that she develops social connections with other participants, and perhaps by looking for a highly structured yoga class rather than one that is more flowing in orientation.

The logic of this process does not take into account ingrained attitudes, athletic competencies, cultural values, or actual opportunities to

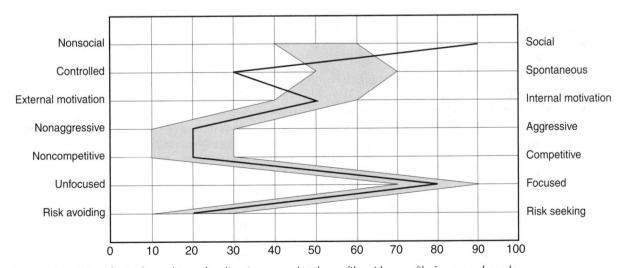

Figure 10.2 Hypothetical matching of a client's personal style profile with a profile for group-based yoga.

participate. Ice hockey is not popular in southern California, and surfing is less popular in Canada than it is in the United States. Moreover, a person may be fearful of the water even though swimming may perfectly fit his profile. The MAPS CD-ROM includes another questionnaire that assesses client interest in activities as well as the person's perceived ability to participate in those activities. With the help of this interest and ability questionnaire, activities in which the client has no expressed interest or possibility of participating are eliminated from the tables of results offered for consideration.

The MAPS Model—Getting to the Client's Core Agenda

Recognizing the thousands of hours that an active person will spend in physical activity during his or her lifetime argues in favor of designing fitness programs that reinforce traits that clients want to develop or maintain. Engaging in physical activity over decades of one's life without conscious awareness of how they work on different facets of character or personal habits may represent a missed opportunity. Sport and exercise have traditionally been recognized for their physical development attributes and only in the broadest way for their character-building potential (Danish et al., 1996; Shields & Bredemeier, 1995; Smith, 1999). The MAPS Inventory provides helpful guidance for understanding specific styles that different fitness programs might reinforce (Gavin, 1988, 1992; Gavin & Lister, 2001). The future of fitness advisement will undoubtedly embrace a more comprehensive analysis of sport and exercise that will produce programming recommendations for clients based not only on physiological parameters but also on a host of lifestyle and personal style characteristics.

By using the dimensions in the MAPS Inventory, clients who intend to develop personal competencies along with other beneficial changes that normally accrue as a result of long-term commitments to active living will have opportunities through their programs to

- develop social skills while reducing anxieties that interfere with effective social behavior,

- increase spontaneity while maintaining a strong sense of personal control,

- develop greater emotional hardiness and personal resilience in stressful life situations,

- move out of aggressive or passive reactivity into a more assertive way of interacting with others,

- balance competitive enthusiasm with synergistic ways of working with others,

- direct thought processes in ways that permit the mind to focus or flow as needed in the moment, and

- develop a spirit of adventurousness and risk taking that is framed by awareness of personal boundaries and safety.

People can choose sport and fitness activities with personal change agendas in mind—to create avenues for practice and support of new behaviors. If, for example, someone feels uncomfortable with strong, forceful actions, making a conscious choice to engage in an activity like weight training could be of benefit. An individual striving to increase his personal comfort in social situations might choose to participate in group fitness classes. Because exercise lowers the physiological sensations of anxiety, this person would be able to engage in a more social context with less anxiety. Over time, the increased comfort in the activity would reinforce new ways of interacting.

Adding Value Through Assessment

In the stages of coaching described in chapter 5, the third stage is assessment. This chapter has provided a general overview of some of the factors that coaches might consider in assessing clients during the early stages of the coaching relationship. Certain types of assessments should be considered mandatory, whereas others are more likely to be optional. Knowing a person's medical history and physical capabilities would seem crucial to any coaching process, yet assessing personality would likely be more discretionary.

In sport and exercise psychology, a host of factors have been related to either activity participation or the outcomes of exercise involvement. Whether or not clients are interested in monitoring their changes in mood states or psychological functioning will depend on their intentions and needs. Coaches, however, may choose to advise clients about the relevance of certain kinds of assessments and periodic monitoring.

The MAPS Model, presented toward the end of this chapter, describes a means of creating added value for clients. The model helps them appreciate some of the unexpected and perhaps unknown benefits of active-living engagements. Through its profiling of clients' personal and exercise styles, the model provides coaches with information to promote dialogue with clients about their needs, agendas, and potential strategies for change. The model is best thought of as suggestive rather than precisely diagnostic. It primarily serves an agenda of inquiry and discovery rather than one of prediction and control. In chapter 11 we will learn more about the MAPS Model and its application to the coaching process.

Applications of Guides in Coaching

"The metamorphosis of the self never ends, and we need effective means to get through each phase successfully."

Thomas Moore

As a lifestyle fitness coach you can readily integrate a wide variety of assessments and guides into your practice. You should be aware, however, that using questionnaires or other measures in a coaching relationship affects some of the dynamics between coach and client. For instance, the client is more likely to perceive you as the expert when you function in the role of test interpreter or evaluator. In other words, you should use coaching guides in a way that reinforces a collaborative, nonhierarchical relationship characterized by codetermination of processes and programs.

The material presented in this chapter revolves around the MAPS Inventory as a guide to coaching. As a coach you may learn about other forms of guidance that you may wish to adapt to your work with clients. Although the details about questionnaires will be specific to MAPS, the processes of coaching will apply to other applications of aids to coaching and their interpretations to clients.

Understanding the MAPS Inventory

The CD-ROM version of the MAPS Inventory contains five sections (or questionnaires), each of which provides information to fuel discussion and understanding with clients (Gavin, 2004). The five sections, briefly described in chapter 10, are reviewed here in detail.

Section 1—Self-Description

This questionnaire contains 42 questions, 6 for each of the seven personal style dimensions. The questions pertain to general habits, preferences, and patterns; they are not specific to sport and exercise. Respondents answer questions on a five-point scale ranging from "Almost never" to "Almost always." Some questions are phrased so that "Almost never" reflects more of a particular dimension, whereas others have the opposite construction. For instance, answering "Almost always" to the statement "I have an easy time engaging in casual conversations with strangers" would indicate a high degree of sociability, whereas a similar answer to the statement "I feel anxious when I socialize with people I don't know" would suggest a lower degree of sociability. Accounting for how the questions are phrased (i.e., reversed or not), responses are added together to create a total score. For example, the least sociable answer receives a value of 0, and the most sociable gets a value of 4. Consequently, the range of scores for the sociability dimension will be 0 through 24, as it will be for the other six personal style dimensions. To aid clients' interpretation of these numbers, the numerical scores are converted into percentile scores based on a norm sample of 1,089 members of fitness centers (Gavin, 2004). A percentile score tells you what percentage of individuals from the norm sample had scores the same as or lower than yours. For instance, a percentile score of 25% means that your score is the same as or higher than 25% of the norm sample; conversely, 75% scored higher than you did. To make this more concrete, let's say that your score was at the 25th percentile on the dimension of adventurousness. This score would indicate that 25% of the norm sample have the same degree or less of risk-taking behaviors and attitudes, and that 75% are greater risk takers than you are. Higher percentile scores are not necessarily better; they simply indicate on the dimension in question where you stand in relation to others. On the dimension of aggression, for example, you might prefer to be nonaggressive in your approach to the world; if your score was at the 10th percentile, you would

probably be pleased with the result. On the other hand, you may love being sociable, so a score at the 80th percentile in the social dimension would probably seem an accurate representation of how sociable you are in comparison with others.

Section 2—Activity Style

This questionnaire contains 14 questions, 2 for each of the seven dimensions. In contrast to the questionnaire about personal style, this questionnaire asks clients about their exercise style or habits, preferences, and patterns in relation to training, sport, and exercise. Clients may intuitively realize the opportunity that sports and exercise presents for balancing life patterns. Executives working in high-stress, competitive, aggressive environments may look for opportunities for release and relaxation in their training sessions. People who are isolated all day at work in laboratories or in front of computer monitors may seek fun and social interaction in their exercise programs. Chances are, however, that most people will display the same inclinations and habits in exercise as they do elsewhere in their lives (Hoelter, 1985). To illustrate the emphasis on activity style represented in these questions, an item assessing sociability is "I prefer to have people around when I exercise," and one that measures competitiveness is "Workouts are more exciting and fun when I can compete against someone else." As in the previous section, five answers are possible, ranging from "Almost never" to "Almost always." The range of scores for each dimension is 0 through 8, and like the personal style scores, these are also converted to percentiles for easy interpretation. Rather than seeing numbers like 7 or 8 as scores, your clients will see percentiles that tell them where their scores fall in relation to the norm sample. Percentile scores also offer the advantage of permitting graphic comparison of the two sets of scores (exercise and personal styles).

Section 3—Activity Interest Level

As mentioned in the previous chapter, the measures of personal and exercise styles do not account for client abilities, preferences, cultural factors, and opportunities as they relate to specific fitness programs and sports. A person may have a negative attitude about dance-style fitness classes or about team sports, even though from a profile perspective these activities may be reasonable matches. To account for this and to provide coaches with additional information, this section presents 50 common sport or fitness activities. Clients are asked to indicate their level of interest for each activity on a five-point scale (high, medium, low, none, and unable to do activity). Distinctions are made not only between types of activities but also about how they might be done. For instance, listings appear for running, swimming, and cycling, either alone or with a group. Group fitness classes are divided into a number of popular forms, including dance style, martial arts style, military style, stretch and relaxation, and circuit training. When clients respond to an activity with an answer of "None" or "Unable to do activity," the activity is removed from further consideration in the description of results.

Section 4—Reasons for Exercising

Although coaches will want to explore this area through dialogues with clients, this section provides a quick overview of some of the more customary reasons why people choose to engage in sport and exercise programs on a regular basis. Twenty reasons are presented, including such options as weight control, dealing with a current health problem, preventing future health problems, reducing stress, improving endurance, body shaping or toning, having fun, dealing with moods and anxiety, and developing mental toughness. Clients have three choices of answers: Yes, No, or ? (Not sure or don't know). The report that clients receive tables their answers to each reason so that coach and client can explore motivational patterns for active living.

Section 5—Background Information

The final section consists of 11 questions regarding different aspects of a client's profile and background. These questions encompass age, sex, previous involvement in sports and exercise, and estimated aerobic capacity. Answers to questions about height and weight are converted to a body mass index score (ACSM, 2000). As a general summary of relevant client characteristics, this section provides a useful snapshot at the outset of the coaching relationship.

Client Reports Based on the MAPS Inventory

The questions that clients answer in the MAPS Inventory are integrated with the aid of a computer program so that a meaningful report can be

returned to clients for discussion with their coaches. The report consists of an overview and two main sections.

Overview

The first page of the report summarizes the client's motivations for exercising, background information, and top matching activities (see figure 11.1):

- **Motivations for exercising.** For each of the 20 reasons for exercising, the client's answers of Yes, No, or ? are tabled for review.
- **Background information.** The client's answers to the 11 background questions are summarized, along with the client's body mass index (BMI) computed from a formula involving height and weight.
- **Top matching activities.** Using a combination of information from the client's personal and exercise style profiles and expressed interest (or capability) in different sports and activities, a limited number (approximately five) of activities are listed as choices that seem to offer the best match to the client's interests and profiles.

Section 1—Your Personal and Exercise Style Profiles

Information about interpreting the profiles is provided along with a graph of the client's results, under the heading of "Personal Style and Exercise Style." Scores on each of the seven dimensions are indicated as percentiles with a range of 0% to 100%. Figure 11.2 provides a sample of results from section 1. The more similar the two profiles are, the more the client prefers to exercise in a manner paralleling how she lives in general; conversely, the more dissimilar the two profiles are, the more her exercise patterns will diverge from her general lifestyle patterns.

Section 2—Activity Matches Based on Personal and Exercise Style Profiles

Because seven dimensions are involved in each of the two profiles, seven matches are possible between a client's profile and the profile of any given activity. A table presented in this section lists activities in which the client has expressed some interest according to the number of matches that it has with the

Matching Activity and Personal Styles (MAPS) Reports

Name of client _____

Date _____

Your report contains an overview plus two (2) sections. Parts of the report will help you understand your personal and exercise styles. Other parts will offer recommendations for sports and fitness activities based on a comparison of your styles with the normal social and mental demands of different fitness activities. The results in this report are guidelines, not absolute facts. Use them to help you think about your exercise and sport choices in new ways. Ultimately, you are the best judge of what works for you.

Motivations for Exercising	Yes	No	?
Weight control		x	
Deal with a current health problem		x	
Prevent future health problems	x		
Reduce stress and release tension	x		
Shape my body and increase physical attractiveness	x		
Improve endurance	x		
Be with friends or make new friends			x
Have fun	x		
Deal with moods and anxiety	x		
Enjoy the challenge and excitement of competition		x	
Develop mental toughness	x		
Become more assertive	x		
Live more adventurously			x
Be physically fit			x
Increase feelings of relaxation			x
Build self-esteem			x
Reduce negative habits		x	
Create opportunities for personal achievement		x	
Develop greater focus and concentration		x	
Learn new skills for life			x

Background Information	
Exercise attitudes	don't enjoy exercise
Exercise participation	rarely train
Aerobic capacity	adequate
Strength level	marginal
Flexibility	some flexibility
Physical status	only worries
Nutritional habits	always eat well
Years regular exercise	0
Age	33
Height	5'6"
Weight	135 pounds
BMI	21.79

Top Matching Activities	
1	Stretch and relaxation classes
2	Dance style fitness classes (aerobics, funk, step)
3	Aquaform/Aquafitness
4	Walking with a group
5	Running with a group or Master's class
6	Yoga classes

From the *MAPS Inventory CD-ROM* included with *Lifestyle Fitness Coaching* by James Gavin, 2005, Champaign, IL: Human Kinetics. (www.HumanKinetics.com)

Figure 11.1   Sample overview page of MAPS Inventory report.

Section 1. Your Personal and Exercise Style Profiles

The chart below compares your Personal and Exercise Style Profiles on seven dimensions. Higher scores indicate more of the indicated traits; lower scores suggest lower levels of the trait. High scores are not better than low scores; they are simply different. Different styles work well for different people. Here's a brief definition of each dimension:

Low scores mean	DIMENSION	High scores mean
Like to do things alone. Reenergize yourself in solitary activities.	SOCIABILITY	Like to do things with others. Feel energized in social interactions.
Prefer highly structured, predictable activities. Focus on control.	SPONTANEITY	Prefer spontaneous, unpredictable activities. Highly flexible in lifestyle.
Rely on external rewards and outcomes for motivation.	MOTIVATION	Strongly self-motivating. Rely little on outside influences.
Easy going, accepting, sometimes passive. Prefer non-demanding activities.	AGGRESSIVENESS	Highly assertive, take charge style. Like forceful, charged, aggressive activities.
Avoid competitive activities. Prefer non-competitive ones.	COMPETITIVENESS	Love competition in almost any form.
Unfocused or easily distracted. Prefer activities that allow mind to wander.	MENTAL FOCUS	Focus and concentrate easily. Like activities that keep you focused.
Emphasize safety and caution. Avoid taking chances or risks.	ADVENTUROUSNESS	Like adventure and taking chances. Prefer risky or adventurous activities.

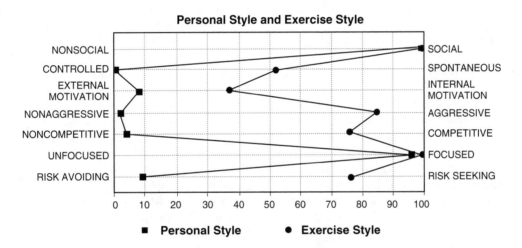

Personal Style and Exercise Style

■ **Personal Style**   ● **Exercise Style**

Personal and Exercise Style Profiles		
Dimension	Personal Profile	Exercise Profile
SOCIABILITY	99%	100%
SPONTANEITY	0%	52%
MOTIVATION	8%	36%
AGGRESSIVENESS	2%	85%
COMPETITIVENESS	4%	76%
MENTAL FOCUS	96%	100%
ADVENTUROUSNESS	9%	76%

From the *MAPS Inventory CD-ROM* included with *Lifestyle Fitness Coaching* by James Gavin, 2005, Champaign, IL: Human Kinetics. (www.HumanKinetics.com)

Figure 11.2 Sample of personal and exercise style profiles from section 1 of MAPS.

client's profile (see figure 11.3). For each listed activity, the client's degree of expressed interest is also shown. This table is constructed in such a way that it combines results for both profiles. If you examine figure 11.3 you will see that the left-most column shows the number of matches between the client's personal style profile and various activities. The sample lists all activities with seven out of seven matches. These activities are placed in subgroups according to how many matches they show with the client's exercise style profile.

Coaches who have other sources of information about their clients may develop ways of integrating it with the results of the MAPS Inventory. The upcoming sections will present suggestions and illustrations for a coaching process that begins with guidance provided by the MAPS Inventory. When reading the dialogues, pay attention to how the coach fosters participation and collaborative decision making in identifying client goals.

Coaching Dialogues Initiated With the MAPS Inventory

Imagine that a new client has been asked to complete the MAPS Inventory early in the process of the coaching relationship. How might this information be integrated into the coaching process, and what role would the coach play in interpreting results to the client? The report produced by the CD-ROM accompanying this book may be self-explanatory. Clients may read their reports and immediately grasp the major implications. But because MAPS is intended as an aid to coaching, coaches should review the results with clients through dialogue so that clients can derive the richness of meaning contained in the report.

Dialogue to Initiate the Review

How would a lifestyle fitness coach begin a dialogue to review results from the MAPS Inventory? Let us assume that the coach and client have met for an introductory session and that the coach recommended that the client complete the MAPS Inventory before the second session. In the following session the coach must convey competence in understanding and applying results from the questionnaires without dictating interpretations or drawing conclusions for the client. A good place to begin is a discussion of the client's motives (see Motivations for Exercising in figure 11.1 on page 230). The dialogue that

follows provides sample exchanges between coach and client, as well as identification of coaching skills and their intended effect (see coaching dialogue 11.1, "Discussion of Janine's Motives" on page 234). To get the most from this dialogue, you should first read the dialogue on the left side of the page without concern for the skills and comments listed on the right. On your second reading, pay attention to the skills and comments along with the dialogue.

The client is a 33-year-old lawyer who works for a large corporate law firm. Janine indicated to her coach during the first session that she needs to reduce her feelings of stress from work as well as commit to a serious training program so that she can eventually compete in a running marathon. She has been moderately active over her lifetime but never in a consistent fashion.

The coach balances the need to demonstrate competency and authority with efforts to share responsibility for the codirection of the coaching process. At different points Janine seeks direction and attempts to have the coach provide reassurance for feelings she has not yet fully expressed. For instance, in segments 4 through 8, a kind of dance occurs between coach and client until it finally becomes clear that the coach is not going to give pat answers but rather will use the questionnaire results in a collaborative way to foster greater understanding. In segments 12 through 16, the client's insecurity becomes more transparent, and only through the coach's ability to resist the temptation of being the expert with all the answers is she able to unveil the client's concerns. Janine's reference to being "normal" signals the possibility that perhaps she has issues that go beyond the competencies of a lifestyle fitness coach. For this reason the coach presses for clarification, as exemplified in segments 30 through 39, in which it becomes apparent that the client's anxiety and mood concerns are highly related to her work stresses and do not represent a generalized pattern of mood disorder. The coach offers her some reassurance in segment 37 with the remark, "That's my understanding, too." An effective coach will keep in mind all the pieces of information that the client reveals over time so that, should there be a need for referral, the coach will recognize it by virtue of having documented indicators of the issue throughout the relationship.

In regard to documentation, the coach will want to take notes for each client session. Depending on your style and the client's comfort level, you may take notes during the session. More likely, you will want to spend a few minutes after each session to make your notes. Your recall of significant interactions during the session will be sufficiently clear

Section 2. Activity Matches Based on Personal and Exercise Style Profiles

Below you will find a table of activities that match your Personal and Exercise Style Profiles. Here's what the information in this table means: Activity matches based on your profiles are formed from scores on the seven dimensions. Each of your scores was compared to the profiles of different activities. For each activity, there was a possibility of seven matches, one for each of the seven dimensions. For example, if your score on the dimension of Sociability is high, any physical activity or sport that requires high levels of social interaction would have been counted as matching your profile. This process was repeated for the remaining psychosocial dimensions: Spontaneity, Motivation, Aggressiveness, Competitiveness, Mental Focus, and Adventurousness. Each time one of your scores matched an activity's profile, you were given one matching point for that activity.

In the table below, activities are listed according to the number of matches they have with your profile. The higher the number of matches, the more like your profile the activity is. This means activities with high numbers of matches (e.g., 5, 6, or 7) should be enjoyable to you. Activities with low numbers of matches (e.g., 0, 1, 2, 3) might be more challenging for you to engage in on a regular basis, especially if you have difficulty keeping to a regular exercise program.

Results for your Personal Style and Exercise Style are presented in the same table so you can make comparisons. Keep in mind that some activities with a high number of matches may not interest you very much. Based on personal history, beliefs about your own abilities, or other reasons, you simply may not choose to take up these activities even though they match your profile. Check the information in the column, "Your Interest Level," to identify your interest in each activity.

Similarity between Personal Style and Activities	Similarity between Exercise Style and Activities	Sports and Fitness Activities	Interest Level
6	3	Walking with a group	High
5	4	Hiking with others	Medium
		Aquaform/Aquafitness	High
	2	Yoga classes	High
		Stretch and relaxation classes	High
		Muscle toning classes with hand held weights	Low
4	3	Stability ball classes	High
		Social dance	Low
	2	Exercising on cardio machines at a fitness center (stair stepper, treadmill, etc.)	Low
3	7	Mountain biking with a group	Low
	5	Tennis	Low
		Squash, racquetball, badminton, or handball	Low
	4	Ballet or modern dance classes	High
		Pilates classes	High
	2	Swimming by myself	Low
2	6	Fitness classes with a martial arts style (e.g., Aerobox)	Medium
	5	Dance style fitness classes (aerobics, funk, step)	High
		Circuit training	Medium
		Martial arts classes (e.g., aikido)	Low
		Martial arts classes (karate, boxing, taekwondo, kickboxing)	Low
		Running with a group or Master's class	High
	4	Cross-country skiing or snow-shoeing with friends or a group	Low
		Non-contact team sports (e.g., volleyball, basketball)	Low
		In-line skating with a group	Medium
	3	Cycling by myself	Low
		Contact team sports (e.g., rugby, football)	Low
		Weight lifting with free weights	Low
	2	Running by myself	Low
1	5	Military style fitness classes (boot camp, etc.)	Medium
	4	Cycling with a team or Master's class	Medium
	3	Swimming with a group or Master's class	Medium

From the *MAPS Inventory CD-ROM* included with *Lifestyle Fitness Coaching* by James Gavin, 2005, Champaign, IL: Human Kinetics. (www.HumanKinetics.com)

Figure 11.3 Sample of activity matches based on personal and exercise style profiles.

Coaching Dialogue 11.1   Discussion of Janine's Motives

Dialogue	Skills	Comments
1. Coach: "Janine, would this be a good time to go over the results from the MAPS Inventory?"	Closed question.	Determines client readiness to deal with the questionnaire results.
2. Client: "Yes, it is. I was looking forward to hearing what you could tell me about my results."		
3. Coach: "Great. I think we will both understand a lot more through this process . . . and hopefully come up with some clearer ideas about directions."	Minimal encourager and information.	Implies the collaborative nature of the relationship and indicates the purpose of the review.
4. Client: "I looked over the report, and I think I understand a lot of it, but I'd be interested in what you have to say."		
5. Coach: "How would you like to proceed? Do you want to go over each section, step by step, or are there specific areas you want to focus on right now?"	Open and closed questions.	Places responsibility for the approach back on the client.
6. Client: "Well, is there a way you normally do this?"		
7. Coach: "It really depends on the client. I can recommend a strategy, but there may be something that piqued your interest that you'd like to get to right away."	Information and advice or suggestion.	Indicates competence while continuing to share responsibility for the process with the client.
8. Client: "Hmm. I have a bunch of questions about the results, but maybe we could just do it your way, and I'll get my questions answered in the process. If not, I can always ask, right?"		
9. Coach: "Of course . . . So, let's go over the report one section at a time. Whenever you have questions, just ask."	Instructions.	Taking leadership, yet indicating the client's co-ownership of the process.
10. Client: "Terrific."		
11. Coach: "The first section of the report is a listing of your reasons for exercising, that is, the ones you checked on the questionnaire."	Information.	Provides obvious information without indicating interpretations.
12. Client: "Yes, I'm not sure why I checked some of the ones I did, but I see I put down 'prevent future health problems,' 'shape my body and increase physical attractiveness,' 'deal with moods and anxiety,' 'develop mental toughness,' and 'become more assertive.' Of course, the ones about improving endurance and reducing stress and releasing tension we talked about last week. What do you think this means?"		
13. Coach: "Are you asking me what it means that you checked these items?"	Closed question.	Serves to verify the client's request and to encourage the client to be clearer about her needs.
14. Client: "Well, yes. Do you have any data about why people check these items?"		
15. Coach: "Each person seems to have a different story behind why they check these reasons. What would be helpful here is for us to explore your reasons for checking them."	Information and advice.	Answers the client's question in a way that encourages her to search for her own meanings.

Dialogue	Skills	Comments
16. Client: "Yeah, I guess that was a silly question. I think I wanted to know whether my answers were normal, or something like that."		
17. Coach: "Well, they are normal—normal for you, so what we need to do is to look at these reasons more closely."	Feedback and instruction.	Reassures the client without examining her concern about being "normal."
18. Client: "'I think I understand the one about preventing future health problems . . . My father died of a heart attack a few years ago. He was only 57."		
19. Coach: "I'm sorry to hear that . . . So, yes, it makes sense you would be concerned about your health."	Immediacy and feedback (or opinion).	Expresses concern for the client and validates her experience.
20. Client: "And I want to look good so—although we really didn't talk about this agenda last week—at 33 I am concerned about losing my sex appeal. Embarrassing to say."		
21. Coach: "So, it feels a bit embarrassing to acknowledge that you want to look your best and that this motivates you to exercise?"	Reflection of content with a minor reframe (interpretation) presented in the form of a question.	Without reassuring the client, the coach offers the client an opportunity to reflect on her meaning.
22. Client: "You know, when you say it that way, it sounds pretty normal . . . like what's wrong with exercising so you can look good?"		
23. Coach: "Sounds pretty normal to me."	Feedback (or opinion).	Validates the client's experience without probing for deeper issues.
24. Client: "Yes, it does to me too . . . I think I know where the 'mental toughness' and 'becoming more assertive' reasons are coming from. I work in a pretty hard-core, competitive, mostly male law firm. You can't show your feelings there without someone taking advantage of you."		
25. Coach: "So, developing mental toughness and becoming more assertive are related to your work, and that might be something we should consider in designing your program?"	Reflection of content in the form of a question.	Demonstrates listening, makes a connection with the coaching agenda, and leaves the issue open for client exploration.
26. Client: "I think so . . . I don't know how to do that, but I know I wear my feelings on my sleeve at work, and it affects how my colleagues look at me."		
27. Coach: "Would you like to explore this issue some more right now or just keep it in mind to work on later?"	Closed question.	Involves the client in taking responsibility for direction of the session.
28. Client: "No, let's move on, but I would like to come back to it sometime."		

(continued)

(continued)

Dialogue	Skills	Comments
29. Coach: "OK, I've made a note . . . What next?"	Information and open question.	Coach shares responsibility for tracking issues and then involves the client again in determining direction.
30. Client: "Well, the only one we haven't talked about is my moods and anxiety. I wasn't even sure why this was on the questionnaire . . . I didn't know this had much to do with exercising, but I think it's pretty important to me."		
31. Coach: "Yes, regular exercise has been shown to have a beneficial effect on moods and anxiety—that's why this reason was on the questionnaire—and so it's important to you."	Information and reflection of content.	Offers input corresponding to the client's query and then brings the focus back to the client's issue.
32. Client: "Well, this is again one of those embarrassing moments . . . You know, whether I'm normal or not . . . But sometimes I really get stressed out, and when the weekend comes, I have little energy for getting out of my PJs and going out."		
33. Coach: "Hmm . . . So your stress gets so high sometimes that you just don't want to go out on the weekend."	Reflection of content.	Emphasizes content rather than feeling to encourage the client to provide more information.
34. Client: "Yeah, I don't think it's serious . . . It doesn't happen very often, but I do know that work takes its toll on me, and I have very little energy left when the weekends come, not to mention the fact that I often have briefs to prepare over the weekend."		
35. Coach: "Sounds like you see this as very work related, and in this respect it ties in closely with what we talked about last week."	Summarizing.	Provides an integration of comments from two sessions, confirming the client's messages.
36. Client: "For sure. I just need to manage my stress better . . . and from what I know when you're stressed, you feel anxious and lack energy sometimes."		
37. Coach: "That's my understanding, too . . . Is there anything else you want to say about this that would help in our work together?"	Information and open question.	Supports the client and inquires about additional meaning.
38. Client: "Well, I think you're getting a better idea of why I really want to make a strong commitment to exercise, and I would like to learn more about some of the benefits I can get from it."		
39. Coach: "Yes, I am getting to understand your interest and commitment better . . . and I do have some things you can read that will help you appreciate all that you might gain from a regular fitness program."	Feedback and information.	Responds to the client's needs and offers support for her agenda.

right after the session for you to write down key points that you want to remember. Note taking during the session can influence the flow of dialogue between coach and client, as well as raise client concerns about what you are writing.

What is interesting about this dialogue is that it begins with a simple review of items checked on a questionnaire, yet it moves to a deeper layer of conversation than the previous one between coach and client. The client had entered the coaching relationship with certain preconceived notions of exercise benefits, which excluded some of her deeper needs. She mentioned reducing stress and training for a marathon in her first session. By representing a wider range of agendas, the MAPS Inventory allowed coach and client to broaden their perspectives of the agenda, while continuing to frame their engagements within the legitimate domain of sport and fitness.

Dialogue Concerning the Profiles

The next section of the report that a client is likely to encounter is the profiling of the seven dimensions. Because this material may be novel for clients, the coach should orient a client to the profile information in a manner that contains its meaning within appropriate boundaries. In the client's report will be a guide to interpreting the seven dimensions in the profiles. One profile will be based on the client's general orientations and patterns; this is referred to as the personal style profile. A second profile is based on how the client prefers to experience training and sport involvements; this is called the exercise style profile.

Results from the two profiles may be similar or different. When they are similar, the client is probably consistent in her approach to life and exercise involvements. When differences are present, the client may be either attempting to balance general life tendencies (personal styles) when she exercises or expressing some desire to develop aspects of herself that are not normally represented in other parts of her life. For instance, an overcautious person may engage in risky sports as a way of nurturing the feeling of adventurousness in life. A highly aggressive businessperson may look for tension release through yoga or Pilates classes as a way of balancing work demands.

In section 1 of the client's report, one graph combines the two profiles (see the Personal Style and Exercise Style graph in figure 11.2 on page 231). In coaching dialogue 11.2, "Discussion of Janine's Personal and Exercise Style Profiles" on the next page, the coach will be reviewing the combined graph.

Now we will continue the dialogue between Janine and her coach in showing how the profile information could be presented.

Coaches may be tempted to interpret profiles to their clients, yet as Janine notes in segment 26, this strategy could backfire. The client is the expert on the meaning of her profile. The coach is the expert on the technical aspects of how the profiles are constructed and the general meaning of the seven dimensions. Bear in mind that no matter how a question is asked, clients will always interpret the question according to their unique understanding. This means that whatever a client's profile is, its true meaning lies within the client, not in some technical manual for interpreting results.

Clients may need encouragement to offer their own interpretations before the coach interjects her opinions and interpretations. The more the client looks to the coach for answers, the more emotional dependency the client displays. When coaches fall into the trap of being the expert and rescuing clients from the struggle of finding their own meanings, they are likely to foster client dependency.

Certainly, coaches should be experts in certain areas and inform clients about techniques, procedures, and even test results when such matters require scientific or other advanced information that clients may not have. But a coach should provide only a general framework for understanding the seven dimensions of the MAPS Inventory and then encourage clients to explore their profiles and interpret the results.

The coach provides Janine with a framework for understanding why the personal style profile and exercise style profile might differ but leaves the task of attributing meaning to these differences to the client. For instance, as Janine begins to explore some of the discrepancies between her two profiles, the coach encourages her to continue (see segment 17). When Janine wants the "expert's" opinion about how she is thinking and feeling, the coach appropriately turns the question back to her (see segments 22 through 26). Even when Janine resists, the coach provides a rationale for why it might be better for her to search for her own answers than to rely on the coach's interpretations.

As the session progresses, the client takes on more responsibility for making interpretations. Her resistance to the coach is minimal, as exemplified in the exchange shown in segments 22 through 24. Notice that the coach does add her expert information to the client's understanding, but only after she has encouraged the client to interpret findings on her own (see segment 25).

Coaching Dialogue 11.2 Discussion of Janine's Personal and Exercise Style Profiles

Dialogue	Skills	Comments
1. Coach: "Janine, are you ready to move on to the profiles you see here on your report?"	Closed question.	Determines the client's readiness to consider the profiles.
2. Client: "Sure thing, but maybe you could tell me what these profiles are all about . . . They seem like a bit of a personality analysis."		
3. Coach: "Be happy to. Research has shown that sport and fitness activities have a lot of relevance to certain aspects of human behavior, and, on the other hand, exercise and sport may have little relevance to other aspects. The seven characteristics that you see here are thought to be more closely tied to the exercise world, so that's why they were focused on in the questionnaire. Clear so far?"	Information and closed question.	Provides an explanation and checks for understanding.
4. Client: "Got it. Please go on."		
5. Coach: "OK. I would rather call these dimensions indicators of your personal style than personality measures. They are mostly about the general ways in which you behave and the ways you prefer to live your life. For instance, do you like competitive situations or not? This isn't exactly personality—it's more about what feels good to you, how you like to spend your time—and that's why it's called your personal style."	Information.	Continues to explain, pacing information at a rate at which the client can comprehend it.
6. Client: "OK, so what is this profile telling me?"		
7. Coach: "We'll get into the details when we look at your profile, but in general your profile gives you indications of how you behave and what your preferences are. The numbers shown in the table under the graph [refers client to table] indicate your percentiles based on how your scores compare with a large group of people involved in exercise. Your scores can be related to different exercise programs to suggest how they might fit your patterns or how they might challenge you."	Information.	Continues to explain.
8. Client: "That makes sense . . . So this profile is designed to show me what sports would suit me. Is that right?"		
9. Coach: "Yes. As we go through the results, I believe things will become clearer. Do you have enough general information about the profile for us to move ahead?"	Advice or suggestion and closed question.	Checks the client's needs and suggests a process for proceeding.
10. Client: "I think so. I just wanted to understand what the intention of all this was . . . Now it makes sense."		
11. Coach: "Great. So let's look at your two profiles here on this graph [refers the client to an image of two profile lines]. There are some definitions right above this [refers the client to the definition section of the report page], but here you can see a profile graph for what's called your personal style and one for your exercise style. The first is about how you behave in general, and the exercise style is about what you prefer when you are exercising. Clear?"	Instruction and information.	Provides direction and general understanding.

Dialogue	Skills	Comments
12. Client: "OK, so I see that the lines are almost the same in a couple places and different in the others."		
13. Coach: "Yes, where they are the same, it means that the way you typically act or prefer to be matches the way you want to be when you are exercising, and where they're different, it means you prefer to exercise in a style that differs from your customary pattern."	Information.	Provides general information without specific details about the client's profile.
14. Client: "Oh, like balancing things out? I see here that my general pattern is pretty nonaggressive, but in fitness I seem to want to be very aggressive . . . Maybe this goes along with my goal of wanting to develop more assertiveness and mental toughness."		
15. Coach: "I think you're getting it, and you seem to be making sense out of your results. What else do you see?"	Feedback and open question.	Confirms the client's understanding and reinforces the client in taking responsibility for attributing meaning to the results.
16. Client: "Well, I see a similar thing on the competitiveness dimension. I don't seem to like competition in general, but I want to be competitive when I am exercising . . . This is very interesting."		
17. Coach: "Tell me more about what you see that's interesting."	Instruction or indirect question in the form of a reflection.	Encourages the client to find her own meanings.
18. Client: "Maybe I recognize that I need to change some things about myself, so I must have answered the exercise questions in a way that would help me change. Is this possible?"		
19. Coach: "I believe so. Sometimes people show differences in their profiles because they want to balance their patterns, for example, doing relaxing exercise programs to balance a very stressful job, and sometimes they use exercise programs to build up their 'mental muscles' in certain areas."	Opinion and information.	Gives the client feedback about how the coach sees her and offers a way of understanding without directly interpreting her results. Encourages the client to draw her own conclusions.
20. Client: "Mental muscles? What do you mean?"		
21. Coach: "Remember, we were talking about personal style. If your style is to be somewhat fearful and ineffective in competitive situations, you can help yourself gain more comfort with competition by getting involved in low-level competitive activities in sports."	Information.	Provides information in a manner that relates directly to the client's issues.
22. Client: "You mean like my desire to run a marathon?"		
23. Coach: "Could be. What do you think?"	Opinion and open question.	Gives the client responsibility for discovering meaning.
24. Client: "Wow. You're making me work hard. I thought I was paying you for answers [laughs nervously]."		
25. Coach: "I could give you my opinions, but I think it makes more sense for you to try to discover what these results mean to you."	Immediacy and advice or suggestion.	Encourages the client to find meaning rather than foster dependency on the coach.

(continued)

Dialogue	Skills	Comments
26. Client: "You're right. I think I wanted you to give me the answers, and then like the lawyer I am, I could cross-examine you [laughs nervously]."		
27. Coach: "OK, so now that we're clear about this, what do you think?"	Open question.	Acknowledges the client and refocuses the dialogue.
28. Client: "Well, as you can see on my personal style profile I'm very social, I don't like competition, and I'm not very aggressive. When I told you last week about wanting to run a marathon, I think I realized I would be pushing the envelope. I knew it would be hard . . . Looking at this profile gives me a better idea of exactly why it will be hard and how it's going to challenge me."		
29. Coach: "So, you can see the challenges in the goal you've set for yourself. How do they feel?"	Reflection of content and open question.	Focuses on client challenges and probes for reactions.
30. Client: "I think I'm OK with them. It's what I want. I usually need a lot of support—that's the social side of me. I won't get that running a marathon, but I can at least get some of it from you. As for the competitive part and developing mental toughness—that's my interpretation of aggression—well, I need to work on that."		
31. Coach: "So, you're hoping to get some support from me—and, yes, that's what part of this relationship is about. And I'm glad to hear that you see the challenges and want to take them on for your personal benefit."	Reflection of content and immediacy.	Confirms the client's message, reinforces the role of the coach, and shows support for the client's goals.
32. Client: "What else can I get from this profile?"		
33. Coach: "From what I'm hearing, you've already got a lot. Your comments confirm the results. Where your exercise profile differs from your personal style profile is in areas that you want to develop. Is there anything else about your profiles that you want to talk about?"	Feedback, summarizing, and open question.	Summarizes overall interpretation of profiles and encourages the client to explore results further.
34. Client: "What I think the profile is saying is that I'm very focused—which I am—and that I have a strong emphasis on control—which I do. Also, I'm not a great risk taker, but, again, in my exercise profile, I show more interest in taking risks."		
35. Coach: "And how do you feel about these patterns?"	Open question.	Encourages exploration of the remainder of the profile.
36. Client: "As I said, I agree with the results, and at least for now I'm OK with them. I like to be in control, and it's important for me to be focused in my work. As for taking risks, 'better safe than sorry'—that's what my mom always told me."		
37. Coach: "So, you feel OK with them."	Reflection of feeling.	Confirms the client's feeling about the profile.
38. Client: "Yes, and with the other areas, I think I'm going to have enough to work on . . . So what's next?"		

Dialogue	Skills	Comments
39. Coach: "Well, that's good. You seem to have identified what you consider a manageable challenge, and one that I think I can help you with . . . What's next? If you're ready to move on, let's look at how your profiles match with different sports and fitness activities. OK?"	Feedback, opinion, information, and suggestion.	Frames the client's agenda and indicates ability to assist. Makes one final check before moving ahead.
40. Client: "I'm ready."		

Sometimes clients may be puzzled by their results and begin to argue that they are inaccurate. In these cases, coaches should help clients create what they believe are accurate profiles rather than defend the accuracy of the MAPS Inventory. The value of guides such as this lie more in the dialogue they foster than in the results they produce.

Dialogue Concerning the Matching Tables

For the two profiles, personal style and exercise style, a single table lists all the sport and fitness programs in which the client has expressed interest according to the degree to which they match the client's profile. In chapter 10 we considered how the profiling of activities represents a band or range of scores on each dimension rather than a single value. When the client's numerical score falls within the range of scores for the activity on one of the seven dimensions, the result is considered a match. With seven dimensions, seven matches between client profile and activity profile are possible. The higher the number of matches, the more closely the activity parallels the client's profile. What the table of results does not describe are the dimensions on which the client's profile matches or mismatches the dimensions of the activity. This absence of this information can create some confusion when clients review the tables.

Take the case in which a client is adamantly opposed to doing any activity that involves aggressive actions. Nonetheless, this client's profile may still show six out of seven matches with an activity like hockey, with a mismatch occurring only for the aggressiveness dimension. Six out of seven matches would suggest that hockey is a good match for this client. The aggressive actions required by this sport, however, would lower its attractiveness to this client and probably cause him to see it as a poor fit. Differences between the tabled results suggesting that hockey is a good fit and the client's internal reaction to the aggressiveness of the sport would likely cause the client to view the results with skepticism.

Fortunately, clients' answers to questions in section 3 of the MAPS Inventory, activity interest levels, minimize this kind of confusion. By asking clients whether they are interested in pursuing certain activities, the MAPS Inventory removes from consideration those in which the client has no interest or is incapable of participating in. In the example, the fact that hockey appears means that the client expressed at least some interest in this activity. Although the table might show a large number of matches between the profile of the client and the profile of hockey, it would also record the client's interest level, which is likely to be low. A valuable discussion might result from helping this client realize ways in which this sport corresponds to other dimensions of his profile.

To gain greater appreciation of ways of helping clients understand their potential programs, let us continue to review Janine's report (see figure 11.3 on page 233) and the dialogue between Janine and her coach about the report (coaching dialogue 11.3, "Discussion of Janine's Activity Matches for Her Personal and Exercise Style Profiles" on page 242).

Not all clients will be as perceptive as Janine is. Although she continues to exhibit dependency on the coach as reflected in such remarks as, "Is that right?" (segment 2), "What do you think?" (segment 16), and "Is that a good idea?" (segment 28), she is not only willing to express her opinions but also seems to have a fundamental understanding of herself and her potential connections to different activities. When clients genuinely struggle with making sense out of their results, coaches may have to provide more interpretations and information.

In reviewing information from the table summarizing matches related to personal style and exercise style profiles, clients may feel overwhelmed by the amount of information available. To some degree, the indications of activity preferences (high, medium, or low) will help them sort out their results. When clients have little interest in an activity, the activity

Coaching Dialogue 11.3 Discussion of Janine's Activity Matches for Her Personal and Exercise Style Profiles

Dialogue	Skills	Comments
1. Coach: "Janine, I know you've read through your report. Do you have a general understanding about what this table is telling you?"	Closed question.	Checks for client understanding and involves the client in process of understanding results.
2. Client: "I think so. It looks like the more matches there are, the closer the activities resemble my own profile. Is that right?"		
3. Coach: "Yes, and because your two profiles were different, the sports and activities that more closely match your personal style may be somewhat different from ones that match your exercise style."	Information.	Provides explanation to assist the client's personal interpretations.
4. Client: "Yes, I think I realized that."		
5. Coach: "Great. So, can you tell me what you think these results are saying to you?"	Minimal encourager and open question.	Involves the client in exploring for meaning.
6. Client: "Wow. That's a big question. There are so many results here."		
7. Coach: "Yes there are. Maybe we can take the results piece by piece starting with the activities with high numbers of matches with your profile. Make sense?"	Information, suggestion, and closed question.	Acknowledges the client's feeling, offers direction for proceeding, and asks for confirmation.
8. Client: "OK . . . Well, what I see here is that 'walking with a group' has six out of seven matches with my personal style, but it looks like it only matches my exercise style on three out of seven of the dimensions . . . There aren't any other activities that match my personal style that much."		
9. Coach: "What sense do you make of this?"	Open question.	Encourages client exploration.
10. Client: "I actually like walking and I like being with my friends. And it's not very risky . . . or competitive . . . or aggressive. So yes, it makes sense . . . and, of course, since my exercise style was different, walking with a group wouldn't match as much."		
11. Coach: "Yes, you're understanding this clearly. What else do you see?"	Feedback and open question.	Supports the client's understanding and moves the session along.
12. Client: "What I see in the next box, five matches, are some other activities that I like."		
13. Coach: "For instance?"	Indirect question.	Continues to encourage the client to make meaning of the results without inserting opinions or interpretations.
14. Client: "Like yoga and aquafitness and stretch classes . . . "		

Dialogue	Skills	Comments
15. Coach: "Uh-huh."	Minimal encourager.	Allows the client to continue directing the dialogue.
16. Client: "All of this makes sense for me . . . Maybe I should look at the activities that don't match. What do you think?"		
17. Coach: "Seems like a reasonable strategy to me."	Opinion.	Supports the client's approach.
18. Client: "Oh yes [looking at the activities with few matches] . . . There's team sports and martial arts and solitary activities like running alone . . . Uh-oh!"		
19. Coach: "Uh-oh?"	Reflection of feeling.	Emphasizes the client's emotional response to the results without attempting to interpret.
20. Client: "Well, the team sports and martial arts are not the problem. I'm simply not interested in doing them, but running alone . . . Isn't that what marathon training is all about?"		
21. Coach: "Well, it can be, but there are ways in which you can train that can make it more suitable to your profile. And remember, we already talked about how your goal would be challenging. You might note that running with a group, while it only has two matches with your personal style, has five out of seven matches with your exercise style."	Information with minor reframe and reflection of content (from earlier segment).	Offers the client a new way of perceiving her training and acknowledges the client's self-selected challenge.
22. Client: "Yes, that's true . . . And you also mentioned I could train with a group, and that would certainly fit my social nature . . . This is great. The questionnaire confirms some of the things I've been feeling."		
23. Coach: "I'm glad to hear that. What else pops out in this section of your report?"	Immediacy and open question.	Offers support to the client and continues to probe.
24. Client: "Well, I didn't indicate very much interest in weight lifting, but could you explain to me why it shows up with only two matches to my personal style profile?"		
25. Coach: "I could, but first what's your guess?"	Information and open question.	Gives the client responsibility for discovering meaning.
26. Client: "I get it. You want me to think for myself . . . OK, that's fair. Let's see . . . It's probably not very social, and it definitely seems hard, and all I ever hear are grunts coming out of the weight room, and that's a bit of a turnoff . . . Yeah, it doesn't seem like me."		
27. Coach: "I think you've answered your own question. In my words, it's not very social, as you said; it takes a lot of determination and personal motivation without a whole lot of support; it involves aggressive energy to get those weights up in the air; but it has some focus, and that is like you; and it involves a lot of control, which is also like you."	Opinion and information.	Supports the client's interpretation and then offers professional information about the activity.
28. Client: "That makes a lot of sense. Thanks . . . Maybe I should pay more attention to what my exercise style profile results are. Is that a good idea?"		

(continued)

(continued)

Dialogue	Skills	Comments
29. Coach: "It could be, and it's also helpful to keep both sets of results in mind. That's why all your results are put into one table so you can see how they relate to both your personal and your exercise styles."	Opinion, suggestion, and information.	Provides the client with guidance about keeping all the information in mind.
30. Client: "Yes, that does make sense because my general pattern may be more ingrained, even though I may want to exercise differently."		
31. Coach: "You definitely seem to have the hang of it."	Feedback.	Supports the client's growing understanding.

will nonetheless appear in the table, but the client can readily dismiss it from further consideration. From the coach's perspective, however, knowing which activities do not match the client's profile or which activities the client has expressed little interest in may be as informative as knowing which activities match well or which activities interest the client most. The coach gains fuller understanding of clients not only by knowing what fits or what the client chooses but also by knowing which activities hold the potential for stretching the client.

We may want to consider one final set of results. In the next part of the dialogue, we will examine what the report offers as top matching activities as well as summarize salient features of the process of reviewing MAPS.

Summary Dialogue

The MAPS Inventory provides other types of information, including a list of top matching activities based on the degree of interest and matching across the two profiles (see Top Matching Activities in figure 11.1 on page 230). Further, the report summarizes the client's self-reported history of fitness involvement, estimated fitness level, and body mass index, an indicator of body composition.

The coaching dialogue concerning questionnaire results may be ongoing, yet there might be some attempt to draw at least temporary conclusions or summaries from the information reviewed. Novice exercisers, in particular, should retake the MAPS Inventory 3 to 6 months after commencing regular exercise. A contrast between their profiles and other results can be revealing.

In the coaching process, decisions about action remain open to revision throughout the relationship as more information and understanding becomes available. Clients are likely to be in a process of transition or evolution as they work with coaches, so coaches must continually seek feedback about how clients are experiencing agreed upon pro-

cesses and commitments. Nonetheless, in fostering engagements with action, coaches need to help clients achieve sufficient understanding from which they can plan and commit action.

In this concluding dialogue with Janine (coaching dialogue 11.4, "Discussion of Janine's Top Matching Activities"), the coach will help her pull together the diverse elements of her review of the MAPS Inventory.

This last segment brings coach and client to some greater understanding of values, needs, and motivations. This section also reflects movement toward action planning. Although clients may enter coaching with some preset ideas about what they should do and the reasons underlying their choices, the MAPS Inventory affords a second chance to reflect and examine motivations and agendas. Moreover, by providing profiles of how the individual functions in life and how she prefers to engage the fitness world, these questionnaires broaden the discussion so that coach and client can incorporate other factors relevant to programming. Clients will not always understand the parameters of lifestyle fitness coaching, and by using the MAPS Inventory they are more likely to recognize the more encompassing domain of fitness challenges and benefits.

Maintaining Rapport in Using Assessments

Lifestyle fitness coaches should develop their own styles and adapt tools and guides to their preferred ways of working with clients. Whether a coach uses the MAPS Inventory or some other means of fostering dialogue with clients about their needs and agendas, the processes of communication will be relatively similar. What is perhaps central to consider is the influence of questionnaires and tests on the coach–client relationship.

Coaching Dialogue 11.4 Discussion of Janine's Top Matching Activities

Dialogue	Skills	Comments
1. Client: "This is a lot of information. So what's the bottom line of it all?"		
2. Coach: "Yes, it is a lot, Janine. I don't know if this will answer your question, but there is a section of the report that attempts to integrate all your interests and both of your profiles."	Reflection of content and information.	Validates the client's experience and provides data relevant to the client's question.
3. Client: "Oh, yes, I saw that part. It's a list of my top matching activities. How did they determine that?"		
4. Coach: "In the section called Top Matching Activities, the computer program listed those activities that showed the highest matches with each of your profiles and also those in which you indicated the highest levels of interest. These activities may well reflect what suits your present styles and interests, but they don't necessarily indicate where you're going, that is, the kinds of challenges you want to undertake because often these challenges don't match with your styles."	Information.	Provides an explanation to assist the client's understanding.
5. Client: "Yes, that makes sense. That's why running alone isn't listed here."		
6. Coach: "Right. So, what do you understand from this section?"	Feedback and open question.	Encourages the client to explore meaning.
7. Client: "Well, I see 'walking with a group' again and also doing a bunch of activities in a group, including 'dance style fitness classes.' They make sense to me. I would enjoy these activities, and I am glad to see that 'running with a group' is there. But as you said, I want to take on something different to push me a bit, and maybe to help me change."		
8. Coach: "So, the results confirm where you are, but not entirely where you are choosing to go."	Reflection of content.	Acknowledges the client's understanding and fosters further discussion.
9. Client: "Exactly."		
10. Coach: "If you were to pull together all we've discussed last week and this week in reviewing the questionnaire, what kinds of implications or conclusions might you draw?"	Open question.	Encourages client exploration.
11. Client: "Hmm . . . I liked what we just did with the questionnaire. Somehow it gives me a better understanding of myself and also what this whole fitness thing is about for me . . .Yes, and it confirms my intuition that I need to push myself in new directions. You know, I hadn't thought about it before we analyzed weight training, but I might want to look into doing that once in a while, too."		
12. Coach: "So, you feel confirmed by this review, and you have some ideas to begin planning your program."	Reflection of content.	Validates the client's experience and encourages her to search for her own conclusions.
13. Client: "Yes, I feel more commitment than ever to start training for a marathon, and I'd like your input on how you think I could get involved in a weight-training program."		

(continued)

(continued)

Dialogue	Skills	Comments
14. Coach: "This is sounding like a decision to me. Is it?"	Feedback and closed question.	Moves the client toward closure.
15. Client: "Yes, it is. I'm going into this with my eyes wide open. Before we talked about all this today, I had impressions but nothing concrete. Now, I have a kind of road map that I know will help me when I'm feeling a bit unmotivated. Thanks. This has been great. So, what's the next step?"		
16. Coach: "I'm glad to hear this. I think you have made the most of this report, and now we can start looking at specifics. So, let's talk about possible scenarios for your training."	Immediacy, opinion, and instruction.	Reinforces the client, offers support, and moves toward action planning.

You will reap significant benefit by gaining some experience with the MAPS Inventory at this time. Learning activity 11.1 suggests a way in which you can begin to develop competencies in the use of questionnaires in a coaching process.

When coaches use tests or questionnaires like the MAPS Inventory, clients may experience concerns about being exposed, evaluated, or vulnerable. After all, the coach now has an extremely personal set of data about the client. Coaches need to approach the dialogue with clients about reports or results with care and sensitivity. When clients seem defensive about the results or argue about the findings, coaches need to give priority to the client's experiences rather than attempt to validate data in the report. Rarely can a coach justify trying to convince a client that she is wrong about her interpretations of information derived from tests or questionnaires that she completed.

The MAPS Inventory serves only as a guide to understanding and planning. The client's experience and the coaching dialogue are real, not the statistical values in the report. As the dialogue concerning the report proceeds, effective coaches will monitor both the process of the discussion and the details being explored. When the process seems to threaten rapport between coach and client, effective coaches will rely on their knowledge of coaching skills, the ebb and flow of attending and influencing, and their adherence to nurturing the core conditions of the relationship.

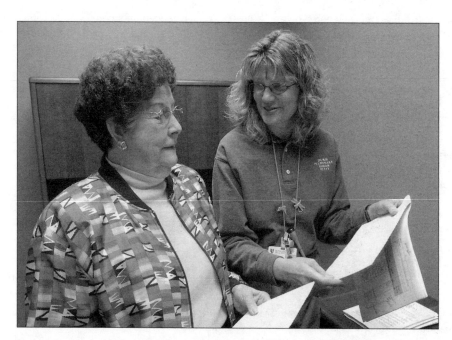

You can gain experience using the MAPS Inventory by having a friend or family member take the inventory and then talk with you about the results.

Learning Activity 11.1   A Practice Coaching Session Based on the MAPS Inventory

Let's assume that you have completed the MAPS Inventory and are reasonably familiar with its results. What would be helpful for you now is to practice engaging in dialogue with someone about his or her results. Try to find someone with whom you are familiar and who is open to taking questionnaires and reviewing results with you—perhaps a friend, family member, or colleague.

Ask the person to complete the MAPS Inventory. Print out a copy of the results and allow the person at least 15 minutes to read the report privately. After your "client" has had sufficient time to gain some understanding of what the report reveals, invite him or her to talk to you about the results.

You can proceed in essentially two ways. The first way models the dialogues in chapter 11 with Janine. In this fashion, you would progressively move through major sections of the report. For instance, you would first look at motivations, then you would review the profiles, next you would look at the matches, and then you would conclude with a summary discussion that could include a review of the top matching activities along with any insights and commitments that your client may wish to share.

The second method of reviewing results is client centered. You might open with a general question about what your "client" understands from the report and then pursue areas of interest or concern as connected to different areas of the report. For instance, your "client" may wish to understand more about the profiles, so that would be your starting point. Or, he or she may want to understand how the MAPS Inventory determined the top matching activities. In this method, any point of beginning will invariably lead to discussions of other areas. If your "client" does not choose to review a section of results, you can always suggest that he or she do so, once all of your "client's" primary concerns have been addressed.

The more practice you have with the MAPS Inventory, the better prepared you will be for lifestyle fitness coaching sessions involving these questionnaires. Over the next few weeks, try to get as much practice as possible. Remember that you should assure even friends and family of the confidentiality of their results and your discussions.

Opportunities and Directions in Lifestyle Fitness Coaching

People want to experience fulfillment and balance in their lives (Whitworth et al., 1998), yet many people have lives fraught with hardships and adversity or they may lack the necessary energy and direction to create these states of being. As much as some people feel the need to go it alone, most of us benefit from social support and competent guidance when things are difficult and we lack critical pieces of information.

Accommodating regular sport and fitness participation in modern lifestyles is rarely simple or easy, as participation rates would suggest. Even when someone has demonstrated commitment to physical activity at one stage of life, changes and transitions may adversely affect participation at other stages. Perhaps when people are younger and their normal routines involve much physical movement, the effects of mostly sedentary lifestyles are modest. As years pass, however, the accumulating effects of inactivity, poor posture, restricted ranges of movement, and biophysical changes in metabolism and body structures increasingly manifest themselves in common ailments (chronic back or neck pain), weight gain, and perhaps disease (e.g., cardiovascular disease, diabetes, osteoporosis). Although not life threatening, low levels of participation in sport, fitness, and other active-living pursuits are missed opportunities for enhancing joy, satisfaction, creativity, and personal growth. While we may consider physical inactivity and its aftereffects a product of our age, it makes little sense to romanticize

*"To live is to change.
To live well is to change often."*
John Henry Newman

249

historical periods when physical activity was an integral part of life. People who worked as manual laborers, farmers, foresters, blacksmiths, or artisans often experienced the wear and tear of what we would now define as overuse syndromes. A carpenter might have hammer elbow, not tennis elbow. An underground miner might have osteoarthritis of the knees not from running too many marathons, but from climbing ladders throughout every workday. Moreover, in any romantic remembrance of the past, we have to factor in significantly shorter life spans with waning years characterized by the ill effects of lifelong imbalanced functional efforts. Few 19th or even early 20th century people knew how to offset the effects of repetitive work habits through stretching, corrective exercises, or core strengthening. If they did know, they likely had little time to devote to such efforts.

When we think of the many blessings of a long life, we implicitly incorporate notions of health and functionality throughout the life span. Yet these are not givens. They are more likely the rewards of active living, healthy eating, moderation, good genes, and a little bit of luck. Although we may be far wiser these days about what we need to do to be healthy and live long, satisfying lives, habits formed before we even knew the word often dominate our intelligence as we follow the path of least resistance through our fast-paced, fast-food, automated, and instantly gratifying new world.

Now for the good news. Modern-day fitness is just that—a recent arrival on the landscape of life. Health fitness professionals are discoverers and explorers, deconstructing myths, mapping new terrain, and creating unforeseen possibilities for participation and active living. As noted earlier, fitness once was jogging, then it was aerobic dance, but now its look is limited only by the imagination. With all the options available, with the magnificent guidance of science, and with a superbly informed cadre of health fitness professionals, the power for change rests mostly in the realm of education and support. Most people need help in initiating and maintaining active lifestyles. As a health fitness professional you have both the power and the motivation to contribute to their health and wellness.

Your Expertise As a Coach

Information is power, but it is too often insufficient to motivate and sustain change. People know that smoking kills, that fast food is nutritionally harmful, that seat belts should be worn—the list goes on. The simple fact is that changing beliefs, values, and behaviors is extraordinarily difficult—no matter what.

Do you smoke? Do you occasionally drink too much? Do you always eat what is right for you? When did you last order the supersize special at a fast-food outlet? Maybe you have most of this under control, or better yet these issues have never arisen in your life. Most people don't always observe healthy habits, even though they may experience guilt each time they finish a bag of chips, feel remorse the morning after, or promise themselves that this time they really are going to stop smoking.

Lou Andreas-Salome, Sigmund Freud's biographer, wrote, "When confronted by a human being who impresses us as truly great, should we not be moved rather than chilled by the knowledge that he might have attained his greatness only through his frailties?" People do amazing things. They overcome unimaginable limitations. They thrive in the harshest of circumstances. What one person is capable of, many more inherently have the capacity to do. Yet, we never do it alone and rarely just for ourselves. Artic explorers, transatlantic voyagers, and pioneers of all kinds may have been physically alone throughout their ordeals, but it is unlikely that they were alone in their thoughts. We are inspired by others, we strive so that others may feel proud, and we may even put ourselves in harm's way for the well-being of unknown others.

We are social animals. For better or worse, our lives are shaped by and directed toward inner and outer human connection. Our rich thought processes are replete with images and conversations, with feelings and the remembrances of touch. As long as we remain willing to understand the difficulties that people have in changing longstanding dysfunctional habits, we can keep our hearts open to helping them in processes of change. Doing so will not always be easy for us, and we know it will not be simple for them—although our efforts will smooth the path, lower the obstacles, and instill hope.

With our abundance of knowledge about health and fitness, we sometimes see too much of what is wrong—poor eating habits, substance abuse, inactivity, problematic relationship styles, lack of self-care. What we need to see more of is the inner flame, the passion for life hidden in the corner of someone's existence, the will to be more than one's self-defined or externally defined limitations. We cannot change it all. No one can. Perfection is not a human reality. Striving is.

Change Expertise

As a health fitness professional you will have already traveled a fair distance along the road toward competency regarding the bio-psycho-sociocultural needs (Johnson, 2003b) of different people in relation to physical activity. This experience is your foundation. Your evolving domain of expertise as a lifestyle fitness coach concerns the processes of change. Discussions of the transtheoretical model (Prochaska et al., 1995) and Taylor's (1986, 1987) learning process model have offered you doorways to an ever expanding literature about what people need in order to change and how you can best serve them (Bridges, 2001).

If we reconsider the explosion of interest in life coaching and its seemingly boundless agendas, we may reasonably ask how any coach could possibly have competencies in addressing the countless interests that clients may have. At least part of the answer is simple. The limitless agendas of clients contain a core similarity—they are all about change. Whether someone wants to lose weight, have a successful marriage, find a new career, raise healthy children, exercise more, train better, think smarter, or focus on a myriad of other issues, the fundamental wish relates to change. Maybe someone wants to go backward in time, to reverse the effects of aging and live as he once did in happier years. No matter what temporal direction or what theme, the seeker pursues change.

Lifestyle fitness coaching depends on your expertise in understanding and facilitating change. Someone who wants to eat better has a similar process agenda as one who wants to exercise more. They both will struggle with their habits, their comfort zones, their beliefs and values, and their motivations. Moreover, they will travel along similar terrain with more or less predictable obstacles, sometimes in daylight, other times in the depth of darkness. And you will be their guide because you will understand what they need and where they are. You will remind them where they are going whenever they forget or pretend not to remember. They will find comfort and support in the knowledge that they can reach out in the darkest moments and find your hand.

Coaching Expertise

Lifestyle fitness coaches need to be themselves, to be natural and authentic, yet what becomes your way of being will be anything but normal. Before you become too concerned by this statement, remember that normal (in terms of average or typical behavior in North America) means being physically inactive, moving rapidly toward obesity, probably smoking, and watching too much violence in films and on TV. In social patterns, it means giving advice, pretending to listen while multitasking, interrupting, trying to fix another's problems, and putting the ego into places where it doesn't belong.

Coaches understand communication processes, the skills that build rapport, and the skills that can destroy it. They know when and how to influence, and they recognize the signals telling them to back off and try later. They intervene at levels appropriate to their competencies and their clients' agendas. They may be astonishingly wise, yet they know that their principal goal will be to draw out the wizard within each client, not to pontificate from years of study and experience.

Although the creation of empathic understanding may occasionally look like a technique, coaches will have incorporated an empathic way of being into how they are in the world, whether working with clients, friends, family, or even strangers. Occasionally they will slip up. Sometimes they will lose sight of what is important, their egos will be caught, they will push too hard or too little, and they will make mistakes. Yet their ingrained ownership of skills and theory related to effective helping will bring them at least part of the way back to where they want to be. The support networks of colleagues, coaches, and supervisors that they have created will help them the rest of the way.

Opportunities and Growth in Lifestyle Fitness Coaching

Lifestyle fitness coaches may have a unique advantage over many other types of coaches by virtue of their focus and venues for work. Most likely, lifestyle fitness coaches will be affiliated with at least one major fitness center in their communities. People who visit or frequent those centers have taken the first step and probably more. Your potential clients are in the right place, and it is your place.

Many life coaches rely on Web sites to advertise their services. Or they may create special events, such as public presentations, to describe the work they do and how they can help. Over time, they may create a network for referrals from colleagues, allied health professionals, and former clients. In contrast, if you already have established yourself in the health fitness field, people will perceive the

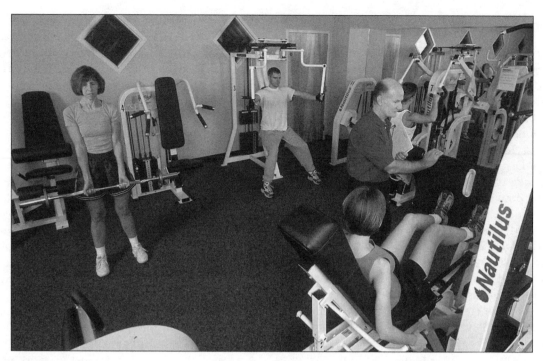

People who work out at fitness centers are potential clients of the lifestyle fitness coach.

expansion of your role to include lifestyle fitness coaching as natural and beneficial. Although you may continue to work in other capacities within the health fitness world, coaching will become an integral part of your professional profile. In time, it may be your primary endeavor.

Reflection and Supervision

Becoming a coach carries with it a profound responsibility to those you serve. No matter how insightful we are, most of us have blind spots about our behaviors and effects on others. As a coach you must reflect on your practice. One of the best ways to do this is to work under the supervision of an experienced coach. Because lifestyle fitness coaching is a relatively new field of professional service, you may encounter some difficulty in finding a supervisor. Fortunately, various options are available. For one, the field of life coaching, although also relatively new, has been around for more than a decade, with thousands of people trained through different certifying organizations. Through an Internet search, you will find the names of many individuals whose Web sites give you information about their specializations and credentials. You can contact some of them until you connect with one who seems to have the skills and styles that suit your own orientation. Another possibility is to contact a local sport or exercise psy-

chologist who has a clinical practice helping clients with such issues as exercise adherence and motivation. You might talk with this psychologist to determine whether her background would enable her to supervise your work. If you are pursuing a coaching career along with friends or colleagues, you could arrange for group supervisory sessions. A third option involves guidance counselors, social workers, or psychologists whose work centers on life adjustment issues. For instance, some of these professionals focus their practice on wellness, stress management, or health promotion. Again, you would want to interview these professionals to determine the compatibility of their styles and processes with those of lifestyle fitness coaching. You might contact local colleges or universities to get the names of professionals who might be suited to your interest in supervision. Finally, you might have read this book in the context of a course on lifestyle fitness coaching. You might invite some of your classmates to form a learning group after you complete the course and arrange with your professor to supervise the group.

Continuing education, reading, reviewing recordings of your sessions, and having discussions with peers and colleagues will also be invaluable. Create an action plan for your ongoing development. Even highly experienced helping professionals recognize the need for continuing professional development and supervision.

Coaching Models As a Form of Education

In our school systems there is deep acknowledgement of the need to incorporate psychological, social, and cultural factors in any process of communication. Education is rarely effective as a one-dimensional conveyance of facts. It must embrace all aspects of the learner.

Similar dynamics apply in the fitness world. Yet rarely do health and fitness centers focus sufficiently on educating consumers. The belief may be that people come to train, not to sit and listen to a lecture. Ironically, this may be true, but at the same time this belief perpetuates the difficulties that people have in making solid, lifelong connections to active living.

Lifestyle fitness coaches can be considered bio-psycho-socio-cultural educators. This book has certainly emphasized their one-to-one work in this realm. What we have not discussed as much is how lifestyle fitness coaches may work with groups using the same set of skills, along with others derived from the field of group dynamics (Kass, 2004). Unique career opportunities exist in creating learning opportunities for groups. The energy generated in group settings can be highly engaging, especially when the group structure encourages participation and dialogue. Using this format, lifestyle fitness coaches may multiply their influence and engage the resources of group members as a support system for one another.

You might, for example, create a program for novice exercisers at the fitness facility where you work. Using tools like the MAPS Inventory, you might initiate the program by reviewing a structure for interpreting the report. Then you could invite participants to pair up with a partner and discuss any aspect of their reports that they are willing to share. Of course, you would want to make yourself available to participants for any private matters that they wish to discuss. Through structured activities and dialogue, you might then guide group members toward the formulation of action plans related to active living. In a follow-up session you could review some of the material on change processes, especially those related to the transtheoretical model and Taylor's learning process model. Again, you would invite participants to share perspectives and information with other group members. Topics for other sessions might include relapse prevention, benefits of exercise, creating social support for active living, and so forth. Through engaging participants in group dialogue and guiding discussions, you would have created a group-based method of lifestyle fitness coaching.

Although some people will prefer personal coaching, others may enjoy the interactions of group sessions. Moreover, because of its lower cost per participant, a group-based method of lifestyle fitness coaching can reach people who otherwise would not have access to such services.

A vast amount of information is available about health, fitness, and active living. Passive processes of reading, viewing, or listening may be insufficient to stimulate action, whereas engaged processes of dialogue coupled with expert guidance and education may tip the scales for many people who formerly struggled on the boundary of healthy and active living.

Becoming a Generalist or a Specialist

Lifestyle fitness coaching is a subset of the larger field of life coaching. We have adequately discussed the advantages of such specialization. Your career path, however, may evolve toward broader or narrower focus. You may choose to specialize even further in working with such groups as postcardiac rehabilitation patients, children and adolescents, or individuals in recovery from substance abuse problems. The more focused your work, the more training will be involved. Broadening your scope of work will have similar implications. Perhaps as you gain experience and knowledge, you may wish to pursue the wider agendas of life coaching or even consider graduate education in counseling and psychotherapy.

Other paths are possible. When clients come to you with interests in active living, they may also have other related issues. These might include nutritional concerns or substance abuse problems. You may find that many of your clients are also trying to give up smoking, eat better, or manage their stress. Each of these concerns represents a career development possibility that you can pursue through additional education and training.

Lifestyle fitness coaching falls under the wide umbrella of the helping professions, as do most roles in the health fitness professions. Although coaching may be a new direction for you now, your experiences in this field may direct you toward greater concentration or toward wider application. The choice will always be yours.

Your Life As a Coach

How you want your career to develop and how much emphasis you choose to give to coaching will be informed partly by your desires and experiences and partly by your personal evolution. We cannot easily predict the future, although we may nonetheless plan for it. Once you embark on a course of learning and development associated with coaching, certain outcomes will become more likely. Understanding the skills and processes of coaching has the power to change you—predictably for the better. As you learn to listen well to others, you will likely learn to listen to yourself better. As you express care and concern for the dilemmas that clients experience, you will most likely become more empathic to your own struggles and challenges.

As you accompany your clients along the path of change, you will probably develop an intuitive understanding of how you can better manage your own passages and transitions.

Becoming an outstanding coach is about becoming the best of yourself. You are a work in progress, and the course that you have chosen will nurture and advance your growth and development as surely as it does that of your clients. May you realize your dreams and may all life's surprises be transformed into new opportunities for personal actualization.

Glossary

behavior rehearsal strategy—A technique used widely in sport psychology whereby athletes are encouraged to practice mental imagery of successful or enhanced sport performance under conditions of alert relaxation.

bio-psycho-socio-cultural—A reference to significant dimensions of human behavior encompassing biological, psychological, social, and cultural factors.

boundary crossing—An ethical matter in which a coach engages in some behavior with the client that holds the potential for jeopardizing the integrity of the relationship, e.g., attending a social event at the client's home.

boundary violation—An ethical matter in which a coach engages in some behavior with the client that jeopardizes the integrity of the relationship, e.g., going on a date with the client.

closed question—A type of questioning in a coaching process that limits the requested response from the client and thereby enables the coach to gather specific information and control the communication flow.

closure—In the context of coaching, refers to the process of ending or terminating the formal or contracted relationship with the client. Closure ideally involves a dialogue and may evolve over a number of sessions.

confrontation—A coaching skill whereby the coach presents to the client evidence of his or her discrepant or inconsistent behaviors or types of information for consideration in service of the client's developmental goals.

containment—Refers to the coach's ability to create safety for the client as the client expresses difficult personal issues or even intense emotions toward the coach.

core relationship conditions—Those qualities often including trustworthiness, expertise, genuineness, and empathy that coaches need to demonstrate in relationship to clients so that clients can effectively engage the process of coaching.

counterdependent—A term referring to a client's behavior pattern indicating resistance to direction or any form of influence by the coach.

countertransference—Indicates the projection onto the client by the coach of feelings, attitudes, or behaviors originating in the coach's relationship with another significant individual in the coach's personal history. Also described as an unreal aspect of the relationship.

dyadic relationship—A term from social psychology referring to behaviors occurring between two individuals who have some sort of temporary or ongoing relation.

ecologically valid goals—Refers to the integrity and validity of goals when considered from diverse perspectives of a person's life. Goals of this nature make sense by addressing multiple needs and fitting into the person's framework for life.

emotional intelligence—In contrast to the classic notion of IQ, this term encompasses a person's wisdom in emotional and social contexts. Similar to the concept of common sense.

espoused theories of action—What people believe or say they do in certain situations, as distinguished from what they actually do.

extrinsic motivation—A type of motivation seen in situations where individuals pursue action in order to achieve some valued outcome (e.g., weight loss) rather than for the experience of the activity itself.

feedback—A coaching skill whereby the coach sensitively presents to the client information, observations, or results of client behaviors to support the client's development and reinforce patterns.

holding environment—A phrase borrowed from counseling and psychotherapy encompassing the safety and trustworthiness of the relationship created by the coach for the client.

identification—A process whereby coaches experience clients' reality in such a manner that they take on the clients' issues as if they were their own.

immediacy—Combining such skills as confrontation and self-disclosure, this coaching skill focuses on the expression of what is happening in the moment in the coaching process, either with the client, within the coach, or in their relationship.

implicit personality theory—Refers to the ideas that individuals have about why people do what they do. It is an informal or personally developed theory about human behavior that most people have generated from their own observations and experiences.

indirect question—A coaching skill whereby the coach requests information from the client in a declarative sentence that implies to the client that certain information is needed in the dialogue.

interpretation—A coaching skill whereby the coach provides new perspectives or ways in which the client can understand issues through a variety of techniques including identifying unstated feelings, reframing, metaphors, or story telling.

intervention—In the context of coaches' engagements with clients, refers to any intentional action to address issues and influence client behavior in a desired direction.

intrinsic motivation—A type of motivation seen in situations where individuals pursue action for pleasure, learning, mastery, or aesthetic enjoyment. Motivation of this nature is associated with the activity itself rather than with outcomes achieved from the activity.

kinesics—The formal study of body motions including but not limited to all forms of nonverbal communication.

life coaching—A relatively new field of assisting normally functioning individuals to address needs and pursue goals through supportive dialogue and structured methods of facilitating change.

lifestyle converter—Someone who is so convinced about the value of certain attitudes, beliefs, or behaviors that he or she actively attempts to make others conform to what he or she believes to be right.

mind methods—Approaches to personal development, change, or therapy that rely on verbal behaviors, imagery, or other thought processes.

Mind methods can be explored with the aid of another person, such as a counselor, or can be self-guided.

minimal encouragers—An aspect of coaching behaviors whereby coaches acknowledge clients' verbalizations or behaviors with brief reference or audible expressions such as "Mmmm hmmm" to reinforce client expression and openness.

neurolinguistic programming, or NLP—A method of understanding human behavior and interpersonal communications focusing on individual patterns that can be used in processes of behavior change.

open question—A type of questioning in a coaching process in which the coach invites the client to expand on a theme or subject so that salient issues can be explored in depth.

outcome goals—Goals that typically focus on the result or end of some activity such as physical training. Outcome goals may include weight loss or winning a contest.

paradigm shift—Refers to instances in which a significant new perspective arises in an area of knowledge, skill, or understanding and brings about questioning or reevaluation of old models or approaches.

paralinguistics—The study of nonverbal aspects of speech including tone, volume, speed, and pauses.

performance goals—Goals of behavior or performance that are independent of others' actions. Examples include learning how to swim or running a distance in a specified time.

personality—The sum total of all the characteristics that makes each person unique. Personality is the characteristic ways in which people behave, especially in relationships with other people. Personality also shows itself in a person's habitual emotional responses to life.

process goals—Goals that emphasize the actions or even the qualities that one wishes to characterize behavior, such as enjoyment or pleasure while engaged in certain actions.

proxemics—The study of physical distances of individuals in social settings and their implications for and effects on these individuals.

psychosocial—A characteristic of thoughts, feelings, or actions that represents both psychological and social dimensions. Psychosocial behaviors, for example, are thought to reflect intrapsychic or internal processes along with social ones.

reflection of content—A coaching skill involving the coach's sensitive mirroring of information provided in a segment of a client's communication to the coach.

reflection of feeling—A coaching skill involving the coach's sensitive mirroring of the emotional or feeling elements of a client's communications to the coach.

reflection of meaning—A coaching skill that relies on such skills as questioning to help the client uncover a deeper appreciation and awareness of issues.

reframe—A form of the coaching skill of interpretation whereby the coach reorganizes the client's messages and communicates them back in a way that offers more options and potential for change.

relapse—Behavioral incidents in which a person reverts to a previous pattern of action that he or she had deliberately altered, usually in the pursuit of some health or wellness goal. For instance, relapse would be seen in a person smoking a cigarette after having stopped for a period of months.

self-disclosure—A coaching skill whereby the coach strategically reveals personal information or tells personal stories to support the client's progress and goal attainment.

self-fulfilling prophecy—Based on a theory that suggests that when people expect themselves to behave in certain ways, typically reinforced by the feedback and opinions of others, their behavior conforms to these expectations—for better or worse.

sport personology—The research and theory relating personality typologies with choices of or participation in different sports.

summarizing—A coaching skill whereby the coach mirrors back to the client key elements of a lengthy segment of communication or similar themes in client communication across a series of sessions.

theories-in-use—What people actually do in situations, as distinguished from what they believe or say they do.

transference—Indicates the projection onto the coach by the client of feelings, attitudes, or behaviors originating in the client's relationship with another significant individual in the client's history. Also described as an unreal aspect of the relationship.

working alliance—A phrase popular in counseling and psychotherapy referring to the agreement and collaboration of coach and client in engaging necessary tasks and patterns of relationship toward the attainment of desired outcomes.

worldview—An individual's personalized perspective incorporating beliefs about why things are the way they are, why people function as they do, how situations evolve, and what matters in life.

References

Abernathy, B. (2001). Attention. In R. Singer, H. Hausen-blas, & C. Janelle (Eds.), *Handbook of sport psychology* (2nd ed., pp. 53-85). New York: Wiley.

American College of Sports Medicine. (2000). *ACSM's guidelines for exercise testing and prescription* (6th ed.). Philadelphia: Lippincott, Williams, & Wilkins.

American Psychological Association (2002). Ethical principles of psychologists and code of conduct. *American Psychologist, 57*(12), 1060-1073.

Argyris, C. (1970). *Intervention theory and method: A behavioral science view.* Reading, MA: Addison-Wesley.

Argyris, C., & Schon, D.A. (1974). *Theory in practice.* San Francisco: Jossey-Bass.

Armbruster, B., & Gladwin, L.A. (2002). Who exercises and who doesn't? New report gives insights. *Club Success: Successful Strategies for Fitness Industry Professionals, 8*(6), 18-21.

Arms, R.L., Russell, G.W., & Sandilands, M.L. (1979). Effects of viewing aggressive sports on the hostility of spectators. *Social Psychology Quarterly, 42,* 275-279.

Arnot, R.B., & Gaines, C.L. (1984). *Sportselection.* New York: Viking Press.

Atkins, D. (2002). Know your role. *American Fitness, 20*(4), 34-36.

Baker Miller, J. (1991). The development of a woman's sense of self. In J. Jordan, A. Kaplan, J. Baker Miller, I. Stiver, & J. Surrey, (Eds.), *Women's growth in connection* (pp. 11-26). New York: Guilford.

Baker Miller, J., Stiver, I., & Hooks, T. (Eds.). (1998). *The healing connection: How women form relationships in therapy and in life.* Boston: Beacon.

Bandura, A. (1969). *Principles of behavior modification.* New York: Holt, Rinehart, & Winston.

Bandura, A. (1977). *Social learning theory.* Englewood Cliffs, NJ: Prentice-Hall.

Barak, A., Patkin, J., & Dell, D.M. (1982). Effects of certain counselor behaviors in perceived expertness and attractiveness. *Journal of Counseling Psychology, 29,* 261-267.

Baron, R.A., & Richardson, D.R. (1994). *Human aggression.* New York: Plenum Press.

Beauchamp, T.L., & Childress, J.S. (1983). *Principles of biomedical ethics* (2nd ed.). New York: Oxford University Press.

Beck, A.T. (1976). *Cognitive therapy and the emotional disorders.* New York: International University Press.

Beck, J.S. (1995). *Cognitive therapy: Basics and beyond.* New York: Guilford.

Belf, T. (2002). *Coaching with spirit: Allowing success to emerge.* San Francisco: Jossey-Bass/Pfeiffer.

Benefits of a working relationship between medical and allied health practitioners and personal fitness trainers. (2001, September). *IDEA Health and Fitness Source, 19*(8), 48-54.

Bennis, W.G., & Shepard, H.A. (1956). A theory of group development. *Human Relations, 9,* 415-437.

Benson, H., & Stuart, E.M. (Eds.). (1992). *The wellness book: The comprehensive guide to maintaining health and treating stress-related illness.* New York: Birch Lane.

Berger, B.G., & Owen, D.R. (1992). Mood alteration with yoga and swimming: Aerobic exercise may not be necessary. *Perceptual & Motor Skills, 75*(3, pt. 2), 1331-1343.

Berne, E. (1961). *Transactional analysis in psychotherapy.* New York: Grove.

Berne, E. (1964). *Games people play.* New York: Grove.

Binswanger, L. (1963). *Being-in-the-world: Selected papers of Ludwig Binswanger.* New York: Basic Books.

Birdwhistle, R.L. (1970). *Kinesics and context.* Philadelphia: University of Pennsylvania Press.

Blair, S.N., & Brodney, S. (2000). The economic burden of physical inactivity in Canada. *Canadian Medical Association Journal, 163*(11), 1435-1440.

Bohm, D., & L. Nichol, (1996). *On dialogue.* New York: Routledge.

Bordin, E.S. (1979). The generalizability of the psychoanalytic concept of the working alliance. *Psychotherapy: Theory, Research & Practice, 16*(3), 252-260.

Brammer, L. (1985). *The helping relationship.* Upper Saddle River, NJ: Prentice-Hall.

Brammer, L., Abrego, P., & Shostrom, E. (1993). *Therapeutic counseling and psychotherapy* (6th ed.). Upper Saddle River, NJ: Prentice-Hall.

Brammer, L., & MacDonald, G. (1999). *The helping relationship: Process and skills* (7th ed.). Boston: Allyn and Bacon.

Brems, C. (2001). *Basic skills in psychotherapy and counseling.* Belmont, CA: Brooks/Cole.

Bridges, W. (2001). *The way of transition: Embracing life's most difficult moments.* Cambridge, MA: Perseus.

Brown, D., & Srebalus, D.J. (2003). *Introduction to the counseling profession* (3rd ed.). Boston: Allyn and Bacon.

Brownlee, S. (2002, January 21). Too heavy, too young. *Time Magazine,* 60-62.

Bruhn, J.G., Levine, H.G., & Levine, P.L. (1993). *Managing boundaries in the helping professions.* Springfield, IL: Charles C Thomas.

Buckworth, J., & Dishman, R.K. (2002). *Exercise psychology.* Champaign, IL: Human Kinetics.

Bugental, J.F.T. (1965). *The search for authenticity.* New York: Holt, Rinehart & Winston.

Byrnes, J.P., Miller, D.C., & Schafer, W.D. (1999). Gender differences in risk-taking: A meta-analysis. *Psychological Bulletin, 125,* 367-383.

Cantwell, S. (2003, Feb./Mar.). Lifestyle coaching. *Fitness Trainer Canada, 3*(1), 10-15.

Cantwell, S., & Rothenberg, B. (2000, July/Aug.). The benefits of lifestyle coaching. *IDEA Personal Trainer, 11*(7), 24-35.

Capuzzi, D., & Gross, D.R. (2001). *Introduction to the counseling profession* (3rd ed). Boston: Allyn and Bacon.

Carkhuff, R.R., & Berenson, B.G. (1977). *Beyond counseling and therapy.* New York: Holt, Rinehard and Winston.

Carson, R. (1990). *Never get a tattoo: Simple advice on the art of enjoying yourself* (p. 13). New York: Harper and Row.

Cashdan, S. (1988). *Object relations therapy: Using the relationship.* New York: W.W. Norton.

Cattell, R.B. (1965). *The scientific analysis of personality.* Baltimore: Penguin.

Centers for Disease Control and Prevention (2003). CDC surveys physical activity levels. *Journal of Physical Education, Recreation & Dance, 74*(7), 12.

Chapman, D.Y., & Osterweil, D. (2001, June). Working with clients with Alzheimer's disease. *IDEA Health and Fitness Source, 19*(6), 56-66.

Chodzko-Zajko, W. (2000). Successful aging in the new millennium: The role of regular physical activity. *Quest, 52*(4), 333-343.

Clark, A.J. (1995). An examination of the technique of interpretation in counseling. *Journal of Counseling and Development, 73,* 483-490.

Compton, B., & Galaway, B. (1984). *Social work processes* (3rd ed.). Homewood, IL: Dorsey Press.

Coonerty, S.M. (1991). Change in the change agent's growth in the capacity to heal. In R.C. Curtis & G. Stricker (Eds.), *How people change: Inside and outside therapy* (pp. 81-97). New York: Plenum.

Cooper, K.H. (1977). *The aerobics way.* New York: Bantam.

Corey, G., Corey, M., & Callanan, P. (2003). *Issues and ethics in the helping professions* (6th ed). Pacific Grove, CA: Brooks/Cole.

Corliss, R. (2001, June 4). The power of yoga. *Time Magazine, 157*(22), 34-45.

Cormier, W.H., & Cormier, L.S. (1991). *Interviewing strategies for helpers: Fundamental skills and cognitive behavioral interventions* (3rd ed). Pacific Grove, CA: Brooks/Cole.

Cormier, S., & Nurius, P.S. (2003). *Interviewing and change strategies for helpers: Fundamental skills and cognitive behavioral interventions* (5th ed). Pacific Grove, CA: Brooks/Cole.

Cotton, R.T., & Andersen, R.E. (Eds.). (1999). *Clinical exercise specialist manual.* San Diego: American Council on Exercise.

Coven, E. (2003, March). Helping seniors cope with illness and loss. *IDEA Health and Fitness Source, 21*(3), 58-61.

Covington, C. (2002). The myth of pure analysis. *Journal of Analytical Psychology, 47*(1), 101-111.

Cozby, P.C. (1973). Self-disclosure: A literature review. *Psychological Bulletin, 79,* 73-91.

Dalleck, L.C., & Kravitz, L. (2002, January). The history of fitness. *IDEA Health and Fitness Source, 20*(1), 26-33.

Danish, S.J., Nellon, V.C., & Owens, S.S. (1996). Teaching life skills through sport: Community-based programs for adolescents. In J.L. Van Raalte & B. Brewer (Eds.), *Exploring sport and exercise psychology* (pp. 205-225). New York: American Psychological Association.

Day, J. (1995). Obligation and motivation: Obstacles and resources for counselor well-being and effectiveness. *Journal of Counseling and Development, 73,* 108-110.

de Shazer, S. (1985). *Keys to solutions in brief therapy.* New York: Norton.

Diamant, L. (Ed.). (1991). *Mind body maturity: Psychological approaches to sports, exercise, and fitness.* New York: Hemisphere.

Dishman, R.K. (1985). Medical psychology in exercise and sport. *Medical Clinics of North America, 69* (January), 123-143.

Dishman, R.K. (Ed.). (1988). *Exercise adherence: Its impact on public health.* Champaign, IL: Human Kinetics.

Dishman, R.K., & Buckworth, J. (1997). Adherence to physical activity. In W.P. Morgan (Ed.), *Physical activity and mental health* (pp. 63-80). Washington, DC: Taylor and Francis.

Dishman, R.K., Sallis, J.K., & Orenstein, D.R. (1985). The determinants of physical activity and exercise. *Public Health Reports, 100*(2), 158-171.

Dollard, J., Doob, J., Miller, N., Mowrer, O., & Sears, R. (1939). *Frustration and aggression.* New Haven, CT: Yale University Press.

Donatelle, R.J., Davis, L.G., Munroe, A.J., & Munroe, A. (2001). *Health: The basics.* Toronto: Allyn & Bacon.

Donley, R.J., Horan, J.J., & DeShong, R.L. (1990). The effect of several self-disclosure permutations on counseling process and outcome. *Journal of Counseling and Development, 67,* 408-412.

Douillard, J. (1988). *Body, mind and sport.* Santa Monica, CA: Hay House.

Douillard, J. (1994). *Body, mind and sport.* (p. 33). New York: Crown Trade.

Dowda, M., Ainsworth, B.E., Addy, C.L., Saunders, R., & Riner, W. (2003). Correlates of physical activity among U.S. young adults, 18 to 30 years of age, from NHANES III. *Annals of Behavioral Medicine, 26*(1), 15-23.

Downs, C.W., Smeyak, G.P., & Martin, E. (1980). *Professional interviewing.* New York: Harper & Row.

Durand, V.M., & Barlow, D.H. (1997). *Abnormal psychology: An introduction.* Pacific Grove, CA: Brooks/Cole.

Dunn, J.G. (1994). Toward the combined use of nomothetic and idiographic methodologies in sport psychology: An empirical example. *Sport Psychologist, 8*(4), 376-392.

Durrett, A. (2002, June). Opportunities in postrehab. *IDEA Personal Trainer, 13*(6), 18-25.

Dychtwald, K. (1977). *Bodymind.* New York: Pantheon.

Dym, B., Jenks, R.S., & Sonduck, M. (2002). Coaching entrepreneurs. In C. Fitzgerald & J.G. Berger (Eds.), *Executive coaching: Practices and perspectives* (pp. 325-344). Palo Alto, CA: Davies-Black.

Edwards, C., & Murdock, N. (1994). Characteristics of therapist self-disclosure in the counseling process. *Journal of Counseling and Development, 72,* 384-389.

Egan, G. (1998). *The skilled helper* (5th ed.). Monterey, CA: Brooks/Cole.

Egan, G. (2002). *The skilled helper* (6th ed.). Pacific Grove, CA: Brooks/Cole.

Eickhoff-Shemek, J.A. (1997). Closing remarks: Progress, potential, and problems in the holistic study of physical activity. In J.E. Curtis, & S.J. Russell (Eds.), *Physical activity in human experience: Interdisciplinary perspectives* (pp. 267-277). Champaign, IL: Human Kinetics.

Ekman, P. (1982). Methods for measuring facial action. In K.R. Schereer & P. Ekman (Eds.), *Handbook of methods in nonverbal behavior research* (pp. 45-135). New York: Cambridge University Press.

Ekman, P. (1993). Facial expression and emotion. *American Psychologist, 48,* 384-392.

Elinor, L., & Gerard, G. (1998). *Dialogue: Rediscovering the transforming power of conversation.* New York: John Wiley and Sons.

Ellis, A. (1994). *Reason and emotion in psychotherapy* (Rev. ed.). New York: Birch Lane Press.

Epidemiology of mental illness. (1994, February). *Medical Sciences Bulletin.* Pharmaceutical Information Associates.

Evans, U.R. (1979). *Essential interviewing.* Belmont, CA: Wadsworth.

Eysenck, H.J., & Eysenck, S.B.G. (1968). *Eysenck personality inventory manual.* London: University of London Press.

Farley, F. (1986). The big T in personality. *Psychology Today, 20*(5), 44-52.

Farrell, P.A. (2001). Hear this: Sharpening your communication and listening skills. In S. Cullari (Ed.), *Counseling and psychotherapy: A practical guidebook for students, trainees, and new professionals* (pp. 59-91). Boston: Allyn & Bacon.

Fast, J. (1989). *Body language.* New York: Pocket Books.

Fay, T., & Doolittle, S. (2002). Agents for change: From standards to assessment to accountability in physical education. *Journal of Physical Education, Recreation and Dance, 73*(3), 29-33.

Feldman, R.S. (2000). *Development across the life span* (2nd ed.). Upper Saddle River, NJ: Prentice-Hall.

Festinger, L. (1957). *A theory of cognitive dissonance.* Stanford, CA: Stanford University Press.

Filby, W., Maynard, I., & Graydon, J. (1999). The effect of multiple-goal strategies on performance outcomes in training and competition. *Journal of Applied Sport Psychology, 11,* 230-246.

Fitzgerald, C., & Berger, J.G. (Eds.). (2002). *Executive coaching: Practices and perspectives.* Palo Alto, CA: Davies-Black.

Flippin, R. (1987, March). Are runners better lovers? *Runner,* pp. 32-36.

Frank, J.D., & Frank, J.B. (1993). *Persuasion and healing: A comparative study of psychotherapy* (3rd ed.). Baltimore: Johns Hopkins University Press.

Frank, R. (2001). *Body of awareness: A somatic and developmental approach to psychotherapy.* Cambridge, MA: GestaltPress Book.

Frankl, V. (1969). *The will to meaning: Foundations and applications of logotherapy.* New York: New American Library.

Fraser, S.N., & Spink, K.S. (2002). Examining the role of social support and group cohesion in exercise compliance. *Journal of Behavioral Medicine, 25*(3), 233-249.

Frauman, D.C. (1982). The relationship between physical exercise, sexual activity, and the desire for sexual activity. *Journal of Sex Research, 18*(1), 41-46.

French, J.R.P., & Raven, B. (1959). The bases of social power. In D. Cartwright (Ed.), *Studies in social power* (pp. 150-167). Oxford, England: University of Michigan.

Freud, S. (1964). *The standard edition of the complete psychological works of Sigmund Freud* (Ed. J. Strachey). Oxford, England: Macmillan.

Friedman, M. (1996). *Type A behavior: Its diagnosis and treatment.* New York: Plenum Press.

Fuller, J.R. (1988). Martial arts and psychological health. *British Journal of Medical Psychology, 61*(4), 317-328

Furnham, A. (1990). Personality and demographic determinants of leisure and sports preference and performance. *International Journal of Sport Psychology, 21*(3), 218-236.

Gabbard, G.O. (1995). Countertransference: The emerging common ground. *International Journal of Psychoanalysis, 76,* 475-485.

Garvin, C.D., & Seabury, B.A. (1984). *Interpersonal practice in social work: Processes and procedures.* Englewood Cliffs, NJ: Prentice Hall.

Gavin, J. (1988). *Bodymoves: The psychology of exercise.* Harrisburg, PA: Stackpole Books.

Gavin, J. (1991). If Sigmund Freud were a personal trainer . . . World IDEA: The Health and Fitness Source. Los Angeles.

Gavin, J. (1992). *The exercise habit.* Champaign, IL: Human Kinetics.

Gavin, J. (1997, October). The psychology of movement. *IDEA Today,* pp. 52-58.

Gavin, J. (2000, May). Understanding psychoanatomy. *IDEA Health and Fitness Source, 18*(5), 61-66.

Gavin, J. (2002). The emotional shaping of human anatomy. *IDEA Personal Trainer, 13*(5), 18-27.

Gavin, J. (2003). Fitness personality: Fact or fiction. *Fitness Business Canada, 4*(6), 45-51.

Gavin, J. (2004). Technical manual for MAPS: Matching activity and personal styles. Unpublished manuscript. Montreal, Quebec, Concordia University.

Gavin, J., & Gavin, N. (1995). *Psychology for health fitness professionals.* Champaign, IL: Human Kinetics.

Gavin, J., & Gavin, N. (2004). Put on your game face. *IDEA Fitness Journal, 1*(2), 38-43.

Gavin, J.F., & Lister, S. (2001). The strategic use of sports and fitness activities for promoting psychosocial skill development in childhood and adolescence. *Journal of Child and Adolescent Care, 15-16,* 325-343.

Gavin, J., & Spitzer, A.M. (2002). The psychology of exercise. *IDEA Health and Fitness Source, 20*(9), 46-53.

Gavin, J., & Taylor, M.M. (1990). Adaptation to sports injuries: Phases of the rehabilitation process. Annual Convention of the American Psychological Association, Boston.

Gazda, G.M., Asbury, F.S., Balzer, F., Childers, W.C., Phelps, R.E., & Walters, R.P. (1999). *Human relations development: A manual for educators* (6th ed.). Needham, MA: Allyn & Bacon.

Gelso, C.J., & Fretz, B.R. (1992). *Counseling psychology.* Fort Worth, TX: Harcourt Brace Jovanovich.

Gendlin, E. (1981). *Focusing.* New York: Bantam Books.

Gibson, R.L., & Mitchell, M.H. (2003). *Introduction to counseling and guidance* (6th ed.). Upper Saddle River, NJ: Merrill Prentice Hall.

Gill, D. (2000). *Psychological dynamics of sport and exercise.* Champaign, IL: Human Kinetics.

Gilliland, B.E., & James, R.K. (1998). *Theories and strategies in counseling and psychotherapy* (4th ed.). Needham Heights, MA: Allyn & Bacon.

Gladding, S.T. (2000). *Counseling: A comprehensive profession* (4th ed.). Upper Saddle River, NJ: Prentice Hall.

Goldman, C. (2001). *Healing words for the body, mind and spirit: 101 words to inspire and affirm.* New York: Marlowe.

Goldstein, A.P., & Higginbotham, H.N. (1991). Relationship-enhancement methods. In F.H. Kanfer & A.P. Goldstein (Eds.), *Helping people change* (4th ed., pp. 20-69). New York: Pergamon.

Goleman, D. (1995). *Emotional intelligence.* New York: Bantam

Gorman, C. (2001, February 5). Repairing the damage. *Time Magazine,* pp. 47-52

Green, H. (1986). *Fit for America. Health, fitness, sport, and American society.* New York: Pantheon Books.

Greenson, R.R. (1967). *The technique and practice of psychoanalysis* (Vol. 1). Madison, CT: International University Press.

Greist, J.H., Klein, M.H., Eischens, R.R., Faris, J., Gurman, A.S., & Morgan, W.P. (1979). Running as treatment for depression. *Comprehensive Psychiatry, 20,* (1), 41-54.

Griffin, J. (1998). *Client-centered exercise prescription.* Champaign, IL: Human Kinetics.

Grinder, J., & Bandler, J. (1976). *The structure of magic: I & II.* Oxford, England: Science & Behavior.

Hackney, H.L. (2000). *Practice issues for the beginning counselor.* Boston: Allyn & Bacon.

Hackney, H.L., & Cormier, L.S. (2001). *The professional counselor: A process guide to helping* (4th ed). Boston: Allyn and Bacon.

Hall, E.T. (1966). *The hidden dimension.* Garden City, NY: Doubleday.

Hall, E.T. (1976). *Beyond culture.* New York: Anchor Press.

Hansen, C.J., Stevens, L.C., & Coast, J.R. (2001). Exercise duration and mood state: How much is enough to feel better? *Health Psychology, 20*(4), 267-75.

Harrison, R. (1970). Choosing the depth of organizational intervention. *Journal of Applied Behavioral Science, 6*(2), 181-202.

Hays, K. (1999). *Working it out: Using exercise in psychotherapy.* Washington, DC: American Psychological Association.

Hays, K. (2002). *Move your body, tone your mood.* Oakland, CA: New Harbinger.

Hellmich, N. (2003, May 15). Fifth of Americans report exercise in daily routines. *USA Today,* p. D12.

Helms, J., & Cook, D. (1999). *Using race and culture in counseling and psychotherapy.* Needham Heights, MA: Allyn & Bacon.

Hendrick, S.S. (1988). Counselor self-disclosure. *Journal of Counseling and Development, 66*(9), 419-424.

Hendrix, H. (2001). *Getting the love you want: A guide for couples.* New York: Owl Books.

Heppner, P.P., & Heesacker, M. (1982). Interpersonal influence process in real-life counseling: Investigating client perceptions, counselor experience level, and counselor power over time. *Journal of Counseling Psychology, 29,* 215-223.

Hepworth, D., Rooney, R., & Larsen, J.A. (1997). *Direct social work practice: Theory and skills* (5th ed.). Pacific Grove, CA: Brooks/Cole.

Hepworth, D., Rooney, R., & Larsen, J.A. (2002). *Direct social work practice: Theory and skills* (6th ed.). Pacific Grove, CA: Brooks/Cole.

Herlihy, B., & Corey, G. (1997). *Boundary issues in counseling: Multiple roles and responsibilities.* Alexandria, VA: American Counseling Association.

Heyward, V.H. (2002). *Advanced fitness assessment and exercise prescription* (4th ed.). Champaign, IL: Human Kinetics.

Hoelter, J.W. (1985). A structural theory of personal consistency. *Social Psychology Quarterly, 48*(2), 118-129.

Holland, J.L. (1985). *Self-directed search manual.* Odessa, FL: Psychological Assessment Resources.

Hubble, M.A., Duncan, B.L., & Miller, S.D. (Eds.). (1999). *The heart and soul of change: What works in therapy.* Washington, DC: American Psychological Association.

Hutchins, D., & Vaught, C.C. (1997). *Helping relationships and strategies* (3rd ed.). Pacific Grove, CA: Brooks/Cole.

IDEA Code of Ethics for Personal Fitness Trainers. (2002, July/Aug.). *IDEA Health and Fitness Source, 20*(7), 110.

Ivey, A.E., & Ivey, M.B. (2003). *Intentional interviewing and counseling* (5th ed.). Pacific Grove, CA: Brooks/Cole.

Ivey, A.E., Ivey, M.B., & Simek-Downing, L. (1987). *Counseling and psychotherapy: Skills, theory and practice* (2nd ed.). Englewood Cliffs, NJ: Prentice-Hall.

Ivey, A.E., Ivey, M.B., & Simek-Morgan, L. (1997). *Counseling and psychotherapy: A multicultural perspective* (4th ed.). Boston: Allyn & Bacon.

Jackson, S., & Csikszentmihalyi, M. (1999). *Flow in sports.* Champaign, IL: Human Kinetics.

Jacobson, E. (1938). *Progressive relaxation.* Chicago: University of Chicago Press.

Johnson, D.W. (2003a). *Reaching out: Interpersonal effectiveness and self-actualization* (7th ed.). Needham Heights, MA: Allyn and Bacon.

Johnson, L. (1997). *ACSM's health/fitness facility standards and guidelines* (2nd ed). Champaign, IL: Human Kinetics.

Johnson, N.G. (2003b). Psychology and health. *American Psychologist, 58*(8), 670-677.

Jones, F., & Bright, J. (Eds.). (2001). *Stress: Myth, theory and research.* Upper Saddle River, NJ: Prentice Hall.

Jourard, S.M. (1958). *Personal adjustment: An approach through the study of healthy personality.* New York: Macmillan.

Jourard, S.M. (1964). *The transparent self: Self-disclosure and well-being.* Princeton, NJ: Van Nostrand.

Jourard, S.M. (1968). *Disclosing man to himself.* Princeton, NJ: Van Nostrand.

Kass, R. (2004). *Theories of small group development* (3rd ed.). Montreal, QC: Centre for Human Relations and Community Studies.

Katzmarzyk, P.T., Gledhill, N., and Shephard, R.J. (2002). Exercise as medicine: Convincing evidence. *IDEA Health and Fitness Source, 20*(9), 11-13.

Kazdin, A.E. (2001). *Behavior modification in applied settings* (6th ed.). Pacific Grove, CA: Brooks/Cole.

Kazdin, A.E., & Wassell, G. (1998). Treatment completion and therapeutic change among children referred for outpatient therapy. *Professional Psychology: Research and Practice, 29* (4), 332-340.

Kelly, G. (1955). *The psychology of personal constructs* (Vol. 1 and 2). New York: Norton.

Kepner, J. (1993). *Body process: Working with the body in psychotherapy.* New York: Jossey-Bass.

Kleinke, C.L. (1994). *Common principles of psychotherapy.* Pacific Grove, CA: Brooks/Cole.

Knapp, , M.L., & Hall, J. (1997). *Nonverbal communication in human interaction* (5th ed.). Orlando, FL: Holt, Rinehart & Winston.

Knox, S., Hess, S., Petersen, D., & Hill, C.E. (1997). A qualitative analysis of client perceptions of helpful therapist self-disclosure in long-term therapy. *Journal of Counseling Psychology, 44,* 274-283.

Kohut, H. (1984). *How does analysis cure?* Chicago: University of Chicago Press.

Koocher, G.P., & Keith-Speigel, P. (1998). *Ethics in psychology: Professional standard and cases* (2nd ed.). New York: Oxford University Press.

Kottler, J.A. (2000). *The nuts and bolts of helping.* Boston: Allyn and Bacon.

Krueger, D.W. (2002). *Integrating body self and psychological self: Creating a new story in psychoanalysis and psychotherapy.* New York: Brunner-Routledge.

Kurz, R., & Prestera, H. (1976). *The body reveals: An illustrated guide to the psychology of the body.* New York: Harper & Row.

Lamb, W., & Watson, E. (1994). *Body code: The meaning in movement.* Princeton, NJ: Princeton Book Company.

Larsen, K. (2002, July). What is lifestyle coaching? *Attendee Handout Book* (pp. 46-51), IDEA Personal Trainer International Summit West. San Diego: IDEA Health and Fitness.

Lawrence, S.A. (2002). Behavioral interventions to increase physical activity. *Journal of Human Behavior in the Social Environment, 6*(1), 25-44.

Lazarus, R.S. (1999). *Stress and emotion.* London: Free Association Books.

Lecomte, C., Bernstein, B.L., & Dumont, F. (1981). Counseling interactions as a function of spatial-environmental conditions. *Journal of Counseling Psychology, 28,* 536-539.

Lee, I.M. (1995). Exercise and physical health: Cancer and immune function. *Research Quarterly for Exercise and Sport, 66*(4), 286-291.

Leith, L.M. (1994). *Foundations of exercise and mental health.* Morgantown, WV: Fitness Information Technology.

LeUnes, A.D., & Nation, J.R. (2002). *Sport psychology: An introduction* (3rd ed.). Pacific Grove, CA: Wadsworth.

Levin, F.M., & Gergen, K.J. (1969). Revealingness, ingratiation, and the disclosure of self. *Proceedings of the 77th Annual Convention of the American Psychological Association, 4*(1), 447-448.

Levinson, H. (1976). *Psychological man.* Oxford, England: Levinson Institute.

Lidane, L. (2003, July/Aug.). The certification balance: How should certifications evolve? *IDEA Health and Fitness Source, 21*(7), 22-29.

Locke, E.A. (1968). Toward a theory of task motivation and incentives. *Organizational Behavior and Human Performance, 3,* 157-189.

Locke, E.A., & Latham, G.P. (1985). The application of goal setting to sports. *Journal of Sport Psychology, 7,* 205-222).

Locke, E.A., & Latham, G.P. (1990). Work motivation and satisfaction: Light at the end of the tunnel. *Psychological science, 1*(4), 240-246.

Locke, E.A., Shaw, K.N., Saari, L.M., & Latham, G.P. (1981). Goal setting and task performance: 1969-1980. *Psychological Bulletin, 90,* 125-152.

Lofshult, D. (2003, July/Aug.). Program trends: The 2003 IDEA trendwatch. *IDEA Health and Fitness Source, 21*(7), 70-74.

Luft, J. (1969). *Of human interaction.* Palo Alto, CA: National Press.

Markova, D. (2000). *I will not die an unlived life: Reclaiming purpose and passion* (p. 125). York Beach, ME: Conari Press.

Marlatt, G., & Gordon, J.R. (1985). *Relapse prevention.* New York: Guilford.

Martens, R. (1977). *Sport competition anxiety test.* Champaign, IL: Human Kinetics.

Martin, C. (2001). *The life coaching handbook.* Carmarthen, Wales: Crown House.

Martin Ginis, K.A., Latimer, A.E., & Jung, M.E. (2003). No pain no gain? Examining the generalizability of the exerciser stereotype to moderately active and excessively active targets. *Social Behavior and Personality, 31*(3), 283-290

Maslow, A.H. (1954). *Motivation and personality.* New York: Harper & Row.

Masters, K., & Ogles, B. (1998). Associative and dissociative cognitive strategies in exercise and running 20 years later: What do we know? *Sport Psychologist, 12,* 254-270.

May, R. (1977). *The meaning of anxiety* (Rev. ed.). New York: Norton.

McCarthy, P. (1982). Differential effects of counselor self-referent responses and counselor status. *Journal of Counseling Psychology, 29,* 125-131.

McMillan, S. (2001, June). Help clients get motivated. *IDEA Personal Trainer, 12*(6), 32-40.

McWilliams, J.R. (1991). *Do it! Let's get off our buts.* New York: Bantam.

Meara, N.M., Schmidt, L.D., & Day, J.D. (1996). Principles and virtues: A foundation for ethical decisions, policies, and character. *Counseling Psychologist, 24*(1), 4-77.

Mehr, J.J. (1998). *Human services: Concepts and intervention strategies* (7th ed.). Boston: Allyn and Bacon.

Mehrabian, A., & Bekken, M.L. (1986). Temperament characteristics of individuals who participate in strenuous sports. *Research Quarterly for Exercise and Sports, 57*(2), 160-166.

Melamed, S., & Meir, E.I. (1995). The benefits of personality-leisure congruence: Evidence and implications. *Journal of Leisure Research, 27*(1), 25-40.

Miars, R.D., & Halverson, S.E. (2001). The helping relationship. In D. Capuzzi & D.R. Gross (Eds.), *Introduction to the counseling profession* (3rd ed). Boston: Allyn and Bacon.

Monk, G., Winslade, J., Crocket, K., & Epston, D. (1997). *Narrative theory in practice: The archaeology of hope.* San Francisco: Jossey-Bass.

Montoye, H.J., Kemper, H.C., Saris, W.H., & Washburn, R.A. (1996). *Measuring physical activity and energy expenditure.* Champaign, IL: Human Kinetics.

Moore, T. (2004). *Dark nights of the soul* (p. 24). New York: Gotham Books.

Morgan, W.P. (1979). Negative addiction in runners. *Physician and Sportsmedicine, 7,* 57-70.

Morgan, W.P. (Ed.). (1997). *Physical activity and mental health.* Washington, DC: Taylor and Francis.

Morgan, W.P. (2001). Prescription of physical activity: A paradigm shift. *Quest, 53,* 366-382.

Morgan, W.P., & Goldston, S.E. (1987). *Exercise and mental health.* Washington, DC: Hemisphere.

Murphy, P., Cramer, D., & Lillie, F.J. (1984). The relationship between curative factors perceived by patients in their psychotherapy and treatment outcome: An exploratory study. *British Journal of Medical Psychology, 57,* 187-192.

Murphy, S., & Martin, K. (2002). Athletic imagery. In T. Horn (Ed.), *Advances in sport psychology* (2nd ed., pp. 405-440). Champaign, IL: Human Kinetics.

Murray, E. (1951). Toward a classification of action. In T. Parsons & E.A. Shils (Eds.), *Toward a general theory of action* (pp. 434-464). Cambridge: Harvard University Press.

Nash, J.M. (2003, August 25). Obesity goes global. Reports 37% of children and adolescents in the US are overly fat. *Time Magazine, 162*(8), 39-40.

Neenan, M., & Dryden, W. (2002). *Life coaching: A cognitive-behavioural approach.* East Sussex, UK; Brunner-Routledge.

Nideffer, R.M. (1976). Test of attentional and interpersonal style. *Journal of Personality and Social Psychology, 34,* 394-404.

Nideffer, R.M. (1985). *Athlete's guide to mental training.* Champaign, IL: Human Kinetics.

Nideffer, R.M., & Sagal, M. (2001). Concentration and attention control training. In J.M. Williams (Ed.), *Applied sport psychology: Personal growth to peak performance* (4th ed., pp. 312-332). Mountain View, CA: Mayfield.

North, N. (1972). *Personality assessment through movement.* London: MacDonald and Evans.

O'Brien Cousins, S. (2000). "My heart couldn't take it": Older women's beliefs about exercise benefits and risks. *Journals of Gerontology: Series B: Psychological Sciences & Social Sciences. 55B*(5), 283-294.

O'Connor, J., & Seymour, J. (1990). *Introducing neuro-linguistic programming.* Wellingborough, UK: Aquarian.

O'Hanlon, B., & Weiner-Davis, M. (1989). *In search of solutions: A new direction in psychotherapy.* New York: Norton.

Okun, B.F. (1982). *Effective helping: Interviewing and counseling techniques* (2nd ed.). Monterey, CA: Brooks/Cole.

Oldfield, S. (1983). *The counseling relationship: A study of the client's experience.* London: Routledge & Kegan Paul.

Orlick, T. (1978). *The cooperative sports and games book.* New York: Pantheon.

Parrott, L. (2003). *Counseling and psychotherapy* (2nd ed.). Pacific Grove, CA: Brooks Cole.

Pate, R.R., Pratt, M., Blair, S.N., Haskell, W.L., et al. (1995). Physical activity and public health: A recommendation from the Centers for Disease Control and Prevention and the American College of Sports Medicine. *Journal of the American Medical Association, 273,* 402-407.

Peck, M. Scott (1978). *The road less traveled: A new psychology of love, traditional values and spiritual growth.* New York: Simon & Schuster.

Pekarik, G., & Finney-Owen, K. (1987). Outpatient clinic therapist attitudes and beliefs relevant to client dropout. *Community Mental Health Journal, 23*(2), 120-130.

Pennebaker, J.W. (1990). *Opening up: The healing power of confiding in others.* New York: William Morrow.

Perina, K. (2002). Mastering their domain. *Psychology Today, 35*(6), 15-16.

Perls, F. (1947). *Ego, hunger and aggression: A revision of Freud's theory and method.* Winchester, MA: Allen & Unwin.

Peterson, C., Maier, S.F., & Seligman, M.E.P. (1993). *Learned helplessness: A theory for the age of personal control.* London: Oxford University Press.

Peterson, J.A., & Bryant, C.X. (2001). More than fitness for older adults: A "whole-istic" approach to wellness. *ACSM's Health and Fitness Journal, 5*(2), 6-12, 28.

Piedmont, R.L., Hill, D.C., & Blanco, S. (1999). Redirecting athletic performance using the five-factor model of personality. *Personality and Individual Differences, 27,* 769-777.

Prestera, H., & Kurz, R. (1976). *The body reveals.* New York: Harper & Row.

Prochaska, J.O., & DiClemente, C.C. (1984). *The transtheoretical approach: Crossing the traditional boundaries of therapy.* Homewood, IL: Dow Jones-Irwin.

Prochaska, J.O., & Norcross, J.C. (2003). *Systems of psychotherapy: A transtheoretical analysis* (5th ed.). Pacific Grove, CA: Brooks/Cole.

Prochaska, J.O., Norcross, J.C., & DiClemente, C.C. (1995). *Changing for good.* New York: Avon.

Quenck, N.L. (2000). *Essentials of Myers-Briggs type indicator assessment.* New York: John Wiley & Sons.

Rakos, R.F. (1991). *Assertive behavior: Theory, research, and training.* Florence, KY: Taylor & Frances/ Routledge.

Ray, R., & Weise-Bjornstal, D.M. (1999). *Counseling in sports medicine.* Champaign, IL: Human Kinetics.

Reddy, W.B. (1994). *Intervention skills: Process consultation for small groups and teams.* San Diego: Pfeiffer and Company.

Reich, W. (1949). *Character analysis.* New York: Farrar, Strauss, & Giroux.

Reis, B.B., & Brown, L.G. (1999). Reducing psychotherapy dropouts: Maximizing perspective convergence in the psychotherapy dyad. *Psychotherapy, 36*(2), 123-136.

Resnick, B., Orwig, D., Magaziner, J., & Wynne, C. (2002). The effect of social support on exercise behavior in older adults. *Clinical Nursing Research, 11*(1), 52-70.

Reynolds Welfel, E., & Patterson, L.E. (2005). *The counseling process: A multitheoretical integrative approach.* Belmont, CA: Brooks/Cole.

Roazen, P. (1974). *Freud and his followers.* New York: Random House.

Robinson, T.L., & Howard-Hamilton, M. (2000). *The convergence of race, ethnicity, and gender: Multiple identities in counseling.* Upper Saddle River, NJ: Prentice-Hall.

Rogers, C.R. (1951). *Client-centered therapy: Its current practice, implications, and theory.* Boston: Houghton Mifflin.

Rogers, C.R. (1961). *On becoming a person.* Boston: Houghton Mifflin.

Rogers, C.R. (1967). *Person to person: The problem of being human.* Moab, UT: Real People Press.

Rogers, C.R. (1980). *A way of being.* Boston: Houghton Mifflin.

Rupp, J.C., Campbell, K., Thompson, W.R., & Terbizan, D. (1999). Professional preparation of personal trainers. *Journal of Physical Education, Recreation & Dance, 70*(1), 54-56.

Ryan, R.M., & Deci, E.L. (2000). Self-determination theory and the facilitation of intrinsic motivation, social development and well-being. *American Psychologist, 55,* 68-78.

Sachs, M.L., & Buffone, G.W. (Eds.). (1984). *Running as therapy.* London: University of Nebraska Press.

Sadella, E., Linder, D., & Jenkins, B. (1988). Sport preference: A self-presentational analysis. *Journal of Sport Psychology, 8,* 214-222.

Sage, C. (1977). *Introduction to motor behavior: A neuropsychological approach* (2nd ed.). Reading, MA: Addison-Wesley.

Sage, G. (1998). Does sport affect character development in athletes? *Journal of Physical Education, Recreation and Dance, 69*(1), 15-18.

Sallis, J.F., & Owen, N. (1999). *Physical activity and behavioral medicine.* Thousand Oaks, CA: Sage.

Santana, J.C. (2002, February). Four pillars of human movement. *IDEA Personal Trainer, 13*(20), 20-28.

Schon, D.A. (1983). *The reflective practitioner: How professionals think in action.* New York: Basic Books.

Schultz, P.W., & Searleman, A. (2002). Rigidity of thought and behavior: 100 years of research. *Genetic, Social, & General Psychology Monograph, 128*(2), 165-207.

Seligman, M. (1995). *What you can change, what you can't.* New York: Simon and Schuster

Senge, P.M. (1994). *The fifth discipline: The art and practice of the learning organization.* New York: Doubleday.

Sexton, T.L., & Whiston, S.G. (1994). The status of the counseling relationship: An empirical review, theoretical implications, and research directions. *Counseling Psychologist, 22,* 6-78.

Sexton, T.L., Whiston, S.G., Bleuer, J.C., & Walz, G.R. (1997). *Integrating outcome research into counseling practice and training.* Alexandria, VA: American Counseling Association.

Shebib, B. (1997). *Counseling skills.* Victoria, BC: Province of British Columbia, Ministry of Education, Skills and Training.

Shebib, B. (2003). *Choices: Interviewing and counseling skills for Canadians.* Toronto: Prentice Hall.

Shields, D.L.L., & Bredemeier, B.J.L. (1995). *Character development and physical activity.* Champaign, IL: Human Kinetics.

Silva, J.M. (1979). Assertive and aggressive behavior in sport: A definitional clarification. In C.H. Nadeau, W.R. Halliwell, K.M. Newell, & G.C. Roberts (Eds.), *Psychology of motor behavior and sport* (pp.199-208). Champaign, IL: Human Kinetics.

Simone, D.H., McCarthy, P., & Skay, C.L. (1998). An investigation of client and counselor variables that influence the likelihood of counselor self-disclosure. *Journal of Counseling and Development, 76,* 174-182.

Skinner, B.F. (1938). *The behavior of organisms.* New York: Appleton-Century-Crofts.

Smale, G.G. (1977). *Prophecy, behaviour and change: An examination of self-fulfilling prophecies in helping relationships.* Oxford, England: Routledge & Kegan Paul.

Smith, D., & Fitzpatrick, M. (1995). Patient-therapist boundary issues: An integrative review of theory and research. *Professional Psychology: Research and Practice, 26*(5), 499-506.

Smith, E.W.L. (1985). *The body in psychotherapy.* Jefferson, NC: McFarland.

Smith, H.W. (1994). *The 10 natural laws of successful time and life management: Proven strategies for increased productivity and inner peace.* New York: Warner.

Smith, R.E. (1999). Generalization effects in coping skills training. *Journal of Sport and Exercise Psychology, 21,* 189-204.

Solomon, H.A. (1984). *The exercise myth.* New York: Harcourt Brace Jovanovich.

Spinath, B., Spinath, F.M., Riemann, R., & Angleitner, A. (2003). Implicit theories about personality and intelligence and their relationship to actual personality and intelligence. *Personality & Individual Differences, 35*(4), 939-951.

Stalikas, A., & Fitzpatrick, M. (1995). Client good moments: An intensive analysis of a single session. *Canadian Journal of Counselling, 29*(2), 160-175.

Stalikas, A., & Fitzpatrick, M. (1996). Relationships between counsellor interventions, client experiencing, and emotional expressiveness: An exploratory study. *Canadian Journal of Counselling, 30*(4), 262-271.

Stamford, B.A., & Shimer, P. (1990). *Fitness without exercise.* New York: Warner.

Strean, H.S. (1986). Why therapists lose clients. *Journal of Independent Social Work, 1*(1), 7-17.

Strong, S.R. (1968). Counseling: An interpersonal influence process. *Journal of Counseling Psychology, 39,* 215-224.

Strong, S.R., Welsh, J., Corcoran, J., & Hoyt, W. (1992). Social psychology and counseling psychology: The history, products, and promise of an interface. *Journal of Counseling Psychology, 39,* 139-157.

Sue, D.W., & Sue, D. (1999). *Counseling the culturally different* (3rd ed.). New York: Wiley.

Suinn, R.M. (1986). *Seven steps to peak performance: The mental training manual for athletes.* Lewiston, NY: Huber.

Sullivan, H.S. (1953). *The interpersonal theory of psychiatry.* New York: Norton.

Sweet, C., & Noones, J. (1989). Factors associated with premature termination from outpatient treatment. *Hospital and Community Psychiatry, 40*(9), 947-951.

Tamminem, A.W., & Smaby, M.H. (1981). Helping counselors learn to confront. *Personnel and Guidance Journal, 60,* 41-45.

Taylor, J. (1994). On exercise and sport avoidance: A reply to Dr. Albert Ellis. *Sport Psychologist, 8,* 262-271.

Taylor, M. (1986). Learning for self direction in the classroom: The pattern of a transition process. *Studies in Higher Education, 11*(1), 55-72.

Taylor, M. (1987). Self directed learning: More than meets the observer's eye. In D. Boud & G. Griffin (Eds.), *Appreciating adults learning: From the learner's perspective* (pp. 179-196). London: Kogan Page.

Taylor, M. (1990). Learning and chronic illness behaviour: A new frontier for adult education. *Proceedings: Canadian Association for the Study of Adult Education.*

Taylor, M. (1999). Process ethics for a process world. Presentation to the Organization Development Network Professional Meeting, Ottawa, Ontario, October 5.

Taylor, M.M., & Gavin, J. (1983). *A model for understanding personal change through the learner's perspective*. Dallas: Academy of Management.

Tedeschi, R.G., Park, C.L., & Calhoun, L.G. (Eds.). (1998). *Posttraumatic growth: Positive changes in the aftermath of crisis*. Mahwah, NJ: Lawrence Erlbaum.

Teyber, E. (2000). *Interpersonal processes in psychotherapy* (4th ed.). Pacific Grove, CA: Brooks/Cole.

Top 10 reasons why people don't exercise. (2003, July/Aug.). *IDEA Health and Fitness Source, 21*(7), 18.

Truax, C.B., & Carkhuff, R.R. (1967). *Toward effective counseling and psychotherapy: Training and practice*. Chicago: Aldine.

Turock, A. (1980). Immediacy in counseling: Recognizing clients' unspoken messages. *Personnel and Guidance Journal, 59*, 168-172.

Vallerand, R.J., & Losier, G. (1999). An integrative analysis of intrinsic and extrinsic motivation in sport. *Journal of Applied Sport Psychology, 11*, 142-169.

Vealey, R. (1989). Sport personality: A paradigmatic and methodological analysis. *Journal of Sport and Exercise Psychology, 11*, 216-235.

Vealey, R. (1992). Personality in sport: A comprehensive view. In T. Horn (Ed.), *Advances in sport psychology* (pp. 23-59). Champaign, IL: Human Kinetics.

Wachtel, P.L. (1993). *Therapeutic communication: Principles and effective practice*. New York: Guilford Press.

Walker, P. (2001, Nov./Dec.). The trainer's role on the treatment team. *IDEA Personal Trainer, 12*(10), 30-37.

Walsh, J. (2003). *Endings in clinical practice: Effective closure in diverse settings*. Chicago: Lyceum.

Watkins, C.E., Jr. (1986). Transference phenomena in the counseling situation. In W.P. Anderson (Ed.), *Innovative counseling: A handbook of readings*. Alexandria, VA: American Association of Counseling and Development.

Watkins, C.E., Jr. (1990). The effects of counselor self-disclosure: A research review. *Counseling Psychologist, 18*, 477-500.

Weinberg, R.S., & Gould, D. (2003). *Foundations of sport and exercise psychology* (3rd ed.). Champaign, IL: Human Kinetics.

Whitworth, L., Kimsey-House, H., & Sandahl, P. (1998). *Co-active coaching*. Palo Alto, CA: Davies-Black.

Willensky, H. (1960). Work careers and social integration. *International Social Science Journal, 12*, 543-560.

Williams, P., & Davis, D.C. (2002). *Therapist as life coach*. New York: W.W. Norton.

Willis, J.D., & Campbell, L.F. (1992). *Exercise psychology*. Champaign, IL: Human Kinetics.

Winnicott, D.W. (1958). The capacity to be alone. *International Journal of Psycho-Analysis, 39*, 416-420.

Wolpe, J. (1990). *The practice of behavior therapy* (4th ed.). Elmsford, NY: Pergamon.

Yalom, I.D. (1980). *Existential psychotherapy*. New York: Basic Books.

Yankelovich, D. (1999). *The magic of dialogue: Transforming conflict into cooperation*. New York: Simon & Schuster.

Young, M.E. (2001). *Learning the art of helping: Building blocks and techniques*. Upper Saddle River, NJ: Prentice Hall.

Zastrow, C.H. (1999). *The practice of social work* (6th ed.). Pacific Grove, CA: Brooks/Cole.

Zautra, A.J. (2003). *Emotions, stress, and health*. London: Oxford University Press.

Index

Note: The italicized *f* and *t* following page numbers refers to figures and tables, respectively.

About the Author

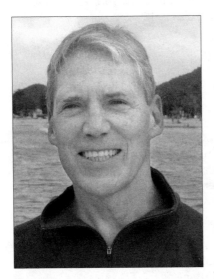

James Gavin, PhD, has been designing and delivering training programs in lifestyle fitness coaching to health fitness professionals since 1998. Gavin, a professor and graduate program director in the department of applied human sciences at Concordia University in Montreal, Canada, has been a consultant to health fitness centers for 20 years and a practitioner of counseling psychology for more than 30 years. Dr. Gavin was awarded a Diplomate in Counseling Psychology by the American Board of Professional Psychology, the highest award in counseling psychology recognizing achievement and excellence in the practice of psychology. He has written and researched extensively concerning fitness personality matching since the early 1980s and has presented around the world at health fitness conferences since 1985. Dr. Gavin is also the author of *Psychology for Health/Fitness Professionals*.

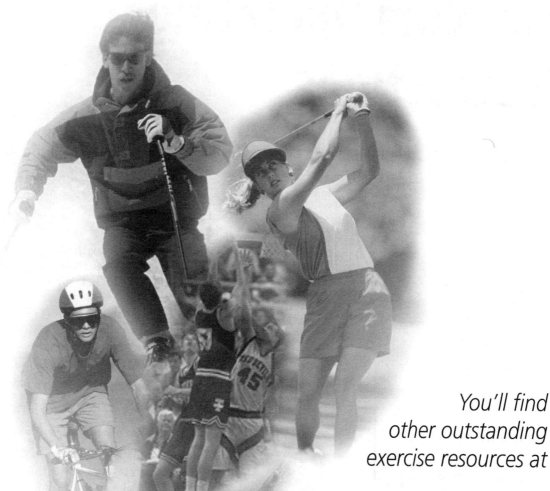

CD-ROM Operating Instructions

Minimum System Requirements

The *MAPS Inventory CD-ROM* can be installed on either a Windows®-based PC or a Macintosh computer.

Windows

- IBM PC compatible with Pentium® processor
- Windows® NT 4.0/2000/XP
- Pentium® processor or higher
- Adobe Acrobat Reader®
- At least 32 MB RAM
- 50 MB hard drive space
- 4x CD-ROM drive
- Printer
- Mouse

Macintosh

- * Power Mac® recommended
- * System 10.2/10.3 or higher
- * Adobe Acrobat Reader®
- * At least 32 MB RAM
- * 50 MB hard drive space
- * 4x CD-ROM drive
- * Printer
- * Mouse

Installing the Software—Windows Installation

1. Insert the CD in the CD-ROM drive.
2. Go to "My Computer" and select your CD-ROM drive.
3. Double-click on the "setup.exe" file
4. The Install Wizard will take you through the installation process. Please be patient as this process occurs. Click through the screens, including the license agreement screen and the location of the MAPS files. You can accept the default location of the MAPS files or you can designate an alternate location.
5. Complete the installation process.

Installing the Software—Mac Installation

1. Insert the CD in the CD-ROM drive.
2. Double-click on the CD icon on your desktop.
3. Double-click on the "MAPS_Install.command" file.
4. The Install Wizard will take you through the installation process. Please be patient as this process occurs. Click through the screens, including the license agreement screen and the location of the MAPS files. You can accept the default location of the MAPS files or you can designate an alternate location.
5. Complete the installation process.

[Note: You must be signed on as an administrator to install this program on a Macintosh.]

Getting Started—Windows Version

1. To access the program, go to the Windows "Start" menu and select the "Programs" option.
2. Select the "MAPS" program group, then the application. The program will launch.
3. Select the "Begin" button from the main screen.
4. Step through the program by selecting the "Continue" button on each screen.

Getting Started—Mac Version

1. To access the program, open your "Applications" folder (default location).
2. Double-click on "MAPS Command" file. The program will launch.
3. Select the "Begin" button from the main screen.
4. Step through the program by selecting the "Continue" button on each screen.

For product information or customer support:

E-mail: support@hkusa.com
Phone: 217-351-5076 (ext. 2970)
Fax: 217-351-2674
Web site: www.HumanKinetics.com